Headaches

Headaches

Dr John Lockley

Complementary Therapy by Karen Sullivan

BLOOMSBURY

ACKNOWLEDGEMENTS
Many thanks to the following for their advice, help and encouragement in the
preparation of this book:
Dr Brenda Bazeley, M.B. Ch. B.
Mr Don Bottoms, I. Eng. M.I.Agr. E., M.Erg.S
Mr Mark Flawn, MRO
Dr A.N. Gale, MD, FRCP
Dr Ninian Thomson
Mr Peter Sykes, LDS., DGDP., RCSEng.
– and especially to my secretary, Nancy Watkin, for all her loyal help.

The complementary therapy material set in italic at the end of each section has
been compiled by Karen Sullivan, and not by Dr Lockley. The advice given is
therefore hers and not his.

First published 1993 by Bloomsbury Publishing Limited,
2 Soho Square, London W1V 5DE

This edition published 1994

Copyright © 1993 Book Creation Services and Dr John Lockley

The CIP record for this book is available at the British Library.
ISBN 0 7475 1462 3

Edited and typeset by Book Creation Services,
1 Newburgh Street, London W1V 1LH

Printed in Great Britain by Cox & Wyman Ltd, Reading, Berks

CONTENTS

	INTRODUCTION	7
1	DIAGNOSIS	12
2	MIGRAINE	24
3	TENSION HEADACHES	55
4	NECK AND SPINE PROBLEMS	63
5	MENINGITIS AND ENCEPHALITIS	92
6	OTHER INFECTIONS	100
7	SINUSITIS	109
8	STROKES	118
9	SUB-ARACHNOID HAEMORRHAGE	127
10	HEAD INJURIES AND CONCUSSION	132
11	HIGH BLOOD PRESSURE	144
12	TUMOURS	150
13	TEMPORAL ARTERITIS	161
14	EYE PROBLEMS	165
15	DENTAL CAUSES	174
16	EPILEPSY	178
17	PSYCHOLOGICAL CAUSES OF HEADACHES	183
18	HEADACHES IN WOMEN	194
19	HEADACHES DURING SEX	205
20	HEADACHES IN CHILDREN	211
21	MISCELLANEOUS CAUSES	215
22	WORK RELATED HEADACHES	221
23	FOOD, CHEMICALS, DRUGS, ADDITIVES & ALCOHOL	226
24	WEATHER, ATMOSPHERE AND HEADACHES	238
25	PULLING IT ALL TOGETHER	243
	FURTHER READING	247
	USEFUL ADDRESSES	248
	INDEX	252

Introduction

Of the symptoms that concern patients most, headaches come high on the list. Headaches are the most common cause of pain seen by family doctors, and although only a small percentage are due to any serious disorder, the fear of underlying disease causes a great deal of anxiety, especially among those who've suffered from headaches for a long time.

Although the vast majority of headaches aren't dangerous, a few are due to serious underlying disease; and the remainder may not go away unless you do something to prevent them. The trouble is, how can you be sure which is which? It's not always easy.

Even when you know the cause of your headaches, there are still many problems. Your headaches may not be lethal, but they still hurt; they're frustrating; they're an inconvenience; they may stop you working properly; and for those who have recurring headaches, coping with the pain and trying to prevent further attacks can be a sizeable and exhausting problem.

Most headaches are like this: not always sinister, but always painful, debilitating and frustrating – a real spoil-sport of a complaint, interfering with both work and pleasure. Sometimes your GP or a specialist can help; for example, in the case of migraine, where a wide range of drugs is now available both to treat the attacks, and to stop further ones occurring.

But, at other times, orthodox medicine seems to have less to offer: there may be no serious underlying cause, but that doesn't mean the headaches will necessarily go away. Often headaches are related to aspects of your lifestyle that your doctor has little or no knowledge of – the type of pillow you use; your dentures; the car you drive; or the lighting conditions at work.

Sometimes your doctor is able to reassure you that there is nothing seriously wrong and that you 'only' have a tension headache. Unfortunately, this doesn't take away the pain, but it does leave you confused, thinking it's your fault you've got headaches, yet perhaps not wanting to bother the doctor any further.

Many patients with chronic headaches end up like this – suffering, but not always able to get any real, lasting or satisfying help, and puzzled because what seems to trigger off the headaches on one occasion doesn't always trigger them off on another.

In short, headaches can be a real pain – and that's where this book comes in. We'll show you *why* you're getting headaches, explain *what* is going on, and, most importantly, *tell you what you can do to stop them*. And believe me, there's a lot that can be done.

Let's get things straight from the start – a headache is a *symptom*, not a disease. Headaches can occur for many different reasons and each type needs to be treated according to its cause. A few of the underlying causes are dangerous – meningitis or stroke, for example. Headaches like these need prompt diagnosis and treatment. But don't become alarmed; most headaches aren't life-threatening, just painful and annoying. If you've suffered from headaches for a long time it's much more likely that your headache is unpleasant, without being serious. On the other hand, it's very important to sort out which kind of headache you have, and to make sure that if urgent treatment is needed, you get it.

We all know people who say they've never had a headache in their lives. Lucky, aren't they? For many others, a headache is merely an occasional annoyance – unpleasant, but nothing more. Unfortunately, some people are affected much more than this. Either they get headaches more often, or their headaches are so intense and debilitating that they affect the quality of their life. It's no joke to have regular migraines. With a headache of this intensity work is impossible and enjoyment out of the question. The knowledge that next week may bring the start of *another* attack merely adds to the unpleasantness.

A few statistics will show the extent of the problem. Nineteen out of twenty of us get headaches at some time or other. Men and women of all races are equally affected, but, interestingly, older people seem to get them less often. Every fortnight, one in four of us will have a headache bad enough to need painkillers. One in three attacks begins at work, and headaches are a common cause of absenteeism. At least one third of migraine sufferers have to stop work when an attack begins, and most migraine sufferers think that their quality of work and their careers have suffered as a result of their migraines.

Most headaches are caused by one of three things: minor viral infections, migraines and tension. Because minor headaches (those that respond quickly to painkillers) are so common, most of us don't go to the doctor when we get one; but of those patients whose headaches are serious or persistent enough to make them consult their GP, one in five will be referred to hospital.

As well as being painful, and in some cases debilitating, headaches are upsetting. If you frequently suffer from headaches, there may be a nagging thought at the back of your mind. Is this the tip of the iceberg? What does it mean? Is there something seriously wrong? Uncle Jim had a headache and he was dead in three months from a brain tumour. How do I know I haven't got one, too?

Even if the cause of your headaches has been sorted out satisfactorily, there is still the problem of living with the frequent pain and the disruption to your lifestyle that they can cause. What *do* you do when you have migraines associated with your menstrual cycle, when you know that *every month* you'll have another three days of misery, vomiting your guts out, with what feels like a piledriver inside your head threatening to split your brain apart? How do you cope emotionally with this, never mind hold down a job, with the frequent absences from work that having migraines implies?

And what about the man or woman who gets frequent tension headaches? Knowing that they're 'only' caused by tension helps – to a point. At least you know you're not dying. Small consolation, because you often feel as though you are, with that nagging pain that goes on for days at a time, apparently totally resistant to painkillers. Nothing the doctor gives seems to help, except perhaps tranquillisers. How do you feel about being on those all the time? Or not having the tranquillisers, and getting the pain instead? Is there an alternative?

If you have recurrent headaches, then this book is for you. It will help you to sort out what's likely to be causing them; why headaches like yours occur; and what you can do to stop them. With patience, most headaches can be treated very effectively. Some are helped by orthodox medical or surgical treatment, others with self-help techniques; some can be alleviated with complementary therapies, and some types of headache are best treated using a combination of all three methods.

A FEW MISCONCEPTIONS

Let's start off by getting rid of a few misconceptions. *Migraines* are not just severe headaches, they're a specific type of headache, with special features. Clinically, migraine is a specific disease of the nervous system which produces a one-sided headache, vomiting and sometimes flashing lights in front of the eyes; in addition, the intensity of the headache can vary from unpleasant to absolutely appalling. Think of the headaches you get with a common bout of the flu – pretty awful. Bad migraines are about ten times worse. So yes, migraines can be very severe headaches, but they are quite different to 'ordinary' headaches.

The second misconception is that high blood pressure is *often* a cause of headaches. It isn't. Although there are some people whose headaches are related to blood pressure, they are in the minority.

The third misconception is that headaches are a sign you have a brain tumour; less than three per cent of brain tumours cause headaches at the time they are diagnosed. Most brain tumours don't start causing headaches until long after other symptoms (personality change, paralysis and so on) have confirmed the diagnosis.

The final misconception is that the longer you've had your headache, the more likely you are to have something seriously wrong with you. In fact, exactly the opposite is true. It's the sudden, severe, one-off headache caused by meningitis, sub-arachnoid haemorrhage or a stroke that poses the biggest threat. The longer-term headaches are more likely to be due to conditions that are unpleasant, but not life-threatening; for example, neck injuries and tension headaches.

HOW TO USE THIS BOOK

There's a pithy medical aphorism which runs like this: *'Diagnose* first – *treat* second.'

It's all too easy to get it the other way round, trying to treat the symptoms before working out why they are there in the first place. Treating only the symptoms is the sloppy way to help, and often it doesn't work.

A headache is a symptom, not a disease. Headaches are associated with a large number of quite different diseases and, especially with long-standing headaches, the best treatment is not to tackle the headache (the symptom) but to treat the underlying condition itself.

The reason it isn't possible to treat all headaches identically is because different causes of headache require different types of treatment; for example, the headache caused by a sub-arachnoid haemorrhage (a bleeding artery inside the skull) needs completely different treatment from that used to cure a sinus headache or a migraine.

What about paracetamol or aspirin? I hear you ask. Aren't these treating the symptoms? And don't they work? Well, yes, they do; and for the occasional headache, a couple of paracetamol may work wonders. But more intense, and more long-term headaches need a much more careful approach. Painkillers like aspirin or paracetamol may help, but they won't sort out the underlying cause, which is the real problem.

Diagnosing the source of a headache is the first stage in getting you better, but accurate diagnosis is not always easy. There's a lot of overlap between symptoms: muscle spasm in the neck can sometimes imitate a migraine; temporal arteritis (an inflammation of the arteries in the temple which may go on to cause blindness) can cause the same type of pain as a tension headache. Sometimes the cause of the headache is obvious, but in others it is only by analysing all the symptoms, and perhaps doing some laboratory tests, that it is possible to make a diagnosis with certainty.

A complicating factor is that there may be several different types of headache occurring in the same person; for example, coming partly from arthritis of the neck, partly from muscular tension and partly from migraine.

Once you know which type (or types) you've got, your next task is to understand more about what's causing it. Look under the relevant chapter in this book for treatment of each condition. Each chapter is set out under the following headings:

- The condition itself: what goes wrong, and the symptoms it produces
- The type of headache
- What else could it be?
- Orthodox treatment
- Self-help techniques
- Complementary treatment
- Associated problems

The earlier chapters in this book cotains information on internal problems: the things that can go wrong inside your body. Later chapters are about external influences, such as the weather, drugs, chemicals, and problems that occur in or from your workplace.

One of the most important concepts in treating headaches is to understand the vicious circle that so often gets set up, in which neck pain causes a spasm in the surrounding muscles. This spasm only serves to ram the neck joints more firmly together, which causes more pain, which in turn causes more muscular spasm. And so the cycle goes on. This vicious circle is a major cause of muscular and tension headaches, and it significantly worsens headaches from other causes.

We've mentioned complementary therapies quite a lot in this book, because they can often help. I'm quite fond of complementary medicine, in general, but the reason why these medicines remain 'complementary' is simply because no one has yet been able to prove scientifically whether or not they work. Although I believe strongly that many complementary techniques will ultimately prove to be valid, and be absorbed into mainstream medicine, we cannot yet be sure which of them will be.

Sometimes complementary medicines can be extremely helpful; however, others can be ineffective, inappropriate or even dangerous. Therefore, when using complementary medicines always consult a registered practitioner. Remember that they are called complementary therapies because they are meant to complement orthodox medical attention, not take the place of it.

Finally, there is no substitute for the advice given to you by your own orthodox medical practitioner. Although a book like this can teach you about headaches, alert you to useful self-help techniques, and show why your doctor is suggesting certain types of treatment, there is just no substitute for your own doctor's examination, diagnosis and advice. He knows you, possibly better than you know yourself; he also knows more about medicine than you do, so don't use any of the suggestions in this book if they contradict the advice he has given.

So, *diagnosis* first – *treatment* second. Let's get on with the diagnosis!

Chapter One

DIAGNOSIS

'*Diagnose* first, *treat* second.' This statement may appear obvious, but it's very easy to make the mistake of treating symptoms (such as pain or nausea) without getting to the root of the condition or disease *causing* the symptoms. Treatment is much more effective if there is an accurate initial diagnosis!

It's all too easy to treat a headache with a couple of aspirins, without stopping to think *why* that headache is occurring. Then, when the headache doesn't go away, you can't help but wonder if you should increase the dose ... and then you've fallen neatly into the trap. *Diagnose* first, *treat* second means that you stop to think *before* you reach for those painkillers, even on the first occasion.

However, diagnosing the cause of your headache may not always be easy, because there can be so much overlap between symptoms. For example, headaches caused by neck problems can sometimes imitate a migraine; temporal arteritis (an inflammation of the arteries in the forehead) can produce a headache similar to one that has arisen from tension; and arthritis in the neck can mimic tension headaches. Unfortunately, there are few hard and fast diagnostic rules: knowing the site or type of pain may not be enough to tell you its cause. Accurate diagnosis of the source of your headaches will probably depend not upon one specific symptom, but on carefully balancing the importance of a number of different symptoms and observations.

Here lies a trap for the amateur doctor! When reading a medical book like this, it's all too easy to come up with the worst possible diagnosis, and then force your own symptoms to fit it. This is the 'medical student syndrome'. When medical students start to learn about disease they often try to self-diagnose their own aches and pains – usually with disastrous results. Every medical school health centre has a constant trickle of students who have convinced themselves (usually erroneously) that they are about to die from some dreadful disease.

Nevertheless, do make sure that you consult your doctor about your fears. He will be able to see things in a much more balanced light. It *is*, of course, possible that you are right in your suspicions – but the vast probability is that you won't be, so don't worry unnecessarily.

The last thing you should do is use this book in isolation, self-diagnosing your own headaches and then blithely self-medicating yourself. If you're having trouble with headaches and you haven't been to your doctor, then *make an appointment*, discuss your problems and *ask for advice*. By all means use this book to point yourself in the right direction. And if you're worried that you have a particular disease, do specifically mention it to your doctor. Once you have discussed the situation and, if necessary, had an examination, listen to the diagnosis and take note of the advice. Doctors have the knowledge, the experience and the objectivity to treat you properly. It's hard to be objective when the patient is yourself!

So let's get down to working out what might be the underlying cause of your particular headache.

Although the site of the pain and its pattern can often point to a particular diagnosis, in practice it doesn't always work out that way; the same source of headache doesn't produce identical types of pain in everyone. For example, tension headaches often produce pain in the forehead, or a feeling of pressure over the top of the skull. On the other hand, some muscle-tension headaches can produce pain centring over one eye (a type of pain which is more usually associated with migraine). So how do you know which is which?

Because headaches can be so variable there is no one symptom which allows us to make a firm diagnosis. Instead, it's a matter of finding the *pattern* of illness which seems to fit most of the facts. The *type* of pain may point towards two or three possible diagnoses; the *time* it comes on may point to a slightly different set of possibilities; the *things that start it off*, to a third group of alternatives; and the *accompanying symptoms* to a fourth.; *put them all together* and you may find a single diagnosis which is common to *all* these groups, and it is this diagnosis which should be top of your list of possible causes.

Obviously, it's nice if everything points in the same direction – and doctors do like to try to make one diagnosis which covers all the symptoms. On the other hand, this isn't always possible in the case of headaches.

Because the symptoms of headaches are so variable, rather than producing just one flow chart to identify the cause of your headaches, I've created several diagnostic charts and lists. Work through them one after the other. If you get some common answers then you're probably heading in the right direction. On the other hand, if you get a group of different possibilities it can mean one of several things:

• Perhaps the source of your headache is producing symptoms in a less common way

• Maybe you've got more than one cause for your headache

• The possible causes of your headache may need to be sorted out by doing some special tests, for which you will need to see your doctor.

Armed with your answers, consult the relevant chapter of this book, describing the causes of headaches in much greater detail. You may well find that this extra detail allows you to pinpoint the cause of your headache more accurately.

But what if you can't? Well, don't forget that several causes of headache can be operating at the same time. Be prepared to have one main diagnosis and one (or even two) secondary diagnoses. It's quite common to find that causes of headaches multiply together – so a patient whose headaches are caused mainly by arthritis of the neck may also find her headaches are made worse by stress and tension; migraine and tension headaches often work together in this way, too; and someone with high blood pressure may also, quite coincidentally, have a bad neck from an old whiplash accident.

But diagnosis doesn't stop here. There is a further diagnostic tool: *if the treatment works it confirms the diagnosis.* (That is assuming, of course, that the treatment is not a catch-all method such as taking high doses of painkillers.) Similarly, if a specific treatment doesn't work, it may mean that the diagnosis is not as accurate as you supposed. However, this advice needs to be handled with care, because people don't always respond to the same treatment in the same way. For example, many migraine sufferers find great relief by using metoclopramide (together with a simple painkiller); others find this of no help at all, and prefer one of the ergotamine preparations. The response to treatment can help us to confirm the diagnosis, but it isn't always specific.

To sum up, try to look at the *overall picture* and see where it *all* leads – symptoms, signs, tests and response to treatment. If the majority of answers point in the same direction, you should look up the details of this illness; only if you find no clear answers should you look at the alternatives.

CHARTS FOR DIAGNOSIS: SITE OF HEADACHE

SITE OF PAIN

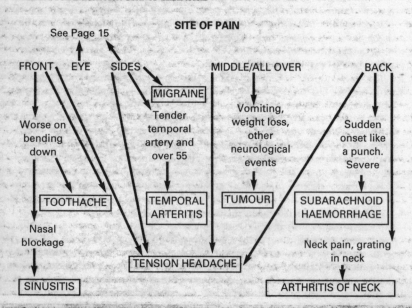

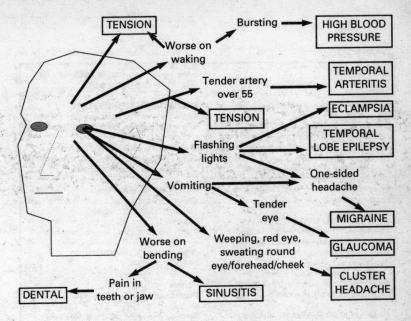

Site of Headache (Eye and Side of Head)

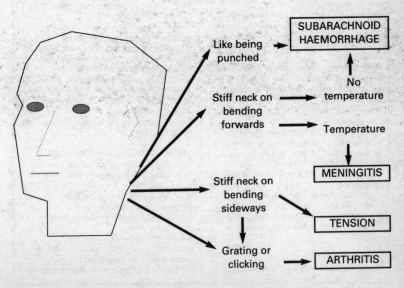

Site of Headache (Neck)

SYMPTOMS:

TEMPERATURE
Viral infection – high temperature (often 101–104°F)
Bacterial infection – lower temperature (98–101°F)
Meningitis – rare, but potentially deadly. Associated with vomiting, light hurting the eyes, and a stiff neck on bending forward
Encephalitis – see meningitis
Malaria – high swinging temperature (104°F), with intermittent shivering attacks, and profuse sweating; usually acquired in the tropics

STIFF NECK ON FORWARD BENDING
Meningitis – temperature, light hurting the eyes, vomiting, altered consciousness
Sub-arachnoid haemorrhage – no temperature, sudden onset, may be vomiting, altered consciousness
Meningism – temperature, slightly stiff neck (difficult to tell apart from meningitis)

STIFF NECK ON SIDEWAYS BENDING
Muscle spasm – tender neck muscles
Neck injury – history of injury to neck; tender neck muscles
Osteo–arthritis – pain in the neck, creaking and clicking in neck on moving head
Cervical 'slipped disc' – pain going into arms, lack of power in hands, numbness or pins-and-needles in arms

VOMITING
Viral infection – raised temperature
Migraine – some cases may have flashing lights in front of eyes, often on one side only, nausea and vomiting
Stroke – paralysis in arm, leg or both, or loss of speech
Sub–arachnoid haemorrhage sensation of blow to back of neck, no temperature, may be altered level of consciousness
Meningitis – raised temperature, light hurting the eyes, neck stiff on bending forward
Glaucoma – tender eye, dim vision
Hydrocephalus – occurs in both children and adults: with vomiting, swelling of skull in infants, convulsions, continuous headache

AFTER INJURY
Whiplash, exacerbation of osteo-arthritis, head injury – concussion, fractured skull and/or bleeding inside skull

WORSE WHEN SLEEPING LATE
Migraine – may be flashing lights in front of eyes, nausea and vomiting, headache on one side only
High blood pressure
Tension headache – sore neck muscles, no temperature, constant headache

WITH PAIN IN ARM
Cervical 'slipped disc' – severe pain in neck and arm, often with tingling or numbness in arm
Neck muscle spasm – sore neck muscles

DISORIENTATION/VAGUENESS/ DELIRIUM
Migraine – one-sided headache, may be visual changes, vomiting
Depression/anxiety – early waking, low mood
Stroke – one-sided paralysis, loss of speech
Sub-arachnoid haemorrhage – sudden onset, like a blow to the back of the neck, no temperature
Meningitis – temperature, stiff neck, light hurting the eyes, vomiting
Tension headache – sore neck muscles, no temperature, constant headache
Raised pressure inside the brain (tumours, hydrocephalus, intracranial hypertension) – vomiting, no temperature
Head injury and/or concussion
Uraemia (kidney failure) diagnosed with blood tests
High blood pressure
Encephalitis – temperature, stiff neck, light hurts the eyes

VISUAL CHANGES/EYE PROBLEMS
Focusing problems – worse with reading or studying, and especially with really close-up reading
Migraine – may be flashing lights in front of eyes, 'blind' spots in visual field, vomiting, one-sided headache, light hurting the eyes
Cluster headache – one eye only, penetrating pain, one eye weeps and is red, pupil small, lid droops
Temporal lobe epilepsy – usually with fits

High blood pressure – blurred vision
Brain tumours – inability to see part of the visual field (often a sector)
Temporal arteritis – sudden blindness in one or both eyes; pain in the temples, tender artery in the temple region, over the age of fifty-five
Glaucoma – inability to see part of the visual field (round the edges); or sudden loss of vision with intense pain
Pituitary tumour – inability to see part of the visual field (at the edges). This is often called 'tunnel vision'
Uraemia – blurred vision
Eclampsia (pregnancy only) – flashing lights

HEADACHE WITH BLINDNESS IN ONE EYE
Temporal arteritis – over the age of fifty-five, tender artery in the temple region
Glaucoma – severe eye pain, vomiting
Brain tumour – may be vomiting, weakness, changes of personality, speech problems
Retinal migraine – vision only temporarily cut off; vomiting, one-sided headache; light hurts the eyes

WORSE ON STRAINING
Tension headache – sore neck muscles, no temperature, constant headache
High blood pressure
Tumour – with vomiting and constant severe headache

WITH NUMBNESS
Stroke – paralysis down one side only, which doesn't go away
Transient Ischaemic Attacks (TIAs) – in the elderly, rather like a stroke but it goes away
Neck injury – with severe pain down affected arm and in neck
Migraine – one-sided reversible paralysis

IN GROUPS OR CLUSTERS
Migraine – may be seeing flashing lights in front of eyes, nausea and vomiting, headache on one side only
Cluster headache – pain round one eye, red and weeping eye, sweating round forehead
Trigeminal neuralgia – pain in side of face, triggered by touch

SEVERE HEADACHE
Migraine – one-sided headache, nausea and vomiting, may have visual changes
Cluster headache – round one eye, red and weeping eye, sweating round eye, occurs in clusters
Trigeminal neuralgia – in cheek, triggered by touching affected area
Sub-arachnoid haemorrhage – like a blow to the back of the neck, vomiting
Stroke – sudden onset, with weakness on one side of the body
Tumour – constant pain, vomiting
Acute glaucoma – tender eye, pupil cloudy, dimness of vision, vomiting
Hydrocephalus – fits, vomiting, constant pain

RELATED TO TIMED EVENTS
At weekends – caffeine withdrawal – migraines from withdrawal of work stress or sleeping in late – blood pressure headaches – tension headaches
Late nights – migraine
Jet lag – may be migrainous or non-migrainous
Night duty – may be migrainous or non-migrainous

RELATED TO EXERCISE
Exercise headache ('True coital headache') – worsening of tension headache

IN WOMEN
Premenstrual (before the period) – irritability, bloating, breast swelling/tenderness
Menstrual (during the period) – May be migrainous or non-migrainous
Eclampsia (pregnancy only) – blood pressure rise, weight, protein in the urine and flashing lights in the eyes
Menopausal – relationship to the menopause and/or hysterectomy, hot flushes, sweats, 'woolly-headedness'. Migrainous or non-migrainous

Related to the contraceptive pill
First migraine on the contraceptive pill – stop the pill immediately
Worsening of type of migraine – stop the pill immediately

SITE:

FOREHEAD
Tension headache – sore neck muscles, no temperature
Sinusitis – stuffed-up nose, pain in face, worse on putting head down
Temporal arteritis – older age group; prominent tender arteries across the temples
High blood pressure
Glaucoma – tender, hard eyeball; may be hazy pupil

FACE
Sinusitis – temperature, pain worse on bending down, stuffed-up nose
Toothache – pain on banging a specific tooth
Trigeminal neuralgia – sharp frequent pains over cheek, triggered by touch
Glaucoma – hazy pupil, vomiting, tender hard eyeball

TEMPLES
Tension – sore neck muscles, no temperature
Temporal arteritis – older age group; prominent tender arteries across the temples

EYE
Migraine – headache usually on one side of face only, with vomiting, and sometimes flashing lights in front of the eyes, no temperature
Cluster headache – round one eye, redness and weeping of eye; running nose, in clusters
Sinusitis – stuffed-up nose, pain in face, worse on putting head down

Neck muscle spasm – sore neck muscles
Glaucoma – tender, hard eyeball; may be hazy pupil; may be vomiting

EAR
Neck muscle tension – pain in neck muscles
Temporo-mandibular joint problems – click on opening jaw

BACK OF HEAD/NECK
Tension – sore neck muscles, no temperature
Osteo-arthritis – creaking and clicking on moving head and neck
High blood pressure
Sub-arachnoid haemorrhage – feels as if there was a blow to the back of the head; may be altered level of consciousness; no temperature

ALL OVER
Viral infection – high temperature, but no stiff neck
Tension – sore neck muscles, no temperature
Migraine – with vomiting and dislike of light; no temperature; may be visual disturbance
Tumour – bursting headache, weight loss and other symptoms
Uraemia (kidney failure) – diagnosed with blood test

ONE SIDE
Migraine – may be flashing lights in eyes, vomiting, dislike of light
Cluster headache – round one eye, occurs in clusters, redness and weeping of eye

MADE WORSE BY:

BENDING DOWN
Sinusitis – stuffed-up nose, pain in face, worse on putting head down
Toothache – pain on banging a tooth
Tension – sore neck muscles, no temperature
Menopausal problems – hot flushes, sweats, 'woolly-headedness'

SEX
Tension – sore neck muscles, no temperature

Neck or spine injury – sore neck muscles
Coital headache/Exertion headache – with exertion
Sub-arachnoid haemorrhage – feels as if there was a blow to the back of the head; may be altered level of consciousness; no temperature

LIGHT
Migraine – may start with flashing lights or blind spots in front of eyes, vomiting, one-sided headaches, dislike of noise

Tension – sore neck muscles, no temperature
Meningitis – temperature, stiff neck on forward bending

NOISE
Migraine – may have started with flashing lights or blind spots in front of eyes, vomiting, one-sided headaches, dislike of light
Tension – sore neck muscles, no temperature

WORK
Postural – working in a fixed, awkward, or unnatural position; working with computers
Chemical – exposure to chemicals in manufacturing; also duplicator fluids, printing ink, paint and non-carbon paper
Tension – sore neck muscles, no temperature
Migraine – from stress and other trigger factors. One-sided headaches with nausea and vomiting. May be visual changes

LENGTH OF TIME YOU HAVE HAD HEADACHES:

In general, the longer you have a headache the less likely it is to be serious.
Sudden (minutes)
Stroke
Sub-arachnoid haemorrhage
Exercise headache
Coital headache
Recent (hours or days)
Viral
Sinusitis
High blood pressure
Head injury
Toothache
Hydrocephalus
Sub-arachnoid haemorrhage
Meningitis
Tumour
Temporal arteritis
Glaucoma
Encephalitis
Eclampsia

Medium term (days or weeks)
Hydrocephalus
Head injury/concussion
Sub-dural haemorrhage
High blood pressure
Tempero-mandibular joint problems
Tumours
Long term or recurrent (months or years)
Tension
Neck problems
Migraine
Depression
Post-traumatic
Eye strain
Bite imbalance
Trigeminal neuralgia
Psychiatric problems
Cluster headache

THE EXAMINATION

Of course, your doctor will diagnose your headaches in a slightly different way, because he or she has the advantage of being able to examine you as well.

However, don't be misled. Many patients think (wrongly) that the examination tells the doctor everything, and that a diagnosis without one means it's probably wrong. In fact, almost the reverse is true. With headaches it is mainly careful, painstaking questioning that leads to the most accurate diagnosis. Perhaps your doctor finds out the critical information that the headache came on *suddenly,* like a blow to the back of the head; or else that the headache comes on if you miss a meal; or, maybe, there's a background of marital discord or stress at work. It's a bit like detective work, piecing information together until it all clicks into place.

Having said this, the importance of the physical examination should be stressed, because there are one or two items that your doctor will certainly want to check. What the doctor examines will vary according to the answers you've given to the questions asked. For example, if the history is highly suggestive of sinusitis, then your doctor may only need to press on the bone overlying the sinus to confirm the diagnosis. A thorough examination of the muscles or nerves would be unnecessary. On the other hand, these will need to be examined if your story points towards a slipped disc in the neck.

The sort of examination your doctor gives you depends upon the symptoms and the history. Some or all of the following may be necessary – blood pressure measured, temperature taken, examination of the movements of your neck to see if you can bend your neck properly, not just forwards but also from side to side. You may be examined for trigger spots and painful areas in the muscles of the neck and back, and your spine may be checked. Your doctor may also examine your temples – to discover whether or not there are prominent pulses and tender arteries – investigate the power you can develop in your arms and legs, tap your reflexes, and even tickle the bottom of your feet! (This is a very quick way to tell whether you have had a stroke or a similar brain injury.) Finally, your doctor may look into your eyes, test your pupil reflexes, press against the bones in your face to see if they're tender, look at your teeth, and check the way your mouth closes.

The combination of history-taking, examination and appropriate prescription may deal with your headaches fully. As we discussed earlier, your response to the treatment is also an important diagnostic pointer. In just a few cases the doctor may be unsure of the diagnosis and under those circumstances will use the resources of the hospital laboratory and X-ray department.

Taking it further

Blood tests may be necessary, although these are usually only helpful in the diagnosis of a few specific types of headache.

One common investigation is the blood count: your doctor will be interested in two aspects of this. The first is the white cell count. The white cells are those blood cells which attack infections. A rise in the white cell count indicates the presence of an infection, and can also indicate whether it is viral or bacterial. A more general, less specific, but often more helpful parameter is to measure the Erythrocyte Sedimentation Rate (ESR). Basically, this test measures the speed with which red cells in the blood settle as they separate from the fluid of the blood serum in which they are suspended. A sample of blood is sucked up into a long thin tube and the laboratory technician records how far the red cells have settled in an hour. Normally the level falls by about twenty or thirty millimeters but in certain types of illness – particularly infections, tumours and the auto-immune diseases – the ESR can be very high: perhaps 60 or more. The ESR test acts more as a pointer to illness rather than a diagnosis. If the doctor finds you have a high ESR he will undoubtedly want to do further investigations to ascertain why. Don't forget, of course, that a high ESR doesn't necessarily relate to your headaches; if you already have rheumatoid arthritis or a viral infection then your ESR may be high anyway.

Other blood tests can be useful, such as testing for abnormal levels of growth hormone in those with a pituitary tumour; and checking for altered hormone levels in those with headaches relating to the menopause or the menstrual cycle. In addition, in one rare type of raised blood pressure caused by a tumour called a *phaeochromocytoma*, urine tests may be useful to spot abnormal levels of a substance called Vanillymandelic Acid (VMA).

X-rays, surprisingly, are often of little value in headaches. Like the myth that the examination is the most important part of the consultation, there's also a myth that X-rays will always find out the cause of illness and that the doctor isn't doing the job well if one hasn't been arranged. Again, this is far from the truth. With the exception of dental, sinus and neck problems, there are only a few specific and often quite rare causes of headache that an ordinary X-ray will help to diagnose: even rarer are those cases where X-rays alone can spot a diagnosis that isn't obvious from the history and examination.

Don't be too eager to press your doctor to give you an X-ray if he or she seems reluctant, because an X-ray may well provide no extra information over and above what is already known. It's important to remember that X-rays are a form of radiation, which provides its own risks. This *particularly* applies to those who are in the early stages of pregnancy, where a single X-ray can *double* the chances of the baby getting leukaemia, even when the abdomen itself is not being X-rayed.

There *are* a few occasions in which X-rays of the head and neck can be helpful. They include the following: sinusitis, where the blocked sinuses can be seen; cervical spondylosis; after head injuries; osteo-arthritis of the spine, where the degeneration of the neck joints can be observed; dental X-rays to spot decay or temperomandibular joint problems; Paget's disease, which thickens the bones of the skull; and tumours of the pituitary gland, where the enlargement of the pituitary gland can be measured as it presses into the bones of the skull.

While brain tumours show up as calcified specks on some occasions, most are *not* visible on X-rays. On the other hand, secondary deposits from tumours can sometimes be spotted as they erode the bones of the skull. In most cases the X-ray merely corroborates a diagnosis that has already been made clinically.

There are, however, specialised X-ray tests that may help. Where there is a clear indication that something particularly unpleasant may be going on – such as a brain tumour, a blood clot inside the skull, high pressure within the fluid surrounding the brain, or a leakage of blood from the arteries within the brain..

One of the limitations of ordinary X-rays is that in one picture you see everything at all levels, super-imposed one on top of the other – rather like trying to read the middle of three sheets of a newspaper by holding them, unopened, up to the sun. The question then arises: is a particular mark within the brain, outside the brain, in the skull, or on the surface of the skin?

Special X-rays called *tomograms* can get round this to some extent by blurring everything except a narrow band of tissue at a particular depth from the X-ray plate; however, an even better method is Computerised Axial Tomography (CAT for short) which can pick up and analyse structural problems that ordinary X-rays cannot separate out properly. In this, many X-rays (up to a hundred) are taken in different planes; the images are received, not on an X-ray plate, but in an ionisation chamber, from where they are sent to a computer and converted into a sequence of detailed cross-sectional images of the part of the body being studied.

A more useful test, increasingly coming into general use, is Magnetic Resonance Imaging (MRI scan). It's otherwise known as an NMR, which stands for Nuclear Magnetic Resonance, but the name frightened off a lot of people, so it's more commonly called MRI. In fact, the procedure doesn't involve radioactivity at all! MRI scans enable the soft tissues of the body (which don't show up very well on X-ray) to be seen in quite immaculate detail. It is, however, a very expensive technique, and not one that is used unless there is a clear clinical need to establish what is going on within the skull.

As well as showing up the soft tissues of the body very clearly, an MRI scan can, to some extent, analyse the chemical make-up of the body, and provide images in the form of 'slices' of the area being examined. In addition, whereas CAT scans can only produce a cross-sectional image of the part of the body being studied, an MRI scan can produce an image in *any* plane.

An MRI investigation is very simple, the machine is a large metal cylinder with a central hole in it, rather like a giant cotton reel. You lie prone on a trolley, which is then inserted into the six-foot-long hole in the centre, where you wait, staying as still as possible. The only problem is that those who are claustrophobic sometimes find it difficult to tolerate the procedure, and in such cases it may be necessary to be sedated or even anaethetised. This is particularly the case with small children, especially as they have to lie stock-still for some time.

The whole procedure is totally non-invasive: totally painless, and completely harmless. Moreover, it can produce pictures of the soft tissues of the most surprising clarity, which can be used to localise the tiniest structural problems within the body. Using MRI scans we can pick up tumours, clots in the brain, strokes, and increased pressure within the cerebro-spinal fluid (CSF).

There is a further radiographic technique that can be used to find out why we are getting headaches. The difficulty with ordinary X-rays is that while they show the bones and denser tissues within the body, they often can't distinguish between the various types of soft tissues such as blood vessels, brain substance, and so on. So the soft tissues in an X-ray tend to show as an indistinguishable grey haze, bereft of any detail. However, if we can put a radio-opaque dye (a compound that won't let X-rays through) into various cavities of the body, we can outline them in a way that enables us to see them on an ordinary X-ray picture. It's a bit like having a small glass bottle full of water placed inside a big glass bottle full of water. Looking from the outside it's very difficult to tell where the small bottle is because glass in water looks very much the same as water on its own. However, if you fill the inside glass bottle with some ink, it then stands out very clearly.

We use this technique with X-rays; it's called contrast radiography, but it can only be used where the doctor can manage to fill a chamber (such as the heart) or surround an object (such as a gallstone) with a kind of ink. Contrast radiography is used in the skull in three special ways – firstly, to see if there is any bleeding from one of the arteries in the brain; secondly, to show up soft tissues within the spinal column, and thirdly, by injecting air into spaces (called ventricles) deep within the brain, we can use it to show whether there is enlargement of the ventricles due to excess pressure of the cerebro-spinal fluid (CSF).

To work out whether there's a bleeding artery inside the skull, or to see if there are little balloon-like blebs on the arteries (see Chapter Nine) dye is injected into one of the arteries travelling up into the head, and a swift sequence of X-rays is taken to see where it gets to. The dye outlines the inside of the arteries and quickly shows up any leak or bleb. We can also use dye in the spinal cord. Sometimes one of the discs between the vertebrae bulges or bursts, and the contents squeeze out, pressing against one of the nerves as it leaves the spinal cord (see Chapter Four). The spinal cord, the fluid surrounding it, the discs and the nerves all look much the same under ordinary X-ray.

To get more information about the size and position of the troublesome disc, we can insert dye into the spine by doing a lumbar puncture The doctor inserts a needle at the base of the spine, draws off a little of the cerebro-spinal fluid which bathes the spinal cord, and inserts some dye. The patient is then tilted so the dye flows up towards the neck, outlining the spinal cord and the bony canal in which it runs. It is now easy to use X-ray pictures to outline those places where a disc is pushing into the area normally occupied by spinal cord and cerebro-spinal fluid.

Lumbar punctures can be used on other occasions for different reasons. In meningitis the cerebro-spinal fluid (CSF) bathing the spinal cord can become infected. It's not easy to get a sample of the CSF that surrounds the brain, but putting a needle into the spinal column in the lumbar (lower back) area is convenient and safe and allows a little fluid to be drawn off. The hospital laboratory can culture this to see if any bacteria are growing in it, measure its sugar content, test it for blood. This helps the doctor to know if there is meningitis; in some types of bleed inside the skull (particularly sub-arachnoid haemorrhage, blood-stained cerebro-spinal fluid confirms the diagnosis.

A completely different approach to diagnosis is through measuring the electrical activity of the brain, using a device called the electro-encephalogram (EEG). A number of electrodes are stuck onto the scalp with tape, and then wired up to the EEG machine. Using an EEG the doctor can diagnose different types of epilepsy. In patients with epilepsy, flashing lights can be used to trigger the brain into producing epileptic-type brain waves. EEGs can also point towards other abnormalities, such as encephalitis, brain tumours etc.

We have quite different EEG readings when we're asleep. Sometimes an EEG is performed while the patient is asleep, to see if there are any abnormalities here. Although it involves being wired to a machine, the whole examination is completely painless and no needles are used.

These, then, are the techniques available to the doctor. You will see immediately how some of them are very complex and expensive, and can be used only in the most difficult of cases. On the other hand, some types of examination are very simple – it's easy to rule out blood pressure as a cause of a headache, just by measuring it! A simple observation like this can make or break a diagnosis. Finally, as discussed earlier, unless the problem is extremely complex, a carefully taken history, with minimal extra examination, will tell the doctor what he or she needs to know.

Chapter Two

MIGRAINE

OVERVIEW

Migraine is *not* just a severe headache, but a whole disease process, one part of which is a headache. Nor are the headaches of migraine always severe, though in many cases they are absolutely appalling. I can't emphasise enough that migraine is not a different *strength*, but a different *type* of headache.

Migraine is common – roughly one in ten people suffer from it. It disrupts work, family and social life. It's responsible for missed job opportunities, it diminishes output, and it accounts for about four million lost working days, and a yearly lost income of at least £200 million in Britain alone.

It's not actually accurate to talk about migraine as if it were a single entity, because there are many different types. The commonest form is a one-sided pulsating headache, lasting between one and three days, usually accompanied by nausea and vomiting and a sensitivity to light and noise. There is complete freedom from symptoms in between attacks.

There are many variants:

• *Common migraine* is what I've just described.

• *Classical migraine* is common migraine, but with an *aura* beforehand, which can last up to an hour. An aura is an inexplicable feeling or sensation which warns the sufferer that he is just about to have another attack. Aura symptoms vary, but often consist of flashing lights in front of the eyes. There are other, rarer variants.

Migraine can be split into five separate sections: the *prodrome* phase, where there may be food cravings, yawning, irritability, or euphoria; the *aura*, with flashing lights in front of the eyes, blind spots in the field of vision, numbness, or difficulty in speaking properly; the *headache phase*, during which the headache itself strikes, accompanied by other symptoms such as nausea, vomiting and sensitivity to light and sound; the *resolution phase*, during which the symptoms start to terminate and the patient is able to sleep it off; and the *recovery phase*, where there is exhaustion and a sense of being washed out.

This is what has been termed 'complete' migraine. *Not all migraineurs will experience every single part of this complete description.* Nor will the attacks necessarily follow the same pattern in the same patient – sometimes there may be an aura, sometimes not.

Women are much more susceptible to migraine than men by a factor of about three to one, largely because of the effect of the female hormone oestrogen. The relationship is complex: sometimes it is the lack of oestrogen that precipitates migraine; sometimes extra oestrogen does the damage.

In children, migraine takes two forms. In some cases children get ordinary 'head' migraines, which behave just like the adult variety; but children often get *abdominal migraine*, where the pain is in the stomach area, not the head. Abdominal migraine never has an aura, but otherwise it follows the same over-all pattern as adult migraine, though there are more symptoms relating to the gut.

The best way to treat a migraine is to identify as soon as possible that you're having an attack, and to start treatment straightaway. Prompt treatment can undoubtedly nip an attack in the bud; leave it for any length of time and you may have to suffer the full horrors over the next three days.

We used to think that common over-the-counter pain-killers such as aspirin and paracetamol didn't work particularly well in migraine, and that more powerful drugs like pethidine and morphine were needed to relieve the symptoms of an attack. Now we know this is not the case. The problem was not that these milder pain-killers didn't work, but that they weren't being absorbed properly. Migraine is a disease not just of the brain, but of the gut as well, and it affects the absorption of material in the stomach. Quite simply, aspirin and paracetamol often didn't work because they never got into the bloodstream.

Some of the newer anti-vomiting drugs, such as metoclopramide and domperidone, stabilise the gut, and allow better absorption to take place; once absorbed, the aspirin or paracetamol subdues the pain. In addition, the anti-vomiting drug also acts directly to reduce the nausea and vomiting.

A second important drug in the treatment of migraine is ergotamine. This is successfully used to constrict the dilated blood vessels in the head, that are thought to be involved in the migraine process. However it is a potentially dangerous drug and the dose levels recommended by your doctor must *not* be exceeded.

A new class of drugs has recently been used. These are the 5-HT agonists. 5-HT is a chemical that helps transmit messages within the brain. During a migraine, boosting the effect of 5-HT can help enormously, and may abort an attack. Sumatriptan is one drug that can do this successfully.

Other drugs that are used to abort an existing attack include caffeine, and the non-steroidal anti-inflammatories (NSAIDs) such as ibuprofen. Finally, if all else fails, pethidine or morphine, usually by injection, and often accompanied by an injectable anti-vomiting agent, will usually control the pain.

Prevention of migraine falls into two main areas. Many activities *trigger off* migraine, and the more each individual can identify his own triggers, and avoid them, the fewer attacks he is likely to have. Common triggers include chocolate and cheese, missing a meal, stress, excitement or shock, physical or mental fatigue, change of routine, bright lights or glare, loud noises, and even intense smells. In some cases hidden food allergies and smoking can trigger migraine.

Drugs can also prevent migraine. The beta-blocker *propranolol* is quite effective, and other drugs such as clonidine and pizotifen are frequently used. Continuous, low dose aspirin may also be useful.

There are many complementary methods for reducing the number of migraine attacks. These include adopting a healthy diet, taking adequate exercise, acupuncture, biofeedback, relaxation therapy and homoeopathy. In addition, osteopathic manipulation may correct neck problems that can trigger attacks in certain people. Complementary methods for treating an established attack include all of the above, plus aromatherapy, Bach flower remedies, acupressure and many many more. Gentle massage of the head may also help, particularly over the temple; cranial osteopathy may also assist.

Perhaps one of the more important complementary techniques comes from the herbalist. Feverfew leaves have always been used as a herbal remedy for headaches, but have recently been discovered to be particularly effective in treating migraine – so much so that there was a move afoot to take them away from over-the-counter availability and turn them into a prescription-only drug. Formal pharmaceutical investigations are currently being carried out.

Why do migraines occur? The answer, in a nutshell, is that we really don't know. There have been a number of theories involving constriction and dilation of the arteries, reduction of bloodflow in the brain, abnormalities of blood platelets (tiny cells within the blood responsible for initiating blood clotting), levels of brain magnesium, levels of 5-HT, previous neck injury, and abnormal reactivity of nerve cells. But, although each of these theories explains some of the features of migraine, none of them accounts for all the features of migraine attacks.

Cluster headache, otherwise known as *migrainous neuralgia*, is a further kind of headache linked to the migraine group. This is an excruciating, stabbing pain behind one eye, with weeping and redness of the eye on the affected side, together with sweating of the skin of the forehead and upper face. The attacks last between fifteen minutes and three hours, and, as its name suggests, occur in clusters lasting several weeks, with long pain-free periods in between the clusters of pain.

Although at first cluster headache seems similar to migraine, being a severe one-sided headache, it is actually quite different. It affects men more than women, by a ratio of about four to one, and is treated in an entirely different way.

The pain of a full-blown migraine is one of the most severe types of pain known to mankind. It can incapacitate the sufferer completely. Once you realise a migraine is coming on, you know that you're in for a ghastly period of up to three days, with your head feeling as though it's being split apart with a sledgehammer and a cold chisel, and vomiting until your stomach has long been empty. And even after the attack has waned, it's not over: it's likely to recur in the future.

Migraine is a very generalised brain event – which explains why it affects so many different aspects of the nervous system. But it's not just a disease of the nervous system, for the gut works in a very disordered way, too. And migraines aren't just pain and vomiting; there are other ways in which they can affect you. As discussed earlier, you may have an aura beforehand, in which there is blurred or disordered vision, and flashing lights or blank spots in your field of view. There can be numbness or tingling in various parts of the body, or difficulty in forming sentences and speaking properly. In a few cases the sufferer feels as if he is being shrunk down to a small size; on other occasions he feels that he has suddenly grown too big.

Migraine is one of the two oldest diseases known to man. In 400 BC, Hippocrates (who is commonly regarded as the father of medicine) described migraine clearly. Several centuries later, Aretaeus, a physician who worked in Alexandria circa AD 200, also described the typical intermittent, recurring headache of migraine, though he didn't call it that. Because of its one-sidedness it was soon known as hemicrania.

Not much progress was made over the next one and a half millennia until a fashionable eighteenth-century London doctor, John Fothergill, described some of the visual features, which he called 'fortification spectra' and, interestingly, suggested that his own migraines might be brought on by chocolate. How right he might have been!

Until the middle of the twentieth century, this was all that was known about migraine. We could observe what happened and give morphine for the intense pain, but there was little else that could help, and migraineurs just had to suffer in a darkened room, be patient, and wait for the attack to abate.

We know a lot more now and my feeling is that within thirty years we will have discovered precisely why migraine occurs, and will at last be able to control it completely.

A FEW MISCONCEPTIONS

We need to start by dispelling a few myths about migraine. This important point was mentioned earlier: Migraine is not *just* a severe headache: it is a special type of headache. Nor is it *necessarily* a severe headache; many sufferers have relatively minor headaches, but the associated symptoms indicate that without doubt they are suffering from migraine.

Another misconception is that those with migraine are frequently incapacitated by it. While this may be true for severe cases, there are many who have an attack only once or twice a year. There are also many others whose attacks are not severe or disabling enough to prevent them working. This doesn't mean that those who have frequent severe attacks of migraine are putting it on – far from it. The headache of migraine is one of the worst types of pain known to man, and in its fullest form is completely incapacitating.

Attitudes towards migraine vary according to which part of society you are in. Some groups of society think that migraine is an intellectual's disease. Other groups believe that migraine is a manifestation of psychiatric illness. Both attitudes are wrong! Migraine attacks people of all socio-economic groups. There is no link with having a high IQ and no direct link with being neurotic (though quite understandably, people with frequent severe migraines can become anxious or depressed as a result).

Perhaps the most surprising fact of all about migraine is that probably only fifty per cent of people suffering from it have ever consulted their doctor about it. Almost more remarkable is that a very large percentage of patients with migraine only ask their doctors about it once, and then don't go back. It seems that many migraine sufferers don't realise what can be done for them and resign themselves, unnecessarily, to their fate.

The point of all this is quite simple – the medical profession can now do a great deal to curb developing migraine attacks and to prevent attacks occurring. If you haven't yet consulted your doctor about your migraines, then please do, because it may make a considerable difference to the quality of your life.

WHO GETS MIGRAINES, AND HOW OFTEN?

Estimates vary as to the proportion of people who get migraines, but figures of between eight and twelve per cent are commonly quoted. There is no racial difference. Migraine affects women more than men.

The number of attacks varies in frequency from sufferer to sufferer, with some people having only one or two attacks a year: others less fortunate may have more than three a *week*.

It's difficult to get an 'average' picture, because only those patients with symptoms bad enough to consult their doctor get counted! At one of the UK migraine clinics, nearly one in ten patients were having more than three attacks a week; a quarter were having more than one attack per week, and nearly half had more than one attack per month.

Migraine generally starts before the age of forty, and most frequently begins in the twenty to thirty age group, though figures vary. Interestingly, migraine often occurs in childhood; a fifth of migraineurs began having attacks before the age of ten.

It *is* possible to have true migraines which start above the age of forty, but it's unusual; above the age of fifty it may well be associated with some other more serious abnormalities such as a tumour. Migraines which start after the age of fifty need full investigation by your doctor.

Migraine is not necessarily for life – about half of sufferers no longer have attacks twenty years later, and migraine is relatively uncommon over the age of sixty-five. Reassuringly, when attacks continue, their intensity usually reduces. We used to think that attacks dropped off after the menopause in women, but we now know that some women improve at the menopause and some get worse; some even have their first attack at this time.

TYPES OF MIGRAINE

As we discussed in the overview to this chapter, there are two main types of migraine, and a host of variants. The definitions are as follows:

Common migraine (migraine without aura)

This is the type of migraine described by eighty to ninety per cent of migraine sufferers.

- A headache of between four and seventy-two hours.

- One or more of the following symptoms:
  - nausea and/or vomiting
  - photophobia (dislike of light), and phonophobia (dislike of noise). Photophobia and phonophobia imply not just a dislike, but also discomfort or pain on being exposed to light/noise
- *And* at least two of the following describe the headache:
  - one-sided
  - pulsating
  - of moderate or severe intensity (to a degree which limits your ability to take part in normal daily activities);
  - made worse by normal physical activity

Classical migraine (otherwise known as migraine with aura)

Classical migraine is common migraine plus an *aura*. The most frequent type of aura is disturbance of vision – blurring of vision, flashing lights in front of the eyes, moving zig-zag lines, distortions of vision or blank spots in the field of view. Other aura symptoms include tingling or numbness in fingers, lips or tongue, weakness on one side of the body, and difficulty in forming sentences or speaking properly. In some cases the aura can include one-sided paralysis lasting up to two hours.

Typically aura symptoms occur *before* the headache starts. Only about ten to twenty per cent of migraineurs get an aura, and the side affected in the aura is *not* related to the side on which the headache occurs.

To have an aura you must have one or more of the following symptoms:

- Disturbances of vision, which are often the same in both eyes
- One-sided tingling or numbness
- One-sided weakness
- Inability to speak normally, usually caused by difficulty in forming sentences.

Aura symptoms are reversible, usually going away completely after less than an hour, and there is a distinct order of severity. Most common are the visual symptoms; then disorders of sensation; then (much less frequently) speech disorders, altered level of consciousness, and finally weakness or paralysis.

SYMPTOMS OF AN AURA

Focussing problems	Scalp pain
Blind spots in your field of vision	Tingling or numbness of hands or
Coloured lights	face
Flashing lines or zig-zags	Hunger, thirst, food cravings
Hallucinations	Double vision
Mood swings	Weakness or paralysis on one side
Speech problems	of the body

Abdominal migraine

Abdominal migraine is migraine that is perceived in the abdomen. It has exactly the same time span as common migraine, but never has any visual symptoms, or any other aura symptoms, such as paralysis. It *isn't* due to blood vessel instability, but may well be due to disordered movement and spasm of the muscles in the gut. The symptoms are abdominal pain, vomiting, sometimes with giddiness, and a dislike of bright lights. Disturbances of mood are common. There may be irritability and yawning, and a loss of energy and drive. Some children also experience a 'peculiar feeling' which they can't quite explain. In later life they may associate it with other migrainous symptoms which have only then become obvious – for example, the development of an aura.

Abdominal migraine often disappears by about the age of twelve, and it is not certain whether or not it progresses to common or classical migraine.

Menstrual migraine

Menstrual migraine is defined as a migraine which occurs at the beginning of the period – either on the first two days of the period, or the day before the period starts. It seems to be linked to a drop in oestrogen levels within the body and responds to treatment with hormone replacement therapy (HRT). About one in ten women with migraine experience menstrual migraine.

Other, less frequent, variants of migraine include the following:

Basilar migraine

Basilar migraine occurs mainly in young women, and is often associated with the time of the period. It occurs as a result of disturbances at a low level of the brain, involving a much more generalised upset in the brain's functioning. Rather than having an aura which affects only part of the body or part of the visual field, in basilar migraine the visual aura can involve the whole field of view. There can be ringing in the ears, dizziness, transient deafness, double vision, weakness on *both* sides of the body, uncoordination and clumsy speech. There can also be drowsiness which lasts for a number of hours or, briefly, unconsciousness. Although these symptoms are very dramatic they are fully reversible.

Migraine equivalent

This is when the typical aura of migraine is not associated with any headache.

Familial hemiplegic migraine

This is a rare form of migraine which is followed by weakness on one side of the body which can last up to a week; some close members of the family often exhibit the same problem. This is the only type of migraine that we believe to be fully hereditary. The tendency to have migraine does run in families, but in a much less specific way than in familial hemiplegic migraine, which may be handed down directly from parent to child.

Ophthalmoplegic migraine

In ophthalmoplegic migraine there is weakness of the muscles that control the movements of the eyes. Double vision is likely to occur, as is a drooping eyelid and a widened pupil.

We're not sure whether ophthalmoplegic migraine is true migraine at all. For a start, the headaches last a lot longer – often a week or more – than in other types of migraine.

Retinal migraine
In retinal migraine there is either complete blindness in one eye or alternatively a large patch missing from the visual field of *one* eye. (This is different from the blank spots in classical migraine, in which the blank areas occur in *both* eyes together.) As there are a number of other diseases that cause blind spots to develop in a single eye, further investigation may be needed to rule out other causes, such as clots in the eye itself.

Migraine with prolonged aura
Sometimes the aura can extend for up to a week. In cases like this there may actually be no headache at all! Although this can be true migraine, it can also indicate other neurological problems and full investigation is usually needed. Some doctors think that migraine with prolonged aura isn't true migraine at all.

Migraine with sudden aura
Technically this is called migraine with an acute onset aura. Here the migraine develops fully within five minutes of the aura starting. Again, this is rare, and it is important to make sure that there isn't something else underlying it.

COMPLICATIONS OF MIGRAINE
Status migrainosus
This is a migraine which continues for more than seventy-two hours, whether treated or not.

Stroke with migraine
Very rarely a migraine can end up with a small area of brain tissue losing its blood supply and dying. Only those who have an aura are at risk of this. Severe migraines associated with the contraceptive Pill can cause a small stroke; the dangerous attacks are: a first migraine attack *starting* on the Pill, and a migraine which *changes its nature* on the Pill, for example, changing from common migraine (without aura) to migraine with aura, or the development of numbness, tingling or paralysis, and so on.

TENSION HEADACHE AND MIGRAINE
Tension headache is quite different from migraine; it is related to stress and muscle tension in the head and neck. The pain is on both sides, and feels like a band round the head, across the forehead or like a weight pressing down on the head. Sufferers may have a headache on most days.

Although its symptoms are completely different to migraine, the combination of migraine and tension headaches is common; and, of course, stress triggers migraines in susceptible people.

MIGRAINE IN CHILDHOOD

Migraine in childhood behaves slightly differently from migraine in adults. As we have already seen it can sometimes occur as stomach pain – abdominal migraine.

However, many children get common or classical head migraines, sometimes alternating between the abdominal and head pain; and others get abdominal pain at the time that the aura would occur in an adult.

Even in children with normal migraine, there are differences between childhood and adult attacks. In children, attacks tend to be frequent and severe, though normally slightly shorter than in adults, and there can be long periods in between the bouts. Incomplete attacks are common. There may be many more generalised symptoms – nausea, vomiting, sweating, passing water frequently, or water retention.

In children there is an association between migraine and travel sickness and with dizziness. It is possible also that repeated attacks of unexplained vomiting (the so-called 'periodic' syndrome) actually are a form of migraine. It may develop into full migraine in later life.

Before puberty, migraine occurs more often in males, which is the reverse of the over-all picture, but after puberty the oestrogen levels of young girls rise. It is oestrogen which is the factor responsible for the preponderance of migraine in women. Basilar migraine is most common in adolescent girls, and ophthalmoplegic migraine in young boys.

The relationship between childhood and adult migraine isn't certain; some lose their attacks only to get them back later. However, of those who have migraine in childhood, approximately half will have stopped having attacks by the age of thirty.

MIGRAINE IN WOMEN

Migraine affects women differently from men. Attacks in women last slightly longer than in men, though this difference only becomes apparent after puberty, when oestrogen levels have started to rise.

In eighty per cent of cases, migraine improves during pregnancy, but it can also worsen. Those who have had menstrual migraine tend to lose it during pregnancy because of the raised (and more constant) levels of oestrogen. It is also common for a migraine to occur around the fourth to sixth day after delivery, when the oestrogen levels drop after childbirth.

The level of attacks may also improve at the menopause, when oestrogen levels drop. However, although some women experience a decline in their migraine at this time, others find that this is when their symptoms start or get much worse. Sometimes migraine at the time of the menopause can be helped with hormone replacement therapy (HRT) which provides extra oestrogen. Pizotifen is a non-hormonal drug that can also be used.

About ten to fifteen per cent of women experience migraine occurring at the time of the period. This also responds to extra oestrogen, perhaps as a 'patch' stuck on to the skin. Just to confuse matters, the Pill (which contains oestrogen and progesterone) can make established migraine worse, or even cause an aura to appear where previously the attacks were without one. Remember: if you get a migraine for the first time on the Pill, discontinue taking it immediately, and contact your doctor.

Rapidly worsening migraine when on the Pill is also a signal to stop taking it; this is particularly the case where migraines change from common migraine to classical migraine (with an aura). Both these problems were much more common when the high dose Pill was used.

SHEILA

At the age of twenty-five Sheila had completed her family, and was on the Pill. She'd used the Pill previously for a number of years without incident. Suddenly, and without warning, she had her first migraine; and it was a particularly bad attack, in which she had visual disturbances, one-sided headache and nausea, and also numbness of the right hand. Her doctor immediately told her to stop the Pill.

After the attack, it was discovered that Sheila's mother had had migraines, and had died in her early forties of a sub-arachnoid haemorrhage (see Chapter Nine).

Two weeks after stopping the Pill, Sheila was still having headaches with zig-zag lines at the edges of her field of vision. She was prescribed Migraleve (an analgesic antihistamine), which helped a lot, and for the next nine years this preparation suited her well and kept the migraines under control. But then she had a much more severe attack, which again led to numbness in the left arm. There was no obvious reason why her migraines should suddenly be getting worse. A few years earlier there had been stresses in her life, but these had resolved. Her doctor wondered whether she had developed any food allergies and enquired about her eating habits. She had recently stopped coffee and chocolate, knowing that these tended to cause migraines in susceptible people ... but she was very fond of cheese. Sheila's doctor suggested that she stop eating it for a time, to see what happened. Her migraines were greatly improved; in fact, for a time she had no migraines at all.

Sheila's job was working with chemicals involved with rubber and glue. One day she spilled a considerable amount, inhaling some of it in the process. Again, another migraine was provoked. Gradually her migraines became worse and she wondered whether this was related to her contact with chemicals. Eventually her attacks became so out of control that her doctor referred her to a migraine clinic.

The migraine clinic was anxious to ensure there was no underlying tumour, and gave her a full physical examination, including scans, but everything was normal. Unfortunately, she proved to be allergic to the beta-blocker group of drugs, so these couldn't be used to try to prevent attacks occurring. She tried numerous other drugs – some of which worked, and some of which didn't. Her headaches are now more or less under control, although she has a mild headache which lasts for three days around the time of her period.

Sheila's case is about as complicated a case of migraine as you could expect to find. There is a clear family history; evidence of several trigger factors, with sensitivity to cheese, the Pill and some of the chemicals that she works with. Some of the drugs have worked, but many of them have lost their efficacy. There is an association with her periods.

Sheila also suffered from migraine and tension headaches. When she went to her doctor again, he discovered something that had been buried for years. In the back of her mind Sheila had always worried whether her mother had died from migraine. Her doctor was able to reassure that there is no connection at all between a sub-arachnoid haemorrhage and a migraine, and with that Sheila burst into tears. She had obviously been enormously worried that one day the migraines would progress and kill her. She went out of the surgery a very relieved woman. Following this, her tension headaches reduced considerably.

Occasionally patients find that their migraines occur when they are ovulating, in the middle of the cycle. Finally, and very interestingly, there seems to be no great alteration in migraine patterns after hysterectomy or removal of the ovaries.

In other words, some migraines seem to be related to oestrogen. It must be remembered that oestrogen is not the only female hormone. Progesterone is also a major part of the female hormone cycle and there be other could links which we have not yet discovered. It may well be that the relationship between hormones and migraines in women is much more subtle, being affected by a relative balance of a group of hormones rather than the effects of a single hormone on its own.

Finally the trigger effects of oestrogen can combine with other triggering events. In other words, the effects of a missing meal may be much worse during your period; the triggering of the drop in blood sugar combines with the triggering effect of a drop in oestrogen often causing a migraine.

THE ATTACK ITSELF
Migraine attacks can be split into five separate stages:
- prodrome
- aura
- headache
- resolution
- recovery phase

However, not all migraineurs get an identifiable prodrome, or an aura. Although theoretically these phases are supposed to be separate (especially, the aura separated from the headache) experience suggests that overlap between the phases is actually quite common.

Attacks can begin at any time. Often, of course, they are related to the timing of their trigger factors. It is not unusual for sufferers to wake with a migraine.

The Prodrome. (Present in some patients only.) It may be others who notice the prodromal features more than you because some migraine sufferers develop recognisable patterns of behaviour. You may get excitable and on edge, or be tired and yawning. There may be craving for food (which would fit in neatly with a food allergy as a trigger). You may have fluid retention, or heightened perception. These prodromal features may last as much as twenty-four hours, with an average of ten hours. Recognising the prodrome can be important, because preventive medicines taken at this stage may abort the attack.

RICHARD

Richard is a doctor in his forties who has had migraine without aura (common migraine) for some twenty years. Over the years he has tried practically every preparation that is used in the treatment of migraine. He has found that for him the best cocktail of drugs is a very simple one: three aspirins, taken the minute he is aware that an attack is starting. Often this will stop an attack, but if it doesn't, then he will take two tablets of the pain-killer co-proxamol shortly afterwards. If this doesn't work, then he knows he's in for the full horrors of a migraine; he has found nothing that will relieve the attack once it's into its stride.

When he spots the attacks happening early on he can save himself a lot of misery. Interestingly, his colleagues and staff can tell that he's about to have a migraine before he can, because for about three days beforehand he becomes slightly 'high', rushing around and behaving in a hyper-excitable and irritable fashion; he doesn't even realise that he is doing it.

If his colleagues tell him that he's becoming excitable, and if he makes a conscious effort to calm himself down, taking things a little more slowly, then the impending migraine doesn't progress to a headache and the attack is aborted. On the other hand, if he doesn't make the effort to calm himself down he soon begins to feel the headache of a migraine coming on. Richard is a good example of a migraine sufferer who has a distinct prodromal illness. In him this phase is unusually long – it may take three days before the headache starts, and without any aura or visual changes, Richard goes straight from the prodrome into the headache phase.

The *aura*. (The aura doesn't occur in common migraine.) There may be disorders of vision, flashing lights in the eyes, blank parts of your visual field; or you may have numbness and tingling over parts of your body; or difficulty in speaking, with an inability to string words together properly.

Aura symptoms vary from person to person. In many people the aura consists solely of twinkling lights at the very edges of the visual field, but in more severe cases can involve zig-zag lines, semi-circular blind spots in the field of vision etc.

A typical visual aura can be descrcibed as follows: it will begin with blurred vision, which is actually a small 'blind spot' near the centre of vision, in *both* eyes, and in the same place in both visual fields. This begins to expand within a minute or two, often forming a semi-circle to the right or to the left. The edge of the semi-circle is jagged, like the teeth of a large saw. This effect is called a fortification spectrum because of its similarity to the plan of medieval forts.

On the inside of this enlarging, jagged outline is a blind area. As the semi-circle becomes larger and larger, the saw-tooth edge becomes more angled and more irregular and the scintillations (flashes of light) in it become more obvious. The whole blind spot moves to one side and then disappears (more often to the right). Only then does the headache start.

At first the headache is not always on one side, and interestingly when it *is* one-sided it is not always on the side opposite to the blind area. Inside the brain nearly everything is converted left to right, so your left brain controls the right side of the body, and vice versa. A blind spot in the *right* side of the field of view is related to problems in the *left* side of the part of the brain dealing with vision. Sometimes the visual aura leaves an 'after-image' reminiscent of a shattered windscreen.

The visual aura ranges from a few minutes to over an hour, but most frequently lasts about twenty minutes. It can also include numbness of the hands or face, double vision, and weakness on one side of the body.

The *headache*. Usually the visual symptoms have gone by now, to be replaced by pain on opening the eyes; photophobia (sensitivity to light) and phonophobia (sensitivity to noise) are common. There is often nausea and vomiting. Note again how some of the symptoms change throughout the attack. Food cravings in the prodromal period may be replaced by nausea and then vomiting; this resolves gradually, passing through a phase when there is only limited tolerance to food. Similarly, the visual symptoms of migraine are in the aura phase, and when the headache takes over, these visual symptoms are replaced by photophobia with pain on opening the eyes.

In eighty per cent of cases the headache is one-sided; it is throbbing, and made worse by movement or straining. The face usually goes pale, and you may feel cold, especially in the hands and feet. During this time you will probably want to lie down in a quiet and darkened room. Light and noise may both be painful, and strong smells may cause nausea. During this time you may feel sleepy and yawn.

Intolerance of loud noise and dizziness often accompanies migraine. Sounds may be distorted and other people's voices may sound unnatural and unreal. This magnification of sound is thought by some patients to indicate that their hearing has become more acute but, in fact, probably all they are suffering from is something called noise recruitment. In this case, there is actually a reduced ability to hear soft sounds, but the louder noises are magnified; in other words, a quiet whisper may not be heard at all, but a normal voice may sound as though the person is shouting.

There may be added noises and distortion of sounds, with roaring, rushing or hissing noises. These added sounds may occur during the attack, or during the aura. Very occasionally, deafness can occur, either in the aura, or during the headache. There is the possibility that repeated attacks of this nature can lead on to permanently reduced hearing, but deafness as a result of migraine is *very* rare.

Dizziness and vertigo (distortion in the sense of balance) are frequently associated with migraine. There are two forms: in the first the room appears to spin round (or else you feel as though you're spinning round within the room) in the second, you experience strange and ill-defined feelings of floating or sinking, and of unsteadiness on walking. These sensations may be part of the aura, or during the headache itself. Outside the attack, a good proportion of migraine sufferers also suffer from motion sickness.

The *resolution.* Vomiting and sleep may herald the decline of the attack, but there is still a considerable degree of headache.

The *recovery.* After the main attack has subsided you will feel very fragile. It takes about thirty hours to get through this stage before you feel back to normal.

THE CAUSE OF MIGRAINE

We really don't know what causes migraine. Some doctors think that it is related to abnormalities in the workings of the nervous tissue in the brain; others think that it is mainly due to changes in the blood supply to the brain caused by the irritability and instability of the arteries themselves. The final answer, of course, may well be a bit of each – partly nervous, partly vascular.

One of the first theories about migraine was that it was due to changes in blood vessels in the head: those on the outside are dilated; those on the inside constricted. This would explain what happens in the visual aura. The way that the flickering (and particularly *expanding*) zig-zags of light occur in the visual aura is easy to explain if there is some sort of abnormal effect happening to the nerve cells in the visual cortex, spreading out rather like a ripple from a stone thrown into a pond. If a wave of blood-vessel contraction were to spread out from a central point in the visual cortex at about three millimetres per minute, it would produce exactly the effect migraineurs observe in the aura.

Each visual cortex (where visual information is processed in the brain) deals with visual information from one *side*, not one eye, so the flickering and blind spots seem to occur in *both* eyes together not because the eyes are affected, but because the area *processing* the information is sending off signals that are confusingly not genuine.

The aura can be aborted by using drugs that open up the arteries in the brain. However, most migraines occur without an aura, so how do they fit in? In addition, the way the aura spreads doesn't correspond to the distribution of blood vessels in the brain. It seems to go across boundaries between blood vessels without stopping – not what you'd expect if it were the constriction of blood vessels that starts off the whole process.

The next theory states that it's not the blood vessels that go wrong, but the nerves, and that blood-vessel changes are secondary. This would explain why the visual disturbances of the aura come before the headache. The prodromal symptoms – such as euphoria, food cravings and increased appetite – could be due to abnormal activity in a part of the brain called the *hypothalamus* (a region of the brain with nerve connections to most other parts of the nervous system).

A third theory is that those things that trigger migraine interfere chemically with the blood, creating abnormal levels of a chemical called 5-HT. We've known for a long time that 5-HT levels change during a migraine attack, and an injection of 5-HT can abort migraines. 5-HT-depleting drugs can increase the number of migraines in susceptible people. Most of the 5-HT in the blood is in the platelets, which are the tiny cell-like structures responsible for initiating clotting.

5-HT has effects on the blood vessels; and the lower parts of the brain are rich in nerves which use 5-HT as their transmitter chemicals. These nerves connect extensively with the higher parts of the brain, so a disturbance of these could well trigger off events higher up in the brain. Another theory involves the trigeminal nerve, which senses pain across the side of the face. When this is stimulated it causes blood vessels outside the brain to open up, and the suggestion is that the spreading wave of depression of the nerve-cell activity finally hits the part of the brain where the trigeminal nerve terminates, causing it firstly to give off pain signals, and secondly to cause blood-vessel enlargement.

Magnesium in the brain has recently attracted a lot of attention. During an attack magnesium levels seem to be low in migraine patients. Magnesium is important in controlling the contraction of blood vessels, as well as controlling the release of transmitter chemicals that send messages from nerve to nerve in the brain. It is also connected with platelet stickiness and clumping may well have a part to play.

Yet another theory involves the stellate ganglion. If the stellate ganglion doesn't work properly, it sends nerve signals which make the arteries go into spasm. The brain can't function without blood, so it over-rides this contraction, opening up the arteries in the brain, and increasing the blood-pressure inside the skull and brain. This theory would also explain why women are more susceptible to migraines, because the female hormones cause more fluid to accumulate in the region around the stellate ganglion causing it to function less well (through oedema). Any damage to the neck or spine in the past can later cause spasm in the area which would affect the function of the stellate ganglion.

Explanations for the pain of migraine are just as confusing. At first, it looked as though the headache was due to pain in the blood vessels outside the brain, especially because of its throbbing nature, beating in time with the pulse. Reducing the pressure reduces the headache – but only in about one-third of all patients.

So what is the answer? It may well be an amalgamation of bits from each theory. There is a *Unifying theory*, which tries to pull all these disparate pieces of evidence together; but for the moment the answer is that we really don't know for sure.

TRIGGER FACTORS

Although we don't know the precise biochemical mechanism of migraine, we certainly know a lot about the things that trigger it. The following things are all known to trigger off attacks in some patients. They are in no particular order.

Food

There's a very complex relationship between migraine and food. Insufficient food – such as missing or delaying a meal, or fasting – may trigger a migraine in susceptible people, and about one in five migraine sufferers claims that a particular food or foods will trigger an attack. Chocolate and cheese are high on the list of culprits, but alcohol, citrus fruits and dairy products are all well known triggers.

There are three completely distinct mechanisms by which food can cause problems.

- *A drop in glucose levels in the blood*, caused by a sudden lack of food.

- Direct stimulation of cells in the brain from the *tyramine content* of certain foods. Tyramine is an amino acid (a chemical compound found in protein) and it is present in high concentrations in some foods – particularly chocolate and cheese. The effect of tyramine is directly related to the dose the patient receives. A smal dose might have a small triggering effect, and a larger dose gives a correspondingly larger effect on the brain. Tyramine and related chemicals are thought to trigger migraines because people who are susceptible to tyramine don't have the enzymes to remove these chemicals as quickly from the body; they remain for longer, affecting the blood vessels and triggering an attack.

FOODS CONTAINING TYRAMINE

All cheeses (especially fermented)	Eggs
Marmite and other yeast extracts	Broad beans
Beer, stout, ale	Avocados
Wine (especially red)	Spinach
Pickled herrings	Oranges
Chocolate	Prunes
Beef	Figs
Liver	Plums
Canned meats	Bananas
Fermented sausage or salami	Tomatoes
Hung game	Aubergines
Soy sauce	

- *An allergic reaction*. Food allergies behave in slightly odd and sometimes quite surprising ways. There is an element of addiction in allergy, so that if you're allergic to a particular food you'll probably be eating it very frequently: you may also crave it. After abstaining from a food to which you are allergic for at least five days, eating it for the first time will promptly trigger a migraine. However, if the food is unsuspected as a trigger and is taken on a virtually continuous basis (for example, the way in which we use milk) then from time to time this food will trigger headaches almost randomly.

COMMON FOOD ALLERGIES IN MIGRAINE

Milk	Orange Juice
Cheese	Tomatoes
Coffee	Potatoes
Tea	

In practical terms, the difference between a pharmacological action of a chemical and an allergic response to the same chemical is that in a pharmacological action the effect is dependent on the size of the dose, whereas in an allergic reaction the effect is almost maximal right from the start. It's like the difference between pedalling an electrical generator in order to create electricity to power an electric bulb, as opposed to switching on a light using a switch on the wall. The man generating the light by pedalling is like the pharmacological response – the harder he pedals, the brighter the light. On the other hand, an allergic response is like the man switching on a light – one small movement and the light is fully on.

If you are familiar with the techniques and effects of food allergy then you'll understand that the way in which foods cause migraine can be very complex. For example, abstaining from food can cause a migraine by two completely different routes: firstly, because the blood sugar is lowered; and secondly, because the patient is having a withdrawal reaction from the food to which he is addicted.

Similarly, the patient who finds that cheese triggers an attack may be having a direct pharmacological effect from the tyramine, or alternatively may be allergic to other components of the cheese. Or it could be a combination of both.

Food exclusion results in long-term reduction in migraines in approximately eighty-five per cent of patients. The most common foods excluded are shown in the box below.

FOODS MOST COMMONLY AVOIDED IN MIGRAINE

Chocolate	Some vegetables (especially
Cheese and dairy products	onions)
(especially Brie, Camembert,	Tea
Stilton)	Coffee
Fruit (especially citrus and green,	Meat (especially pork)
unripe apples)	Seafood
Alcohol (especially red wine)	

Although *caffeine* can help control headaches, and is commonly used in anti-migraine preparations, headaches can occur both from too much caffeine, and from sudden withdrawal in those who drink a lot of tea, coffee and cola drinks. Our intake of coffee can drop suddenly at the weekend, away from work, so if you tend to have weekend migraines it might be due to caffeine withdrawal. Often sufferers halve their intake of caffeine at the weekend, without realising it. The cure? Gradually reduce your intake of caffeine over the *whole week*, evening it out and avoiding sudden drops in intake. Weekend migraine may also be related to a reduction in stress when away from work, and also the effects of sleeping in late, both of which are known to trigger migraines in susceptible people.

Migraine from missed meals can be a problem in those who fast for religious reasons; for example, Muslims during *Ramadan*, and Orthodox Jews at *Yom Kippur* (the Day of Atonement). Also, those who are trying to lose weight may precipitate a migraine by dieting, either because the blood sugar falls, or alternatively due to withdrawal of a food to which they are addicted/allergic.

Conversely, putting on weight can reduce or even stop attacks, probably because the blood sugar level has gone up. We know that migraines also reduce in those who develop diabetes, where the level of blood sugar is generally higher than normal.

JOYCE

Joyce is a forty-five-year-old housewife who had migraine for ten years. Her doctor suggested it might be worth testing to see if there were any food sensitivities. Joyce was instructed to take all normal foods out of her diet, instead substituting turkey and rice at all meals. She was to stay on this exclusion diet for five days, after which she would re-introduce foods one by one.

Within a day of starting the exclusion diet she developed another migraine – a typical withdrawal-type migraine. As happens so often in these cases, she rang up her doctor to say that she was suffering a migraine, and since she wasn't eating any of her normal foods could she please stop the diet? Her doctor explained that a migraine which occurs after stopping normal foods often implies that there is a food allergy waiting to be discovered, and encouraged her to keep on with the exclusion diet.

The migraine cleared and after five days Joyce felt very much better. Then she started putting foods back into her diet one by one, keeping a diary, and noting any return of symptoms. Nothing happened. She was still clear of migraines, and had re-introduced most fresh foods into her diet.Then she began to re-introduce foods in processed form and discovered to her amazement that tinned peas seemed to cause the trouble. As long as she misses these out of her diet, she is well; interestingly, she remarked to her doctor some weeks later that since removing the offending food from her diet, her mental processes seemed to be a great deal clearer and her hearing also seemed to be much more acute.

Anything in your diet can cause trouble. Many chemicals are added to foods during tinning, processing, or freezing and these can be just as potent a cause of migraine as the foods

*themselves. It is interesting, too, how Joyce's mental
befuddlement cleared when she was away from the substance to
which she was allergic. This mental befuddlement is well-known
to those doctors who do a lot of work with food allergies. It
even has a special name – brain fag – which aptly describes the
over-all sense of malaise it engenders.*

There are several methods by which you can avoid problems with food triggers:

Sort out any food sensitivities and then avoid those foods to which you're sensitive.

Don't miss meals, especially breakfast. If you don't usually eat breakfast, at least have something to eat in the mid-morning.

Don't snack or have just a salad for lunch. A slightly more substantial meal is better.

Don't wait to eat until after an evening out. Have a snack before going out to the cinema or theatre.

Prepare yourself for cocktail parties. These contain lots of triggers – alcohol, noise, stress, cheese, wine, insufficient real food, as well as the stress of getting there on time.

Children must eat before exercise. An empty stomach combined with exercise can trigger attacks, so don't go to school without breakfast!

Monitor the foods your children are eating. Children often buy just the sort of foods to trigger their attacks – chocolate, crisps, etc.

The stress of examinations can trigger migraines too.

During an attack, try to eat something sugary or starch .

Stress

Stress is probably the most common trigger for migraine. Stress is a blanket term which can also include excitement and anticipation. Like food allergies, stress can also trigger migraine when it is *removed*; for example, causing a 'weekend migraine', when you're away from the busy office. Migraines can also be brought on by the stress of social situations – such as parties, travel, and going to the cinema or dancing.

There is also the stress brought on by a fear of what the migraines might mean (for example, fear of an underlying brain tumour). This merely serves to multiply whatever stress you have, bringing on more migraines.

Too much or too little sleep can precipitate a migraine; for example, lying in bed at the weekend may start off an attack. There is an increased frequency of migraine in anxiety and depression.

Anything which causes excitement – particularly in children – can trigger migraines. Certain types of physical stress, such as jogging or lovemaking can act as triggers, too.

If it is erratic, exercise can trigger migraine. On the other hand, *regular* exercise is beneficial. Bending or stooping (as in gardening) can trigger attacks, as can lifting heavy weights and straining, as well as physical or mental fatigue.

Car journeys
Car journeys can trigger migraines. A lot of other triggers can be involved, too – the stress and fatigue of the journey; motion sickness; flashing lights at night as cars zoom past in the other direction; windscreen wipers flicking across your field of view, especially where there are bright lights in front (causing flicker). And, when the sun is low and to one side, travelling through a treelined avenue can create *immense* flicker.

Hormonal changes
This is exclusively confined to women. Migraines may be triggered by the drop in oestrogen at the time of the monthly period and may be improved (but sometimes worsen) during pregnancy; often improve (but sometimes worsen) at the menopause, and can be made worse by the Pill, which in rare cases can trigger off a most dangerous type of migraine attack.

Environment
Heat, cold, light and *noise* can all precipitate migraine. The weather can also act as a trigger. The most famous account of this is Dr Edward Wilson, who was on Captain Scott's doomed expedition to the South Pole. He invariably suffered a migraine attack ten to twelve hours before a blizzard started.

In most migraineurs it is probably the increased glare which does the damage. This is made worse by high-altitude thin cloud, which heralds a cold front; the cloud causes the glare, and the rain follows the front.

Bright light and especially high contrast can trigger attacks. Even something as simple as sitting talking to a friend who is silhouetted in front of a sunlit window can bring on a migraine. Some people get migraines from staring at computer screens, particularly when they are not set up very well.

Sunlight reflecting or shimmering off water can act as a trigger. Polarised glasses, which selectively cut out reflected light, can help greatly in reducing the amount of reflected flicker.

An excessively dry atmosphere can act as a trigger – dry air tends to contain increased amounts of dust particles, which are thought to start the migraine process in some people. There are more likely to be excessive numbers of charged particles about in dry conditions, which would explain why susceptible people get migraine in dry weather, and also why migraine is associated with certain winds which blow in the eastern Mediterranean and Switzerland.

Positive ions in the atmosphere can also trigger migraines. These ions occur in large quantities before a thunderstorm. As the storm passes, the charge changes from positive to negative, but by then the migraine may have started. Sprays of water fill the air with negative ions, so having a shower may help counter the effects of thundery weather.

Positive ions are also present in large quantities in centrally heated and air-conditioned offices; there are many ions in the air, but the metal ducting used in air conditioning systems tends to attractive negative ions more quickly than positive ones, thereby stripping the air of negative ions and leaving positive ones behind. Opening the windows, or using an ioniser, may help.

Hot baths can trigger migraines in some people.

Dental causes

It is now recognisd that some types of dental problems can trigger migraines. One particularly strange one is that alterations of the bite can lead to different tensions in the muscles on either side of the head, and this in turn can cause migraines. Sometimes the problem occurs when so many teeth have been lost that the jaw over-closes. Altering the angle of the bite can stop the provocative effects.

Unconscious grinding of the teeth often occurs during sleep, causing tension in the muscles that form the cheeks; this may also prompt an attack. Relaxation therapy may help to reduce the over-all level of stress.

Neck pain

Spasm of the muscles in the neck, which often occurs as a result of minor malpositioning of the vertebrae, can set off migraines. Improvement in the care of the neck – sometimes by manipulation, sometimes by better ergonomic planning – may bring dramatic improvements.

Smoking

Smoking can generate migraines, too. There is a cross-over effect with a food allergy to potatoes, tobacco and tomatoes, as these plants are all closely related.

Body clock

Changes to the body clock such as jet-leg, or going on to night shift may trigger migraines; also, holidays and weekends (with relaxation from stress, late rising, and erratic bedtimes) may do the same.

Anaemia

Anaemia can both worsen migraine attacks, and increase their frequency.

WHY ME?

Only one form of migraine is known to be completely genetic in origin. This is *familial hemiplegic* migraine, a specific (and rare) type of migraine. In this form of migraine, the migraineur suffers from transient paralysis of one side of the body; and other close members of the family suffer from an identical type of migraine.

Although a direct genetic link hasn't been established in other types of migraine, migraine does seem to run in families. Nearly half of migraine sufferers have a near relative with the disease, compared to one-sixth of non-migraineurs.

There may be several reasons for this. Firstly, some people have migraines because of food allergies. The tendency to be allergic is probably a single inherited gene, but the allergen to which you are sensitive and how it manifests itself depends on many other things – such as what substances you've been exposed to, especially at certain vulnerable times of your life. Therefore, migraines caused by food allergies are not solely genetic in origin.

The second reason is that there are probably several different genes involved in migraine, and whether you tend to get migraines or not depends upon what mix of genes you receive in your own genetic make-up.

The third reason migraines run in families is that stressed parents often teach their children stressful behaviour by example. Or, more relevantly, they *don't* teach them how to cope with stress, because they don't know how to do so themselves. Stress therefore runs in families, but in a non-genetic way.

There is no relationship between migraines and class, race or intelligence.

A slight statistical relationship exists between migraine and epilepsy. Both share a number of neurological features, such as visual symptoms, and a spread of the effect within the movements of the brain. In particular, temporal lobe epilepsy can share some features with migrainous attacks; and in those with both migraine and epilepsy, a high proportion started their epilepsy in the years immediately after the migraines started.

There is also a relationship with Menière's disease (one-sided deafness, dizziness and tinnitus); people with Menière's disease have a higher-than-average incidence of migraine.

MIGRAINE ATTACKS AT WORK

Half those questioned about their migraines say that their migraine has interfered with their career and job prospects. Migraine has a considerable effect on our ability to work. With minor attacks it's possible to work through a migraine, but in full-blown attacks it's impossible. Not only is the headache so severe that you can hardly think, but it is worsened by excess noise, motion, flickering lights, stress and computer VDUs, to say nothing of strong smells.

Despite the fact that millions of working days are lost each year due to migraine, only about a third of employees have ever told their doctor that they suffer from migraine, even though they may find that it is triggered at work. It is interesting in that the group who are least likely to tell their employers about their migraine are those in middle management, for whom advancement and job prospects are so important.

Migraine attacks at work present two different problems. Firstly, work is more likely to trigger off migraines, simply because so many trigger factors may be present. Furthermore, stress may trigger off migraines in certain people, and work often stresses us more than anything else. Finally allergic triggers, such as chemicals and strong smells may also be present in your workplace.

It's not just stress and over-work that can cause damage, either. Underwork can do it, too. Therefore, if your job consists of mere machine minding, with little to do from hour to hour except to wait for the occasional problem, then you may get more migraines as a result.

Migraines can be quite dangerous at work, for several reasons. Firstly, your attention and concentration is likely to be reduced because of the pain, so you may make mistakes and errors of judgement. Secondly, if you're working near machinery you may not be aware of danger, particularly if you've got distorted vision or a blind spot in your field of view. It also means you shouldn't be driving if you have visual impairment of this sort. Thirdly, if you get paralysis or weakness you may not be able to control your car or your machine properly. Lastly, your mental functioning declines in migraine, and you may not be able to form sentences properly during the aura phase – and this is potentially dangerous if you need to give clear instructions or make complex decisions.

Once the attack has started, work is not a helpful place to be. In a bad attack a migraineur needs quiet and rest, and most factories and offices are anything but restful, quiet places.

If at the beginning of an attack you can get rest and quiet for a time, and take whatever medication you usually need, then you may abort the attack and be able to return to work; but, if there is no rest room or sick room where you can go and lie down, then the attack is likely to continue and you'll be off work for the next day or so.

Type of headache

The headache of migraine is often one-sided (but not always on the same side), pounding, often immensely painful, and with a slow onset, usually taking thirty minutes to an hour to reach its full intensity. Migraines occur repeatedly, with complete freedom from headache between attacks.

The popular image of migraine is of a one-sided headache, often centred on one eye, but this isn't strictly true. Although a large percentage of migraines are one-sided, some aren't – and the early stages of migraine can be on both sites. Please refer to Chapter 1 for diagrams of the many sites at which migraine headaches can appear.

What else could it be?

Cluster headache is one-sided, centring on one eye, and it doesn't change sides. It's of much shorter duration, lasting fifteen minutes to three hours, and is accompanied by weeping and redness of the affected eye, and sweating of the forehead and face. It occurs in clusters, with long periods of respite in between.

Tension headache is more continuous, often for days on end. It can feel like a tight band round the skull, a weight pressing on the head, or pain in the forehead or back of the neck. There is often dislike of noise or sound, but this is mild by comparison with the photophobia and phonophobia of migraine. The pain too is mild in comparison with most migraines. However, it can be difficult to distinguish between migraine without aura (common migraine) and tension headache.

Subarachnoid haemorrhage is a sudden, severe pain, often with loss of consciousness and vomiting. Typically, the pain feels as if you've been hit in the back of the neck.

Meningitis is a severe headache with photophobia and vomiting, but there is usually a temperature, always a stiff neck on forward bending (except in babies) and sometimes a purplish, blotchy rash.

True coital headache comes on intermittently during sexual intercourse, in those people (usually male) who are susceptible to it. There is a possibility that this is a variant of migraine anyway..

Referred pain from neck injuries can appear to be centred over one eye. There is no nausea or vomiting, and usually the pain and muscle spasm in the muscles at the back of the neck show where the cause of the problem lies.

Acute glaucoma can be immensely painful, with vomiting, and with pain radiating out from one eye. The eye is tender, the pupil is irregular and cloudy, and although there is photophobia, there is also dimness of vision. It's often preceded by seeing haloes round bright lights.

Temporal lobe epilepsy usually ends in a fit, which makes the diagnosis easy. Just occasionally it doesn't, and because temporal lobe epilepsy can produce visual hallucinations similar to those of migraine, it can be confused with it. An electroencephalogram (EEG) may help to distinguish between the two conditions.

Tumours can cause severe headaches and vomiting, but the pain is over both sides of the head, and much more continuous. Usually other symptoms (such as weakness or paralysis, or failure to attend to objects on one side of the field of vision), will have brought the problem to the doctor's attention long before the headaches start.

Strokes can give headache and vomiting, with one-sided paralysis. Usually the headache resolves quite quickly, but the paralysis remains.

Temporal arteritis is a disease of the over-fifty age group. There is tenderness of the artery in the temples; if allowed to continue untreated, it can progress to irreversible blindness in one or both eyes.

Orthodox treatment

The therapy of migraines divides neatly into two parts – firstly, prevention; and secondly, treatment of the existing attack. Drug treatments seem to work equally well on migraine with aura (classical) and migraine without aura (common).

Prevention

You can minimise the number of attacks you experience through carefully eliminating or minimising your trigger factors. However, we all live in a real world, and it's just not possible to eliminate all your trigger factors entirely. There will always be those missed meals, the food inadvertently eaten, the exam to be taken, the stress at work.

Don't worry about those trigger factors you can't avoid. Instead, concentrate on minimising whatever you can, especially when you know you'll be exposed to one or more factors. For example, take a leaf from the book of the woman who says she can drink red wine, but not during the week before her period.

A number of medicines can be used to prevent attacks occurring. These drugs are not pain-killers, nor do they work during an attack. They work solely to prevent attacks occurring – by stabilising your systems so that trigger factors are less likely to provoke an attack. Preventative medicine is of greatest value where the attacks are frequent; it is inconvenient (and expensive) to take drugs for attacks that happen infrequently. It also exposes you to the possibility of side-effects for very little gain. A convenient rule of thumb is that if you get more than two attacks a month, preventative drug treatment is likely to be worthwhile.

Various drugs are used to prevent attacks; these include beta-blockers such as propranolol; anti-5-HT agents, such as methysergide and pizotifen; calcium channel-blockers such as nifedepine; and occasionally tranquillisers and anti-depressants such as amitriptyline, though amitriptyline may well be acting in a different way on migraines.

Drugs to prevent attacks have to be taken on a regular basis, and it may take them several weeks to have full effects. No drug is completely effective, but propranolol reduces the number of attacks in about fifty per cent of migraineurs.

In women, especially those with menopausal or menstrual migraine, attacks can be prevented using replacement oestrogen, either as tablets or patches. In menopausal migraine clonidine can also help.

Treatment of the existing attack

Migraine is a syndrome which involves a lot more than just the brain. One of the things it does is stop the absorption of substances from the stomach (in addition to making the patient nauseous and sick). Anything that is in the stomach that isn't vomited up is likely to stay there unabsorbed for a long time.

Now we've found that we can reverse this with certain types of anti-vomiting drugs. Metoclopramide is one, domperidone is another. These are anti-nausea drugs that also stabilise the muscle activity within the gut, on which it can have a most dramatic effect. Giving a small dose of metoclopramide together with paracetamol or aspirin, allows the pain-killer to be absorbed across the stomach wall and – hey, presto! – in many cases the migraine attack is aborted. Metoclopramide and domperidone also have the extra advantage of being anti-vomiting agents, damping down the vomiting centre and reducing what is probably the second most unpleasant aspect of migraine, after the headache.

The use of metoclopramide and similar drugs has revolutionised many aspects of migraine therapy, and has certainly reduced the need for the heavy morphine-based drugs. At the first sign of an attack a sufferer may take a tablet of metoclopramide together with a couple of tablets of paracetamol or aspirin (or, a combination drug combining both of them) and, with a bit of luck, the attack may be halted.

Migraleve Pink tablets contain an anti-vomiting agent of a different type: Migraleve Yellow tablets (the follow-on tablets) don't contain painkillers.

The most important aspect of treating an attack is to start taking the medicines *early*. Nipping it in the bud is one of the most effective ways of dealing with an impending attack; leaving it for several hours may be too late.

There is a wide variety of drugs to select from, and different doctors will have different ideas about the relative importance of each group. Not all drugs are safe to use for children.

The five groups of drugs used to treat an attack are: analgesics, anti-vomiting agents, ergotamine, sedatives and the 5-HT stimulants.

• *Analgesics.* There's no great virtue in taking strong analgesics when simple ones will do, and often paracetamol and/or aspirin are perfectly acceptable, provided that they are absorbed into the bloodstream. Aspirin has the additional advantage that it helps to reduce the stickiness of platelets in the blood; and, as these may have a role in the migraine attack, aspirin may be of added benefit. Don't give aspirin to children, and don't use it in pregnancy, nor if you have stomach ulcers or are on anticoagulants or steroids.

If simple analgesics like these don't work your doctor may well prescribe something stronger, such as codeine, dihydrocodeine or coproxamol: in the last resort it may still be necessary to use pethidine, morphine, diamorphine, or pentazocine. Where you are continuing to vomit it may be necessary to give these very strong drugs by injection.

• *Anti-vomiting Drugs.* We've already dealt with the anti-nausea drugs. These have two effects: reducing vomiting and nausea, and allowing the absorption of other drugs. Obviously, if there is vomiting already then these agents won't work and will need to be given by injection or suppository.

• *Ergotamine.* Ergotamine is a potent vaso-constrictor (causing blood vessels to clamp up tightly) which, bearing in mind that in migraine the blood vessels are often dilated, may be the reason why it helps. However more recent work suggests that its action on blood vessels is a lot more complex than this. Ergotamine isn't absorbed very well in tablet form so it's often used as a suppository, taken under the tongue or inhaled, using a pressurised inhaler. Caffeine helps the absorption of ergotamine, and is often combined with it. The big problem with the use of ergotamine is that the effective dose is very near the toxic dose. *Do not increase* the dose of ergotamine beyond what your doctor has prescribed, or you could lose the blood supply to your extremities, causing gangrene.

Also, ergotamine must *never* be given to a pregnant woman because it can cause the most violent contractions in the womb, leading either to a premature delivery or to suffocation of the baby within the womb. Ergotamine should also not be used in those with heart disease or circulation problems. Ergotamine mustn't be used too regularly – there is an *ergotamine-abuse syndrome*, in which the ergotamine itself causes headaches. Ergotamine headaches are unlike migraines, being more of a generalised dull headache.

• *Sedatives.* Sedatives are sometimes useful in aborting an attack early on. If you are able to relax and go to sleep you may wake up headache-free, and this is particularly useful when stress is a triggering factor. Common sedatives include the benzodiazepine tranquillisers: diazepam, chlordizepoxide etc. but there are others, such as chlorpromazine.

However, many anti-migraine drugs contain caffeine, which will have the opposite effect! It may be better to avoid caffeine-containing drugs if your migraines are linked to stress or anxiety.

• *5-HT Stimulants* (agonists). Transmitter chemicals allow messages to pass from nerve to nerve in the body. One of these chemicals is a substance called 5-HT, otherwise known as serotonin. 5-HT seems to have an important part to play in the workings of the brain, though the exact relationship between 5-HT levels and problems such as anxiety, depression, eating and migraines is anything but simple. However, we do know that 5-HT seems to be reduced in those suffering from depression, and that it is intimately bound up with eating and appetite, and in migraine. There are three different types of 5-HT receptors, and the ones involved in depression are probably not the same type as the ones involved in migraine.

There are various ways to interfere with the workings of these brain chemicals. They can be blocked or their effects can be increased. One particular group of drugs seems to be able to help in the established attack of migraine. These are called 5-HT agonists or stimulants, and they stimulate the 5-HT receptors, just like 5-HT does in its natural role.

However, it isn't a question of simply giving extra 5-HT and thereby preventing migraines; rather, we actually *prevent* the onset of migraine attacks by using 5-HT *blocker* drugs, such as pizotifen. It seems that to *prevent* a migraine you need to *block* the effect of 5-HT, whereas to *treat* a migraine you need to have *more* of it.

5-HT agonists are one of the most recent developments in the treatment of migraine. Sumatriptan has recently been introduced and it seems to be highly effective in the treatment of the established attack. As with many of the other anti-migraine drugs, it is important to give it as early in the attack as possible, and injecting it makes sure that it gets into the bloodstream quickly. There is an ingenious plastic device called an auto-injector, which allows you to give your own injection safely and simply, without the need for professional help.

Sumatriptan is also available in tablet form for those in whom vomiting or poor absorption is not a problem. The efficacy is similar, but the onset of action is slightly slower. The only drawback to Sumatriptan is that it is expensive to make.

Compound preparations

There are many compound preparations (drug cocktails) available for treating migraine attacks. They all contain drugs that help in various different ways; for instance, a pain-killer plus an anti-vomiting agent; or ergotamine and caffeine.

Do make sure you don't inadvertently give yourself a double dose of any of the constituents by using other drugs at the same time; for example, using your own paracetamol as well as taking one of the compound preparations that also contains paracetamol can give you a dangerously high dose.

Self-help

The cardinal rule in migraine is to know what your own trigger factors are, and to minimise them as much as possible. Careful attention to minimising stress, reducing your exposure to extremes of heat and cold, having regular meals, having regular and enough sleep, not letting yourself lie in at weekends, checking out your own food sensitivities, and meticulously avoiding those foods which cause you problems, will all serve to reduce the number of attacks you get.

If you're one of the fifty per cent of migraine sufferers who haven't yet consulted your doctor, then *go*; see what's on offer. You may find your attacks are much more easily controlled on prescribed medicines than on the ones you can get over the counter.

When you do get an attack, treat it *quickly*, to nip it in the bud. Take your medicines as soon as possible, then find a quiet room in which to lie down and rest. Don't try and fight the attack – the migraine will almost certainly win! There is a ninety per cent improvement rate in those who rest as soon as an attack begins.

Because speed in dealing with impending attacks is essential, make sure you have your medicines with you wherever you go – which may mean separate bottles at home, at work, and in the car or in your handbag.

You may find that it helps to apply ice-packs or a cold compress to your head or neck, or else have a cold shower. Some people find warmth is more appropriate. .

If your doctor is having difficulty finding the right cocktail of drugs for you, it may help him if you keep a migraine diary. These are available from your doctor, or from the national migraine societies. A migraine diary is structured so that you can easily take note of your migraine, any associated symptoms, as well as your medication, and this may help your doctor to work out additional trigger factors that you hadn't noticed, or else establish whether a particular drug regime is slightly more helpful than a previous one.

Complementary treatment

One of the most startling successes of herbal medicines *recently has been feverfew. For a long time this has been used as an infusion for the treatment of headaches, but like so many of the drugs in the herbalist's pharmacopoeia it was assumed (for no good reason) that it probably wasn't particularly effective, and so was available for sale over the counter without prescription. However, recent trials have indicated that it is effective against migraine and there have been discussions about making it a prescription drug.*

Acupuncture and acupressure *are both used in the treatment of migraine. Perception of pain is a complex process and we now think that it is far from a passive process. To simplify this process for our purposes it looks as though a 'gate' in the nervous system has to open in order to allow pain sensations to pass through to our consciousness. By stimulating sensory fibres, acupuncture seems to shut this gate so that pain signals cannot get through as they did before. Acupuncture also releases endorphins – the body's own natural pain-killers – and this may help to relieve the pain.*

Probably sixty per cent of migraineurs receiving acupuncture experience some short-term and sustained benefit. Six to eight sessions of acupuncture will be needed, and the benefit may last from twelve to eighteen months, after which the treatment can be repeated.

Acupuncture can also abort migraine attacks by needling local tender spots in the neck or the temples, and the traditional Chinese points. The difficulty, of course, is getting to the acupuncturist quickly enough at the beginning of an attack.

Acupressure points which apply to migraine are: in the web between the thumb and first finger, pressing towards the finger bone; the corresponding place on the toes, pressing inwards towards the centre of the foot; and at the place where the neck meets the back of the head, close to and on either side of the spine. It may help to massage these areas as soon as a migraine starts.

*Relaxation therapy is also of paramount importance. Minimising the
amount of stress you face is half the battle; learning not to over-load yourself
with too much work, too much excitement, or any other form of stress, will
help considerably. To handle stress, disciplines such as assertiveness training
and relaxation therapy are therefore very important.*

*Biofeedback, which is technically supported relaxation training, may also
help, particularly in migraines linked to tension. Further, by monitoring skin
temperature, it measures the state of blood circulation, which is also related to
migraines.*

*Migraine-like headaches can occur as a result of problems in the neck,
especially from injuries to the spine such as a whiplash accident. Cervical
spondylosis and osteo-arthritis of the neck can also cause migraine-like pain.
Osteopaths feel that manipulation of the neck can reduce the number of
attacks of migraine. Cranial osteopathy may decrease the frequency of
migraine attacks. Soft tissue manipulation will also help to relieve spasm and
tension.*

*Cranial osteopathy may be helpful for children suffering from migraine;
even abdominal migraine is said to benefit from this treatment. Chiropractic
may also help.*

*As far as herbal medicines are concerned, for mild or infrequent attacks,
try infusions of balm, feverfew, meadowsweet and skullcap. Or basil leaves
steeped in boiling water, sipped at the onset of an attack – in the case of
classical migraine, when you experience the aura, this may stave it off. Some
people find light massage of pulse points with basil oil in a light carrier oil
helpful. Lavender, taken internally and possibly combined with valerian,
might be useful for stress-related migraines.*

Aromatherapy *may help prevent a migraine attack, or abort it in its early
stages. It is, however, best used preventatively, since any sensory experience
can be intolerable in the throes of an attack. Warm or cold compresses of
lavender, basil, marjoram or melissa might relieve the early stages of migraine
headaches; peppermint and lavender can be mixed with a light oil and
massaged into the temples and neck. Warm compresses with oil of marjoram
can be applied to the back of the head to increase blood flow. Some
migraineurs swear by a drop or two of lavender, applied neat, just inside the
nostrils. Camomile, fennel, lavender, lemongrass, marjoram or oregano can
be added to a very warm bath to provide some relief. The tension-reducing
effects of constitutional aromatherapy can prevent recurring attacks in some
people.*

Homoeopathy *suggests numerous remedies for migraine, but, as always,
your homoeopath will want to prescribe on the basis of an individual
consultation. Belladonna, bryonia, gelsemium, kali bich, nux vomica and
pulsatilla might be suggested. Homoeopathy is ideal for treating migraine in
children, since it is entirely safe, and can never reach toxic levels. For a child,
a homoeopath might recommend iris, lycopodium, pulsatilla or sanguinaria.
Again, individual prescription is the answer. Abdominal migraine can be*

treated with one of bryonia, ipeac or colocynth, and a hot-water bottle applied to the painful area can help soothe the pain.

Interestingly enough, children seem to react more strongly than adults to food additives, and these are often linked to migraine. Some to watch out for are E-factors, 101, 210-19, 32a and 612. Food allergies in children can be a particular culprit, and their often faddy eating habits exacerbate this.

Diet can be important in the successful treatment of migraine. Some supplemental elements may be suggested by a clinical nutritionist. Some doctors report success in using niacin (Vitamin B3) to abort migraine attacks when they first begin. Niacin can also reduce the symptoms of Menière's disease. Vitamins B6, C and E have also been used with some success. Very often tiny clinical deficiencies of a particular vitamin or mineral can cause much larger ramifications in the working of our bodies. Ensuring that you do have an adequate intake of vitamins and minerals may help prevent migraine caused by chemical imbalance (which can often lead to things like hormonal disruption, and circulatory problems, again the forerunners of migraine).

Root ginger and evening primrose oils may help prevent attacks.

DLPA – a form of the essential amino acid phenylaline – can produce and activate the endorphins, which are the body's own natural morphine, or pain-killers. DLPA also has a strong anti-depressant action. Many people who don't respond to conventional pain-killers do respond to DLPA.

Reflexology can help with tension and allergy-related migraines; some sufferers have even claimed relief from those migraines triggered by sinus difficulties and hormonal imbalance. Reflexology is safe for children, as is the Alexander Technique, which will treat adults and children alike for stress- or circulation-related migraine.

CLUSTER HEADACHE

Cluster headache is a one-sided pain centred on one eye. As well as pain there is redness of the affected eye with weeping, a running or stuffed-up nose, sweating of the face and forehead, and sometimes a drooping eyelid with a constricted pupil on the affected side. The headache lasts for between fifteen minutes and three hours and can occur as often as eight times a day.

Cluster headache occurs in groups (called the cluster period) of about six to twelve weeks in duration. This is then followed by a long period of remission, which on average lasts about twelve months. Although the headache is one-sided, the similarity with migraine ends there. In cluster headache it is always the same eye that is affected, while in migraine, although one side may dominate, headaches can occur on either side in individual attacks. Cluster headache affects predominantly men, by a ratio of four to one. The pain of cluster headache is constant; the pain of migraine is throbbing. For some reason cluster headache is more prevalent in smokers and alcoholics. At the moment we don't know what causes cluster headache but it shares a number of features with the neuralgias, so irritability of the nerves supplying the area may be at the heart of the problem.

The treatment for cluster headache falls into two sections: aborting the existing attack, and preventing further attacks. Prevention of future attacks is by using drugs such as amitriptyline, propranolol, ergotamine, methysergide, calcium channel-blockers and lithium. An injection of sumatriptan will abort an existing attack. Some patients can prevent an attack by breathing pure oxygen (this is *not* appropriate for those with chronic bronchitis or respiratory failure, as it stops them breathing). Other methods include inhaling ergotamine.

Type of headache
Constant, sharp excrutiating pain centred behind or around one eye.

What else could it be?
Migraine shares some features, but principally the redness and watering of the eye provides easy distinction between the two. Migraine isn't always on the same side of the face, as cluster headaches are.

   Acute glaucoma is similar in that the pain of both is sharp and very strong, but with glaucoma the pupil is wide, and the central part of the eye greenish-grey and misty-looking. In glaucoma, the eye is tender to the touch, and just before an attack haloes might appear around bright lights. A family history of glaucoma, or known raised pressure inside the eye may also point to the diagnosis. Finally, acute glaucoma usually gives rise to vomiting, while cluster headaches do not.

Chapter Three

TENSION HEADACHES

Tension in the neck muscles is the most common cause of headache and although the pain is often felt in the forehead or over the top of the head, it actually comes from contraction and spasm of the muscles in the neck. Next time you get a tension headache, run your fingers up and down the muscles on either side of the back of your neck, from the angle where your neck meets your shoulders right up to the underside of your skull, at the back. Almost certainly you will find sore spots – areas of muscle that are particularly tender, and feel very solid. Just touching these areas may cause you pain – massaging them makes you go through the roof!

Tense muscles like this cause headaches, and the root cause of tension headache is muscular tension and spasm in the muscles of the head and neck. Sounds ridiculous, doesn't it? Except that the spasm can be so great that it can even imitate a migraine, with pain boring through the eye socket. Usually, however, the headache from muscle tension is much less severe than this; it's a continuous ache, which is upsetting more because of the length of time it continues, than because of its intensity.

WHAT CAUSES TENSION HEADACHES?

Anything that knots up the muscles in the neck or head has the potential to cause a tension headache. Obviously, stress is a potent factor, but neck injuries, poor posture, eye strain, congenital defects and using the neck in awkward positions are all important causes.

For many people, stress causes them to stiffen and hunch up their shoulders, although why this should happen is curious because it doesn't seem to form any particularly useful function. Try this little test yourself: observe where your shoulders are in relationship to your head and the rest of your body. Now shrug your shoulders as hard as you can, holding it for a couple of seconds. Now let go, dropping your shoulders down suddenly. Notice how much further your shoulders drop than before – which means that at the start you were already holding your shoulders tense!

Stress isn't the only cause of headaches due to muscle spasm. Anything that causes injury or irritation to the bones, ligaments and joints of the neck is likely to cause muscle spasm in the area as a secondary effect. Arthritis of the neck, a whiplash accident, or any exercise which involves holding the neck bent back is likely to irritate the neck joints and send the surrounding neck muscles into spasm.

What are these unpleasant exercises that bend the neck backwards? Painting the ceiling, for a start; working with your hands above your head; and swimming, assuming that you're one of the many that can only swim breaststroke, by keeping your head up out of the water all the time!

Holding your head backwards in this way for any length of time tends to irritate the joints in the back of the neck. Because of the reflex reaction, whereby irritated joints cause the muscles around them to go into spasm, painful, irritated joints cause the muscles nearby to go into painful knots; this rams the joints together even further, which hurts even more, which causes the muscles to go into even greater spasms, which rams the joints together ... and·so on.

Holding yourself tense for any reason is likely to exacerbate tension headaches, because artificially raising the tension in certain muscles tends to increase the tension in *all* your muscles. For example: try threading a needle and notice how tense all sorts of other muscles have become. After a period of finicky work the level of muscle tension can rise in all sorts of muscles – especially those in the neck.

Another potent cause of tense muscles is tightly screwing up your eyes – either in harsh sunlight, or because you should really be wearing glasses. It tenses the muscles in the face, and if continued for long periods, will give you a headache.

Bad positioning of the neck and head is another major cause of problems. Chief among the activities that cause this is using a computer which hasn't been set up at the right level, the correct distance away. It is all too easy to sit in slightly the wrong position, with the monitor placed so that your head is either bent far too far forward or too far back, with your back sagging and your chin jutting forward as you peer at the screen; or else typing away like mad and not moving your head from left to right for hours at a time. Wrong positioning like this, with fixing of the posture, is almost guaranteed to produce neck·ache and subsequent headaches.

Just as the joint – pain/muscle – spasm reflex can cause self-perpetuating muscle spasm and headache, so a tension headache tends to self-perpetuate. Tension headaches *hurt*! So what do you do? That's right, you hold your head as still as possible, so the muscles in the neck stay in spasm; now they're *voluntarily* being asked to contract as well.

When you next get a tension headache, notice the position of your shoulders; almost certainly they'll be tense and raised. Now, consciously relax them. Let them drop down. Leave them like this, go back to what you were doing, and, in two minutes, you'll find they've risen of their own accord, back to where they were originally. No wonder tension headaches can be difficult to get rid of – it's that self-perpetuation again.

However, every cloud has a silver lining: this nature of tension headaches actually makes them very vulnerable to attack, because if you can break the pain/spasm/pain cycle, the vicious circle unwinds very quickly. Reduce the pain and you don't need to hold your head quite so still. Reduce the need to contract the neck muscles and the headache lessens, which means the muscle spasm reduces ... Once a tension headache starts to go, it usually goes very quickly indeed, and doesn't come back; at least, not for some time.

Type of headache

Tension headaches can take one of many forms. They can occur over the forehead, behind the eyes, in the temples, as a band round the head, over the top of the head, at the nape of the neck (where the neck joins on to the back of the skull), or passing up from the neck into the ears. As a rule of thumb, the higher up the neck that the muscles in spasm are situated, the more the pain is perceived towards the front of the head. In other words, if muscles high in the neck are in spasm, you'll get pain in the forehead; similarly, if the muscles in the middle of the neck are in spasm, the pain will be centred more over the top of the head. But this isn't a hard and fast rule.

The pain is often constant, but it can be throbbing; it can be worse with movement or exertion, and sometimes keeps time with the pulse. It can also go on for days at a time – which is why tension headaches are so upsetting.

Tension headaches are seldom severe; at least, not by comparison with the sort of headache experienced by a migraine sufferer, but they are prolonged and nagging, like toothache. They can also cause considerable worry. Why am I having the pain? What sinister illness does it indicate? The fact that it won't go away, even with painkillers, is often what frightens people most. They feel that it must be the tip of some deadly iceberg. Just to make things worse, worrying about the cause of your tension headache merely serves to increase your general level of stress and make your tension headache worse ...

Sometimes tension headaches can make you feel sick or nauseous; and because of the way that neck muscles in spasm can affect the blood supply to the upper part of the spinal cord, tension headaches can often make you feel dizzy, woolly-headed, and off-balance. The changes in tension headaches sometimes cause the arteries in the muscles to open up, exposing the smaller arteries to the full force of the blood pressure. Tension headaches of this sort are often pounding, in time with the heartbeat. Typically, straining or exercising exacerbates the headache, as the blood pressure rises even more during these activities.

One of the typical features of tension headaches is that once they go they are usually gone for good (at least for that day). As we discussed above, this is simply because the 'vicious circle' nature of tension headaches means that they are a self-perpetuating mechanism, and once the vicious circle is broken the headaches go away. Tension headaches can often be worse on waking, especially after sleeping in; and are often exacerbated and triggered off by minor degrees of neck injury.

What else could it be?

Minor degrees of tension headache can sometimes be difficult to distinguish from headaches caused by *viral infections*, though viral infections usually cause a raised temperature and/or a sore throat, running nose, or aching limbs. *Neck injuries* also cause muscle spasm and sometimes it can be difficult to be sure if you are dealing with simple muscle tension, or tension as part of a neck injury.

In those over the age of fifty-five, a headache at the side of the head, in the temples, needs to be distinguished carefully (and urgently) from *temporal arteritis*; with temporal arteritis there is often generalised muscle aching, with loss of appetite and loss of weight in the weeks preceding the headache. In temporal arteritis the artery crossing the temple is often tender to the touch, and there is a high ESR whereas in tension headaches the ESR is normal.

Sinusitis causes pain in the face and forehead but is usually accompanied by a raised temperature, alteration in the voice, and an infected nasal discharge. *High blood pressure* can instigate headaches, especially first thing in the morning, but usually only severe blood pressure does this. Really severe tension headaches (usually on a background of a neck injury as well) can cause pain radiating out of one eye socket, exactly as in *migraine* but there will be no preliminary flashing lights before the headache starts, and no vomiting.

Headaches caused by various *substances* – such as drugs, caffeine, carbon monoxide, etc. can cause the same sort of generalised headache, but exposure to the chemical is usually quite obvious – with the exception of caffeine, which nearly all of us take in in some quantity. The *weather* can exacerbate tension headaches, especially when a thunderstorm is about to break or where there's a lot of glare around. And finally *depression* can be responsible for tension headaches, probably as a result of associated anxiety and a general increase in muscle tension.

In other words, practically every cause of headache can imitate tension headache! However, headaches from viral infections and neck injuries are the commonest causes of tension headaches, and for most practical purposes you can be reassured that your headache is unlikely to do you any damage. In addition, once you've worked out that you're getting tension headaches, you'll soon recognise their approach and take measures to prevent them.

In fact, of all the causes of headaches, tension headache is by far the most benign. True tension headache never causes physical damage and can be cured, or at the very least made considerably better, by appropriate relaxation and anti-stress therapy.

Orthodox treatment
Diagnosis of tension headache is usually quite simple. The treatment is also simple – in principle, at least. Take exercise, learn to relax, and regularly put these two things into practice.

Typically, tension headaches don't respond well to simple painkillers – not because they are a particularly severe or dangerous type of headache, or because they are difficult to treat, but merely because the problems of the stiff neck are *not* just of pain, but also of muscle spasm.

If you try to treat this situation with just a simple pain-killer, all it can do is relieve the joint pain. It won't attack the muscle spasm – but the muscle spasm is what keeps the vicious circle going. Spasm causes pain and pain causes spasm.

At this stage it is common for patients to come to their doctor in some alarm, saying, 'I've got a headache that won't go with pain-killers', which implies that it must be very serious indeed. In fact, it isn't. It's quite simple to remove the pain of a tension headache with a pain-killer *and* a muscle relaxant. (Or else use an alternative method of removing the muscle spasm, such as massage, physiotherapy, heat, etc). Taking both a pain-killer and a muscle relaxant can be like waving a magic wand: and the great thing about it is that once the vicious cycle is unlocked it *stays* unlocked.

A favourite over-the-counter combination medicine is Syndol, which principally contains paracetamol to stop the pain, and an antihistamine to relax the muscles. However, it may make you drowsy, so don't drive or use machinery if you're affected in this way. (It's also not a good idea to take any kind of drugs during pregnancy; consult your doctor if you are suffering from tension headache.)

There are many other drugs to choose from: your doctor will have a large number of prescription drugs that can be used to reduce spasm. One of these, surprisingly, is diazepam (commonly known by its trade name, Valium). Normally, diazepam is used to relieve anxiety, but it also has a potent muscle-relaxant effect, and in tension headaches it may be helpful to use it in quite high dosage for a *short* time, together with a pain-killer. Short-term use like this is quite safe and doesn't give rise to addiction (unless you've previously had problems with addiction to diazepam or similar drugs).

Note the reasoning behind the use of diazepam - here it's being used as a short-term muscle relaxant, acting directly directly on the neck muscles. It is *not*, repeat *not* being used to treat the underlying anxiety and mental tension that so often triggers off tension headaches. Diazepam *could* be used in this way - but it would need a much longer course of tablets, and doctors now prefer to avoid using this group of drugs over a long period, as addiction may occur.

Drug therapy is for short-term treatment only. It may abort the headache, which then goes away for some time, if not for good. However, many people have frequent or even constant tension headaches simply because they are constantly stressed and unrelaxed. Dealing with long-term tension headaches like these are quite different, and therapy revolves principally around anti-stress measures and relaxation therapy.

Anxiety and depression are also common causes of tension headaches.

Self-help
Self-help for tension headaches revolves around one word: *stress*. In principle it's simple: get rid of the stress and tension headaches will become a thing of the past.

Start off by *identifying those things which cause you to feel stressed*, and remove or minimise them. *Then learn to deal with the stress that you cannot remove completely*. Assertiveness training, and business stress management can be useful.

As far as physical stress is concerned, try to *identify those situations that strain your neck and back* – especially those actions that put your body in odd positions: decorating, climbing, swimming, using a computer, etc. Poor posture, bad seating, too soft a mattress can all cause problems.

Local application of *heat* reduces the spasm of tense muscles; as does massage applied properly.

Complementary treatment

Tension headaches are ideal candidates for experimentation with some of the complementary therapies on offer and there are literally hundreds to choose from. Because tension headaches have unique causes in every person, the success of the various therapies will also be individual.

Some of the most generally recognised therapies are listed below, but with the guidance of a registered practitioner, it is certainly acceptable to experiment with any therapies you feel comfortable with. Full explanations of all available therapies isn't within the scope of this book, but some of the following, which have been briefly described, may be of some help.

Acupressure helps with many stress-originated conditions, and many of the massage techniques can be taught and self-implemented. Therapists say that acupressure acts as a catalyst for the body's own natural healing abilities.

The main advantage of kinesiology is prevention. Minor imbalances leading to muscle tension and stress can be picked up and dealt with at each session. Biofeedback (and biofeedback training) measures electrical changes in muscle fibres, and changes in skin temperature etc, revealing tension and anxiety. You can then be taught methods of dealing with the conditions that are uncovered, which many tension headache sufferers find helpful.

Auriculotherapy is based on the same principles as acupuncture (which is also recommended for tension headaches) and acupressure, with the ear acting as a crossroad for the various body meridians. This therapy stimulates various acupuncture points in this area, to alleviate pain and ease tension.

Art therapy allows sufferers to move away from stressful, negative situations. You colour, paint, or work with clay as an expression of emotion which releases stress. Colour therapy might be useful. Certainly counselling may help to explore your feelings and release tension that has been built up. Dance therapy offers five different rhythms which can be practised regularly which free the body from tension and move muscles to relax spasm.

Bach flower remedies can work by dealing with negative states of mind. For example, fear, indecision and worry are all negative emotions. If any of these elements are behind your tension, flower remedies might be suitable. Try agrimony for 'those who hide worries behind a brave face', elm 'overwhelmed by inadequacies', or olive 'drained of energy'. Rescue remedy can be used for extreme stress and anxiety.

Manipulative techniques such as osteopathy can restore normal function, reducing spasm through manual stretching and massage. Your practitioner can help you set up a suitable exercise regime. Your osteopath can suggest methods for dealing with stress on a long-term basis, by avoiding occupational strain and altering aspects of your lifestyle.

Herbalists suggest numerous remedies: try an infusion of lavender flowers or camomile, drunk daily as a tea. Or valerian and skullcap while in the throes of a painful tension headache. Herbs that are supposed to act as tonics to feed and strengthen the nervous system include borage, oats, orange blossom, limeflowers, white willow, vervain and verbena. Comfrey or St John's wort, in the form of herbal oils, can be rubbed into the neck and back. There are numerous other sedative and muscle-relaxing herbs.

A homoeopath will want to treat your symptoms after a full consultation: homoeopathy works best when based on individual symptoms and personal characteristics. A homoeopath might suggest arnica, bryonia, hypericum and rhus tox; ruta for a headache associated with fatigue, and ignatia to relieve that tight band across the forehead.

Aromatherapy may help in stress-prevention, and in actually dealing with a painful tension headache. Massage necessarily provides deep relaxation, and can often relieve the spasm associated with tension. Sedative and anti-depressant oils include bergamot, camomile, clary sage and lavender. Rosemary and black pepper stimulate. Analgesic oils are lavender and peppermint; a cold compress of lavender on the temples, or on the back of the neck, may help. Try massage with a blend of the above oils, or warm baths with a few drops added. Black pepper is not suggested for bathing, but has lovely rubefacient effects when used in massage. Calming vapours (in a vapouriser, or just on radiators or a handkerchief) are mandarin, melissa, basil and ylang ylang.

As always diet is important to keep the body fit and fighting, and tension is always less troublesome in a healthy body. Some therapists suggest that alternative supplemental Vitamin B12 can help during periods of stress, fatigue or recovery from illness. They also suggest an increased intake of Vitamin C helps, as they believe that stress and environmental pollutants drain it from the system. L-Tyrosine, an amino acid, is said to restore the balance of your system, but avoid this if you suffer from migraines or high blood pressure.

Reflexology can deal with stress, relaxation, strain and fatigue. You can also try relaxation techniques, flotation therapy, music and sound therapy, cranio-sacral therapy, naturopathy, and NLP (neuro-linguistic programming), among others.

Associated conditions

There is a huge link between *neck injuries* and tension headaches. Neck injuries cause the muscles around the joints to go into spasm, which in turn causes tension headaches. Tension in the muscles can ram the joints together and irritate an already 'tetchy' neck, initiating further neck pain. Tension headache can also be exacerbated by *menstrual problems*, and can make virtually any other cause of headache worse through the tension/pain/pain/tension reflex. It can often be difficult to distinguish between the *viral infections*, which cause direct muscle spasm, and muscle spasm occurring as a result of the pain of a viral headache. *Relaxation therapy, assertiveness training*, and *anti-stress measures* are essential in dealing with the cause of tension headaches. *Poor nutrition, obesity , lack of sleep* and *lack of exercise* will all make tension headache more likely. *Depression* and *anxiety* are likely to be accompanied by increased muscle tension and, of course, general tenseness is thought to increase the degree of *high blood pressure* that we may experience. Finally, there is a relationship between migraine and tension headaches in that the one can trigger the other.

ADRIAN

Adrian had had a bad night. He hadn't slept well and woke up feeling muzzy, with a headache and pain running up the back of his neck and round the side of his head. As the day went on his neck became more and more sore. That afternoon, in a meeting, he noticed that, completely unconsciously, he was tensing up the whole of his neck and face. He could feel the muscles in spasm, high up in the nape of the neck. Whenever he could, he would try to relax his muscles, but each time he started concentrating on what the speaker was saying, his neck and face started tightening up again.

He remarked how strange it was that although he didn't want to have all his muscles tight in this way, the minute his attention went elsewhere, all his muscles would go tight, try as he might to stop them. In fact, he felt quite ill all day with that peculiar empty, hungover feeling caused by having too little sleep, and it was only after the relaxation of the next night's sleep, together with a couple of pain-killers for good measure, that he was able to get the rest he needed, and relax himself sufficiently to stop the headaches occurring.

Chapter Four

NECK AND SPINE PROBLEMS

We've already seen that excess tension in the muscles of the neck alone can cause headaches. Where there is physical damage to the spine as well, the amount of pain will increase. Not only is there now pain from the neck damage itself, but there will also be an overlay of pain from the nearby muscles, which have been triggered into spasm by pain from the neck lesion. As a result, it is often hard to know where tension headaches leave off and true neck troubles begin: there is such an overlap between the two, and as a general rule any physical abnormality of the neck is almost certain to have a tension/spasm overlay.

In this chapter we're going to look at the purely *physical* causes of headaches originating in the neck. However, do remember that whatever direct pain they cause, *all* abnormalities in the neck are likely to have an overlay of spasm and tension. Not only does this extra spasm create more pain, it often exacerbates the underlying injury by clamping the vertebrae together and squashing the structures in between. Furthermore, spasm actually reduces healing, by restricting the flow of blood tissues in the area. So, although we shall be talking about specific anatomical problems, do remember that *all* neck problems are likely to benefit from treatment for muscle tension as well. However, not all exercises for muscle tension are appropriate if there is an underlying neck injury. Don't do anything that will make the underlying neck injury worse; for safety, exercises should be done to the limits imposed by the neck injury, rather than to the levels normally done for tension headaches.

Any abnormality of the muscles, bones or ligaments of the neck can cause pain. This pain has three quite separate causes; firstly, the abnormality itself can be painful. Secondly, because the lesion stops that portion of the neck from working properly, it forces the remainder of the neck to do extra to compensate for its inactivity. Thus the same amount of bending must be shared among fewer joints, which means that each of these joints has to bend more than it is designed to; this over-uses other joints in the neck, which in turn become stressed and painful. Finally, there is an overlay of reflex spasm from the neck muscles associated with the original lesion, which makes the neck even stiffer and yet more painful.

Not only do the neck joints stop working, but the joints of the upper and lower back may also be affected; they in turn can go into spasm. As further joints become over-used and painful they also start to 'fail', and stiffen up, thereby placing an even greater load on the remaining joints. In this way it is quite possible for all the bending in the neck to be carried out by one joint which is over-active and over-bending, the rest having stiffened up completely.

So, from that one slightly suspect neck joint, fixation and spasm has travelled up and down the spine; the spinal column is now sore and tender, with 'hot spots' of pain in the muscles on either side, and the local pain in the neck is frequently accompanied by headaches at the back of the head, caused mainly by the cramped muscles of the neck.

A seized-up neck like this is the end-stage of a process which may start off with only a small amount of anatomical damage to the neck. Perhaps there's a little bit of osteo-arthritis, or else a neck joint that's slightly out of alignment; but this is all it needs to trigger off the whole process.

There are many diseases that affect the neck in this way. They have different origins, but all have, as a final common path, local pain in the neck, with stiffening of the joints and muscle spasm.

CONGENITAL PROBLEMS

It would be amazing if the whole body were always to develop from a single fertilised egg without the occasional defect occurring from time to time. In fact, it's surprising how few problems actually do occur, but in a developmentally complex structure such as the spinal cord, it would be very surprising if abnormalities didn't happen from time to time.

Anything which affects the normal symmetrical development of the skeleton can cause neck problems, such as having one leg shorter than the other, or a pelvis that is twisted or asymmetrical.

As well as these more major structural changes, there can be many other minor changes on the surface of the bones, which means that the bones and muscles don't work quite as they should.

Often the minor abnormalities are not noticed for some time: the damage they do isn't easy to spot, because it isn't obvious. Nevertheless, because of a small anatomical abnormality, the muscles and ligaments surrounding it have to work in a slightly abnormal way – and, after twenty or thirty years, they will start to show signs of strain. Only then will that fused vertebra be noticed, that slightly wide piece of bone be spotted, that slight difference in leg length be observed.

Just occasionally, operations are possible on the grosser abnormalities – to build up missing or abnormally thin bones, or to remove extra bits of bone, such as a cervical rib (an extra rib in the neck area), that are getting in the way – but in the case of congenital abnormalities, these are the exception rather than the rule. Minor, long-standing neck abnormalities are best treated in the same fashion as osteo-arthritis of the neck. A combination of painkillers, anti-inflammatories, muscle relaxants, heat, and gentle exercises to keep the area moving will help considerably.

INFECTION

Nowadays there are very few infections that can damage the neck. This is a welcome change. A hundred years ago the neck was a favourite site for *tuberculosis* (TB), but, with the advent of powerful anti-tubercular drugs, TB has all but disappeared in the Western world. Unfortunately, with the rise of AIDS, which results in increased susceptibility to TB in those who are affected, we may see more neck complications in the future. TB can infect the bones, the joints, and the lymph glands in the neck, causing long-term, slow inflammation and destruction of bones, joints and soft tissues. The treatment is antibiotics, often given for many months at a time.

Of far more importance nowadays are the *viral infections*. Although these don't last long, they can produce very painful neck problems, especially in children. Viral infections of the throat or ear often cause local swelling of the lymph nodes draining the area, as these react to infection, providing extra cells to fight the invading virus. (Lymph nodes are the lumps we feel under the armpits or in the neck when a viral infection strikes.)

When lymph nodes do their job of fighting off infection, they swell and can also become infected and inflamed. This swelling irritates the surrounding muscles and in some cases triggers off localised muscle spasm. The spasm this generates can be all round the neck, causing generalised stiff muscles; more often, however, only a single muscle is infected. When this happens, its spasm pulls the head round awkwardly; this is called a *wry neck*. It's painful – some of the muscles in the neck are taut, and in spasm, and the patient finds it hard to move the neck in a particular direction (the direction in which the affected muscle would have to lengthen).

A wry neck doesn't have to be associated with an infection. Often physical stimulation is enough: perhaps a slight injury to a joint, twisting the neck into such a position that one of the neck muscles over-tightens and develops cramp. A common way is to wake with a wry neck – presumably during the night the head moved into an awkward position, and cramp has developed.

Treatment of wry neck

Wry neck can be immensely painful, but often painkillers don't help all that much because they don't stop the muscle spasm. Muscle relaxants can sometimes be helpful. A particular over-the-counter favourite is a drug called Syndol which is a combination of paracetamol, codeine, caffeine and an antihistamine that has useful sedative properties. Unfortunately, it's not appropriate for children under the age of twelve; nor should pregnant women take drugs without their doctor's advice.

Your doctor you may offer you painkillers and a prescribable muscle relaxant. Diazepam (perhaps better known by its trade name, Valium) is very effective as a muscle relaxant though it can make you very drowsy; there is no problem with addiction when using the short courses needed to treat muscle spasm.

Applying heat to the affected muscle can often be very comforting; and encouraging the patient to move the neck and stretch the muscle that's in spasm can be beneficial. However, it can be exceptionally painful to move a neck against the pull of a muscle which is in spasm and can quite literally bring tears to the eyes. Often neck exercises can be of particular help in loosening up neck muscles. Swimming is particularly good, but don't breast stroke; back stroke is best.

Some osteopaths and chiropractors like to manipulate wry necks; personally, I don't. I usually attempt to unlock them with the simple measures already outlined, and only if there is persisting trouble do I then seek to manipulate. Antibiotics are unlikely to be of use because most swollen lymph glands like this are a result of a viral infection, and viral infections don't respond to antibiotics at all.

Complementary treatment

If osteopathy or chiropractic prove helpful, by all means continue with the treatment. Cranial osteopathy may be of particular use. Aromatherapy is also an option; try light massage with one or a blend of the following oils, all of which are said to have anti-viral properties: bergamot, eucalyptus and tea tree. Baths and vaporisation with the same oils will have a similar effect. Remember that massage should never be undertaken if there is fever.

Extracts of some herbs, such as licorice and St John's wort are said to have anti-viral activity – and Echinacea is thought to stimulate the immune system. By fighting the cause of the inflammation, the neck- and headache will cease to exist. Zinc may also stimulate the immune system, but consult a registered clinical nutritionist, or herbalist, before trying any of these.

To relax and loosen the neck and head muscles, reflexology is often suggested, either by a trained therapist, or by a friend or partner. Self-manipulation is easily learned, and helpful for any number of conditions.

Aconite (30c) can be taken at two-hourly intervals for up to twelve hours; however, if stiffness is not alleviated, do contact your doctor.

Light yoga exercises, and some of the stretching exercises suggested for stress reduction may reduce muscular spasm, facilitating faster healing and providing longer-term pain relief. Certainly acupuncture and acupressure are recommended for pain relief.

There are numerous other complementary therapies which may or may not provide some relief from the pain, and many claim to attack viruses. If you think they could help, try royal jelly, Bach flower remedies (in particular, Rescue Remedy for the onslaught of pain, or olive to increase your energy) and T'ai Chi.

SHIRLEY

Shirley is twenty-eight. She woke one morning with pain in her neck, and her head twisted slightly to one side. What alarmed her most was that every time she tried to tilt her head to the affected side, or even straighten her head so that her chin was pointing forwards she would get intense pain in the back of her neck and up into her head.

This was readily confirmed on examining her. Although she could bend her neck to the right without any difficulty, trying to twist the head round to the left was met with resistance and pain, and trying to bend the head sideways towards the left shoulder was out of the question.

Shirley didn't have a temperature, and hadn't had a recent sore throat or viral infection, so she didn't have a viral type of neck pain, nor did she have neck spasm from the enlarged lymph nodes that follow a viral infection. In fact, Shirley had a simple wry neck – the slight twisting of the head is a dead giveaway.

At first she had been quite worried about it, but as soon as she knew the diagnosis she began to relax. Her doctor explained to her that she had simply got a wry neck. This was caused by a muscle in spasm, and although it would be painful for a time, it wasn't serious. She was prescribed a muscle relaxant and painkiller, and recommended to apply a hot water bottle to the painful muscles.

Stretching muscles that are in spasm can help; for example, with cramp in the calf muscle, the treatment is to get someone to pull the toes up, passively stretching the calf muscle at the same time.

It's possible to do the same sort of thing to the neck muscles, passively stretching them to encourage them to relax. Shirley's doctor told her how to move her head gently in the directions that were uncomfortable, to encourage the muscles to relax and lose their spasm. Unfortunately, this exercise causes some discomfort before the muscles start to relax.

One of the tips her doctor passed on was that she could let gravity do the stretching for her. She should lie on her side, choosing the side that was difficult to move the head towards. Although it would have been more comfortable for her to have two pillows so she could rest her head without pulling on the muscles that were in spasm, if instead she had one pillow (or even none) she could then let her head gradually drift downwards, under the force of gravity, which gradually and persistently pulled on the muscles that were in spasm, encouraging them to lengthen.

Shirley put all these ideas into practice, and three days later was pain-free and back to normal again.

A second cause for neck- and headaches is direct viral infection of a type that has the ability to make muscle fibres more irritable, and therefore more likely to go into spasm on the slightest stimulation. Neck muscle tension like this causes pain in the back of the neck, with headaches at the back, all over, or at the front of the head. As there are seldom any other signs of infection, an outbreak of infection with this type of virus is rather like having an epidemic of tension headaches. Clinically, there's little to distinguish headaches like these from true tension headaches, and it's usually the GP who notices it first, when the sixth patient that day with a 'tension headache' walks through the door. Treatment is exactly the same as for wry neck.

WENDY

One February day, Wendy was in bed with a particularly violent headache, with pain over the whole of the top of her head. She'd recently had flu, but this illness seemed to be different. Not only did she have a headache, but she'd been vomiting and felt nauseous. However, her temperature was more or less normal, so she didn't have flu: that usually gives a temperature of 101°F or more.

Was it meningitis? Thankfully she had no neck stiffness and could easily bend her chin on to her chest, so it wasn't that. However, she did have some spasm in the muscles of the upper and middle part of her neck.

Wendy had one of two things – either a late effect of her previous viral infection, giving muscle stiffness, or else a second viral infection of a type that was particularly prone to cause muscle spasm.

Her doctor prescribed some painkillers, and a muscle-relaxing agent. Her problem soon settled down: she was able to get up a few days later and was back at work within a week, none the worse for wear.

DEGENERATIVE DISEASE OF THE NECK

Where bones meet to form a joint, their ends are covered with smooth cartilage whose function is to allow the ends of the bones to slip easily over each other. The cartilage forms a slippery joint surface that has minimal resistance to being moved or bent.

The two bones are held together firmly in a bag of ligaments which allow movements only in specified directions and inside this bag is a little joint fluid, called *synovial* fluid.

The general term *arthritis* means an 'inflammation of the joints'. There are two main types – rheumatoid arthritis, which is a specific inflammation of the joints and muscles; and osteo-arthritis, which is a degenerative wearing-away of the cartilage. Although to the lay person 'rheumatism' and 'arthritis' are often synonymous, in fact, rheumatoid arthritis and osteo-arthritis are quite different diseases, affecting different types of joints, and with completely different disease profiles. However, both types can cause painful joints that don't work properly; both types can affect the neck, but osteo-arthritis is much more common.

There is a third type of degenerative disease – *cervical spondylosis*. This is essentially weakening and thinning of the 'disc' between the vertebrae.

LOIS

Lois is a twenty-two-year-old with an irritable neck. From time to time one or two of the joints on the left side seize up. When they become painful the vicious circle of pain causing muscular spasm and spasm causing further pain in the joint begins. As a result, she has frequent episodes of neck pain and pain at the back of the head, sometimes with pain radiating down the arm and into the top of the shoulder, and a neck that won't move to the left-hand side as well as it will on the right. However, she never had the 'twisted neck' posture of wry neck – hers was a much less specific source of spasm and pain.

She had already tried one or two standard remedies, including a proprietary painkiller/muscle relaxant combination. Her doctor normally likes to try these first before attempting manipulation.

The first time her neck was manipulated Lois was very apprehensive. Would it hurt? Would it be uncomfortable? Would it do any damage? Her doctor reassured her, and, having examined the neck and felt the places where the muscles were in spasm, he manipulated it.

There were a couple of clicks, and a very surprised-looking Lois sat up to find that the pain had immediately halved in intensity: not only that, but she could move her head almost fully to the left!

Her doctor taught her some exercises, warned her not to try head-rolling, and encouraged her to continue taking the painkiller and muscle relaxant that she had been using. This is important, because often manipulating the neck or back leaves the patient feeling slightly sore for the next twenty-four or forty-eight hours, and using the medicine prevents any further locking up of the joint due to pain.

Local soreness after manipulation is to be expected. If a joint hasn't moved for a time then the muscles and ligaments surrounding it become stiff. It's exactly the same as when you sit slightly awkwardly on the floor.

A mild painkiller and muscle relaxant used for the next day or two stops the pain and spasm syndrome from building up again, and allows the freed joint to continue to move. Lois was delighted with the result and went off happily.

Three months later she was back again, with exactly the same symptoms. Manipulating the neck again brought her back to normal.

Gradually, Lois is beginning to understand her own neck a little better and at the first sign of spasm setting in she gives herself a dose of muscle relaxant plus painkiller; she also exercises and mobilises the neck to stretch the muscles. Much of the time this treatment works on its own; if it doesn't, she knows that it's time to get the neck manipulated again.

Osteo-arthritis

In osteo-arthritis the cartilage covering the bone ends gets rubbed away, so that inside the joint, bone rubs on bone. This makes the joint stiff, creaky and painful (because there's no slipperiness left), giving off clicks and cracks as bits of bone rub against each other.

Because the joints are painful, the reflex effect of local muscle spasm comes into play as the muscles nearby try to protect the joint from further discomfort. As a result, the joint is now painful, eroded, and even stiffer.

Osteo-arthritis frequently doesn't affect a single joint. Often many neck joints are affected to some degree, though there will always be one that is worse affected, one that will 'go down' first. And where more than one joint is concerned, it's all the easier for a problem in one joint to cause the remainder to seize up, simply because they are overwhelmed by the extra stress put upon them because that first joint has stiffened up.

For some reason osteo-arthritis seems to affect the lower joints of the neck more than the upper ones. This is important because the lower joints in the neck do most of the side bending, and in osteo-arthritis stiffness of the neck to side bending is a typical finding.

As we discussed earlier, osteo-arthritis occurs when the cartilage in the joint wears away. Recent research suggests that the quality of the cartilage may have something to do with it; some people seem to produce cartilage which isn't as strong as it could be. This is probably a genetically based flaw in cartilage production.

Whatever the quality of the cartilage, osteo-arthritis can be made worse by a number of factors. *Excess stress* on the joint can cause more wearing-away of the joint surfaces, and *using the joint in an odd way* causes excess stress on the joint surfaces. Excess stress like this can come from various sources, such as congenital abnormalities of the neck bones, poor posture, and a job or activity that concentrates movement on to one joint that is used too much. Jobs which require you to hold your hands up above your head are notorious for causing neck problems – plastering (especially of ceilings) is a good example.

Obesity doesn't cause problems in the neck, but as you might expect, stresses the lower, more weight-bearing joints of the body such as the lumbar (lower) spine, the hips and the knees. Normally the joints in the neck only have to carry the weight of the head, and even if you are so obese that you have large flapping jowls or a very thick neck, the extra weight carried is minimal by comparison with the weight of the skull and the head. However, even if obesity isn't a direct problem in degenerative problems in the neck it can still have an indirect influence. Abnormalities at one spot in the spine have a knock-on effect up and down the spine at every third vertebral joint. In this way a bad back is likely to have definite effects on the neck.

Complementary treatment

There are numerous treatments which are claimed to stimulate the body to repair damaged tissue and surfaces, and to improve the circulation to that area to facilitate quicker healing.

Useful herbs include devil's claw, bogbean, feverfew and celery seed. A poultice from slippery elm, directly on the offending area, may also help. A warm drink made from one teaspoon of vinegar (cider, preferably) and one teaspoon of honey in hot water, taken each morning, is helpful for some people in order to prevent attacks.

Cypress and lemon essential oils help the body deal with toxins; camomile and benzoin kill pain; and ginger or black pepper are rubefacient, increasing blood supply to the area and stimulating the healing process. All of these oils may be used in a light massage, mixed with a suitable vegetable-based oil, like grapeseed or avocado.

The Alexander technique teaches body awareness and correct posture, which provides relief for many sufferers.

Arnica, bryonia and rhus tox help relieve symptoms, as do acupuncture and acupressure (although this particular kind of pain relief is not recommended if you are pregnant). Some gentle yoga exercises will provide relief: they are thought to stimulate healing, and improve circulation and well-being.

A clinical nutritionist would suggest that red meats, alcohol, salt, fats, caffeine and strong-tasting spices be eliminated or cut down. It is sensible to start off any diet with a cleansing fast, although this should always be done under the supervision of a medical or registered complementary practitioner. Increasing your intake of Vitamins A, B, E as well as calcium and magnesium (which are needed to form the synovial fluid) may help prevent recurring attacks but this should always be done under supervision as vitamins can be toxic in excess (especially Vitamins A and D). There are also many vitamins and minerals that are anti-oxidants, which clinical nutritionalists recommend for preventing osteo-arthritis.

Copper bracelets are commonly used in rheumatism; it has been proved that copper, when dissolved in sweat from the contact of the bracelet with flesh, can be absorbed into the skin, which may explain how it appears to bring relief, as it is thought to have anti-inflammatory and anti-oxidant properties.

The Chinese give routine injections of royal jelly (coupled with pantothenic acid – Vitamine B5) which allegedly offers quite rapid relief of osteo- and other forms of arthritis.

T'ai Chi is a good option, combining stretching of the muscles with light exercise.

Cervical spondylosis

The term *cervical spondylosis* is used in different ways by different doctors. Some use it to mean 'any degenerative condition of the neck', using 'cervical spondylosis' interchangeably with 'osteo-arthritis'. Others maintain that there is a significant difference between them, and that osteo-arthritis is a disease of the *joints* at the back of the spine whilst cervical spondylosis is degeneration of the *disc* at the *front* of the spine.

Separating the vertebrae in the spine, at the front, is an *intervertebral disc* (commonly called 'the disc'). It's tough, and has a structure like a flattened squash ball filled with putty. The disc is there to hold the vertebrae apart correctly, to act as shock absorber for the spine, and also to assist the spine in bending. Discs only occur at the front of the spinal column; at the back each vertebrae bends down to form a joint with the vertebra below it. At the level of each disc a pair of nerves comes out from the spinal cord, travelling on their way to distant parts of the body.

All is well, provided that the disc is tough; but, if it isn't, on being squeezed or stressed the disc can squash. At first the disc merely balloons or bulges out, but in more severe cases it ruptures and its contents spill out through a hole in the disc wall. (This is a prolapsed disc, colloquially known as a 'slipped' disc.)

Cervical spondylosis is the name for all degrees of disc disease, from the first minor defects to a full-blown slipped disc. Minor degrees of spondylosis do little damage, other than causing local pain and muscular spasm; in some cases, the disc gradually regains its original shape. However, if the squashing is severe enough, the disc (or its escaped contents) may press against the spinal cord or the spinal nerves that run close by.

This causes a number of problems because the pressure of the disc interrupts the normal flow of information up and down the nerve. It can cause considerable pain in remote parts of the body, such as a leg or hand, numbness, or pins-and-needles, and sometimes weakness of muscles that are normally controlled by the affected nerve. Exactly which parts of the body go numb or weak depends of course upon which nerve is being trapped, and how badly.

Early on, cervical spondylosis is usually intermittent: episodes of pain occur, separated by long pain-free periods. Symptoms vary weekly or monthly, rather than daily, and the more the neck is stressed, the worse the symptoms become. Rest and relaxation may remove the pain entirely.

The doctor will diagnose the condition principally from the patient's history, and the examination, checking particularly for muscle spasm in the neck, muscle weakness in the upper limbs, lack of sensation in the skin of the upper limbs, and alteration in the reflexes at the elbow and wrist. You might think that X-rays would help, but often they don't. The disc isn't visible to ordinary X-rays, so all that can be seen is a narrowing of the gap between two vertebrae where the disc is, showing that it's been squashed.

However, many people have a bit of narrowing like this without any symptoms; equally, this narrowing doesn't always show up, and quite major degrees of slipped disc can occur without any obvious X-ray changes. It is only by performing specialised X-rays and scans that the exact diagnosis can be made with complete certainty. (Most of the time we don't need to be that exact, as the treatment of the less severe cases is the same for both osteo-arthritis and cervical spondylosis.)

Cervical spondylosis and osteo-arthritis are often accompanied by the formation of little outgrowths of bone called *osteophytes* which do show up on X-ray.

We're not sure why it is that some people get cervical spondylosis and others don't. Presumably the genetic make-up of certain people means that they have weaker discs; this becomes more of a problem if they do a lot of lifting, or use their neck and neck muscles in an awkward way that constantly puts stress on the discs. If you've suffered neck injuries, you are probably more susceptible to cervical spondylosis.

Minor degrees of cervical spondylosis are painful, and an annoyance, but are not an emergency. On the other hand, a sudden massive disc lesion (structural change), particularly one causing severe muscle weakness, may need operating on very quickly indeed – otherwise the ensuing nerve damage may be permanent.

The reason for cervical spondylosis and osteo-arthritis being commonly considered as one disease is quite simple – whenever there is pain in a joint, the muscles around it go into spasm. Sometimes this pain and spasm is severe enough to imitate a trapped nerve; in particular, it is quite possible for muscles in spasm to press on nerves, or else deny them their blood supply, and so imitate the far more serious effects of a slipped disc.

Therefore, although cervical spondylosis and osteo-arthritis are actually quite different processes, in practice their effects merge and from a practical point of view it is often easiest to consider them together. They sometimes co-exist in the same person, anyway.

Nerve entrapment
Between adjacent vertebrae, a pair of nerves leaves the spinal cord at the level of the joint between the vertebrae. These nerves have a difficult journey, because the hole they go through is small, and liable to get constricted for several reasons:

• If the disc is bulging or has ruptured, it or its inner contents may press on the nerve. In addition, if the disc has half-collapsed, now that its centre has been forced out, the two vertebrae on either side will come nearer together, trapping the nerves as they exit between them.

• A joint that is suffering from arthritis of any form may swell from internal inflammation and this swelling can press on the nerve.

• In osteo-arthritis or cervical spondylosis, extra pieces of bone called osteophytes can grow out from the bone, causing further obstruction to the workings and movements of the muscles and joints, and pressing on surrounding tissues, including nerves.

• If there is muscle spasm, the bones of the spine are rammed together, narrowing the gap between them to a minimum, and trapping the nerves.

• Because the joint is sore, the muscles around it reflexively go into spasm to try to prevent the joint moving any more (which might cause further injury). The firm belly of these muscles in spasm may press on the nerves; additionally, the extra pressure within and around the muscles may inhibit the flow of blood into the area. This is important because starving a nerve of blood stops it transmitting information properly. It doesn't kill the cell, as it would in the brain, because the nucleus of the cell is well protected inside the spinal cord, and the 'nerve' that passes out from the spinal column is actually just a long extension from the cell rather than the central substance of it. Cutting off the blood supply to that extension causes temporary disruption only.

In other words, these nerves have a pretty hazardous passage from the inside to the outside of the spinal cord! Normally, everything works well – the delicate nerves are protected from external injury by the spine, which is strong, but can still move very freely. It's a good design, and very effective, but like any complex piece of equipment, when it starts to go wrong, it goes *really* wrong.

If a sensory nerve is stimulated somewhere along its length, the signals given off kid the brain into thinking that it's experiencing excess sensation *from the point the nerves normally supply.* The brain interprets signals coming from nerves that supply the fingers as though there is something stimulating the fingers. It doesn't occur to the brain that this pain might be caused by something stimulating the trunk of the nerve halfway along its route to the brain.

You can see this mechanism in action very clearly each time you bang your elbow. The pain is perceived not so much at the elbow, but as a painful, tingling, numb sensation in the little and ring fingers. This is because the ulnar nerve (the one that goes round the outside of the elbow) is being stimulated by the blow. Normally it supplies the little and fourth fingers of the hand and so the brain imagines that the extra signals from the stimulus of the blow must have come from these fingers.

In addition, with extensive nerve trapping, local reflexes (the well-known one is the knee jerk, but ankle, wrist and elbow jerks are all similar) will be minimal or even absent.

This is of direct relevance to headaches that are caused by degenerative disease in the neck. Frequently nerves get trapped as they travel out from the spinal cord in the middle of the neck, to supply the arm or the trunk. Anything which causes trapping of nerves produces pain in the region the nerve normally supplies.

With the exception of the very top nerves in the neck most nerve entrapment doesn't cause headaches directly. More often, headaches are a secondary effect: the muscles in the neck react to the inflammation and pain from the neck joints by going into spasm and this spasm in turn causes headaches. In other words, local pain in the neck, together with headaches, shows there is a problem with the neck – and pain in the arms, reduction in reflexes, or reduction in muscle power shows that the problem is severe enough to trap nerves.

Type of headache
The position of the headache varies in cervical spondylosis, according to which disc(s) is affected. In early cases, the symptoms are intermittent, varying from week to week, or month to month. In more severe disc disease with nerve trapping the pain is constant, and severe, with no relief obtained whatever position the patient puts his neck or arm in.

What else could it be?
Often it is only by using specialised X-rays and scans that the exact diagnosis can be made, and as the treatment of the less severe cases is exactly the same, there is often little point in doing these more complicated tests. However, where the pain cannot be relieved and if there is the possibility that an operation may be needed, these investigations will be necessary to pinpoint the exact site needed for the operation.

Orthodox treatment
Treatment of an established minor cervical spondylosis consists of rest, the avoidance of both lifting and any strong movement of the muscles of arms and neck, painkillers, and muscle relaxants. Physiotherapy is often used.

If conservative measures like these fail then it may be necessary to operate. Over the last five years, techniques for operating on discs have improved greatly. There are various methods, but two operations that are particularly effective include removing the spilled part of the disc at the point where it presses on the nerves; and removing the disc entirely, replacing it with bone transplanted from the pelvis. This is difficult surgery and not without problems, but both types of operation usually succeed very well indeed.

Self-help
To reduce the possibility of getting cervical spondylosis, get into the habit of adopting a good posture, which minimises the strain on the neck. Similarly, avoid lifting excessively heavy weights.

If you've already been diagnosed as suffering from cervical spondylosis, do all of this as a metter of course. Finally, if the symptoms become severe, or you have weakness in your arms, seek advice urgently.

Complementary treatment
Manipulative and soft-tissue therapy may help – physiotherapy is commonly used, but occasionally osteopathy and chiropractic may assist. However, as it is easy to do permanent damage to the nerves in the neck by injudiciously manipulating a slipped disc, be sure to consult a registered practitioner.

Techniques designed to relax the muscle spasm will also help minimise extra stresses on the already weakened disc, so acupuncture and reflexology may be useful.

Homoeopathy may be helpful in the treatment of cervical spondylosis; in particular, you can try any of the following, at 6c, four times daily, for up to a week or ten days: argent nit, picric ac, agariceus. To help with the dizziness that is often a symptom of cervical spondylosis, theridon, borax and kali carb are suggested.

Massage with essential oil of black pepper may help promote healing. To reduce and prevent muscle spasm, try a poultice of peppermint leaves steeped in half a cup of boiling water and cooled slightly. Try drinking peppermint tea to relieve spasm. Remember, however, that peppermint makes ineffective any homoeopathic remedies you might be taking. Gentle T'ai Chi and yoga exercises will also help.

JOHN

John is a thirty-three-year-old mechanic who suddenly developed severe pain between the shoulder blades, particularly on the right side, together with neck pain and weakness of the grip in his right hand. He also had headaches radiating up the right side of his head and neck.

There was a great deal of spasm in the neck muscles, which pulled the neck over to the left side, although he was still able to move his neck to a surprising degree. At this stage his X-ray proved normal.

Because of the severity of the pain his doctor referred him to the local orthopaedic surgeon who gave him physiotherapy and an orthopaedic collar, together with regular anti-inflammatory medication. For a time this kept the symptoms under reasonable control, allowing him to continue at work without too much discomfort. However, the weakness in his right arm continued.

After rather inadvisably doing a workout in the local gym he developed a sore, stiff neck on sideways bending, together with severe pain down the right arm, and numbness in the ring finger of his right hand. John is no wimp, but that night the pain was so intense that he had to call out his doctor. The pain only settled after an injection of morphine.

Now that it looked as though John had 'slipped a disc', the orthopaedic surgeon referred him to a neuro-surgeon to see if the disc could be operated on. By this time there was a one-centimetre difference between the circumference of the right and left upper arms, from muscle wasting caused because the signals travelling from the brain to the arm muscles couldn't pass properly along the trapped nerve.

The neuro-surgeon arranged an MRI (Magnetic Resonance Imaging) scan of John's neck, which showed that the clinical impression was entirely correct – the centre of one of the discs in the neck had been forced out on the right side, compressing one of the nerves as it left the spinal cord to go down the arm. The surgeon planned to remove the disc completely, fusing together the vertebrae above and below using slivers of bone taken from the pelvis. Surgery like this can be difficult and John was told about the possibility that it might not go completely according to plan, but he was anxious to have something done to ease the pain and so the operation was carried out.

It was amazingly successful. You might think that an

operation on the vertebrae would mean an incision at the back of the neck; far from it! The disc is more or less central to the neck, and is easiest to get at from the front and side – so now John has a small diagonal scar on the right side of his throat which will easily be hidden by his shirt collar.

Immediately after the operation he woke up to find out that the pain and headaches which he had had for six months had gone completely. In fact, the sorest place was the side of his pelvis (where the surgeon had made a small nick in order to retrieve some slivers of bone in order to pack the space between the two vertebrae, where the disc had been removed).

For the first six weeks after the operation, the neck is very susceptible to damage so John had a cervical collar, which he had to wear at all times. He had been in the habit of sitting with his collar off for a few moments, and then standing up to put it on. However, like everyone else, when getting out of a chair, as he leaned his body forward he would tilt his head back, keeping it horizontal, but bending his neck back in the process. He had to be reminded of the importance of putting the collar on before he attempted to rise from his seat.

The other problem concerned his dog, Marmaduke, a large and vicious German Shepherd. Marmaduke was likely to fight any potential burglar to the death, but would also leap up and play-fight with John. Often he did this more boisterously than was safe, and John had the scars to prove it.

When his doctor visited John after he returned home following his operation, Marmaduke was there in the back garden, baring his teeth. One of his doctor's first suggestions was that the dog should go to friends or into a kennel until John had recovered fully: all it needed was for Marmaduke to lunge up at John in a play-fight, and before he could stop himself, John would have reflexively jerked his head away, damaging his healing neck in the process.

Rheumatoid Arthritis

Rheumatoid arthritis is another of those conditions about which a whole book could be written. Its relevance to headaches is actually quite limited, except that rheumatoid arthritis can be a source of considerable neck pain, and can also cause inflammation and discomfort at the *tempero-mandibular* joint, which is the hinge joint connecting the jaw to the skull just in front of the ear. Arthritis of this joint can cause local pain shooting up into the top of the head and considerable tension in the muscles surrounding it – particularly the very powerful muscle of the cheek, which closes the mouth.

Rheumatoid arthritis can be a particular problem in the upper part of the neck and can lead to very fragile bones. There is a special bone peg at the top of the second vertebra, called the *odontoid peg*, the soundness of which is vital for the skull to move, yet stay firmly fixed to the neck. In people with severe rheumatoid arthritis this peg can be broken off, in which case the head and neck become unstable and may trap the spinal cord. Because of the vulnerability of this peg to minor degrees of force, sufferers from rheumatoid arthritis should *never* have their necks manipulated: they may become paralysed as a result. Massage and physiotherapy, on the other hand, are quite acceptable.

The effects of rheumatoid arthritis are much the same as osteo-arthritis, as far as production of headaches and reflex muscle spasm are concerned. Rheumatoid arthritis irritates the joint linings, and everything else follows in train: muscle spasm in the muscles surrounding the joint, trapping of the nerves as they come out between the vertebrae, radiation of pain up into the back of the head and sometimes into the forehead area, and generalised stiffness on moving the neck.

We don't really know why rheumatoid arthritis occurs. What we do know, however, is that it is primarily an inflammation of the lining of the joint – called the synovium. The synovium also extends round the inside of the ligaments surrounding the joint so that effectively the synovium is like a microscopically thin bag inside the main ligament bag surrounding the joints.

We *can* detect those who are suffering from rheumatoid arthritis, using a specific blood test for 'rheumatoid factor'; another blood test for a substance called C-Reactive Protein (CRP) has recently become available, and abnormalities in either of these indicate that the joint pain is being caused by rheumatoid arthritis rather than osteo-arthritis.

Clinically, rheumatoid arthritis behaves quite differently from osteo-arthritis. While osteo-arthritis is a disease of the bigger joints – hips, knees, spine – rheumatoid arthritis tends to be a problem in the smaller joints, though any joints can be affected, and in severe cases are. Whereas in osteo-arthritis joints are usually cool to the touch, in rheumatoid arthritis they are typically warm because of the severe inflammation occurring inside them.

Rheumatoid arthritis also has a different disease profile to osteo-arthritis in that osteo-arthritis is a disease of older age, a wearing-out of the joints, which tends to get worse rather than better as time goes on. Rheumatoid arthritis, however, comes in bursts and may well burn itself out; this doesn't mean that the joints go back to normal, because they have often been severely damaged by the inflammatory process, but it does mean that the joints become cool again and cause pain only because of the degeneration of the joint surfaces that has occurred.

Orthodox treatment

The mainstays of medical treatment for rheumatoid arthritis are non-steroidal anti-inflammatory drugs (NSAIDS). These are drugs which behave very much like aspirin, in having not just a simple anti-pain function, but also an anti-inflammatory function.

The non-steroidal anti-inflammatories are notorious for producing side-effects in the stomach – principally gastritis and bleeding – and it is important to take them on a full stomach: otherwise you may bore a hole in your own stomach lining.

Even with these precautions it is quite possible to develop a gastric ulcer in a small proportion of cases, so when taking non-steroidal anti-inflammatories, if you notice that you are beginning to get stomach pains, do tell your doctor immediately. It may be important to stop the drugs and to go on to alternative medication.

There is an unfortunate relationship between the effectiveness of the non-steroidal anti-inflammatory drugs and their ability to produce side-effects. In general, the stronger the drug the more aggressive it is towards the stomach lining. However, don't be alarmed; most people can tolerate these medicines without any problems. Sometimes it helps to give anti-acid drugs as well, in order to reduce the stress on the stomach lining.

The non-steroidal anti-inflammatory drugs include a host of well-known names: aspirin in all its forms, indomethacin, diclofenac, ibuprofen and many, many, many others. Sometimes these drugs can be administered in a long-acting slow-release tablet, to be taken once a day; others can be given by suppository to try to avoid the effects on the stomach.

A cocktail of non-steroidal anti-inflammatory drugs and a straight painkiller such as paracetamol, co-proxamol, or dihydrocodeine is often sufficient to bring rheumatoid arthritis under control. For the more serious cases, referral to hospital will be necessary: the rheumatologist has at his disposal a number of so-called 'disease-altering' drugs which can dampen the inflammatory reaction in a different way. Drugs used in this manner include gold injections, penicillamine, and methotrexate, a drug that was originally used for cancer and which has now found a very useful role in tiny doses for controlling rheumatoid arthritis. However, these drugs are potentially quite toxic and if you are taking them you will need to have regular blood counts to check that your bone marrow has not been affected. Physiotherapy can be enormously helpful in rheumatoid arthritis – especially in a hydrotherapy pool.

Self-help
Self-help in rheumatoid arthritis is much the same as self-help for osteo-arthritis. In general, the object is to lessen the load on the joints and to use the joints carefully – which means making sure your posture is good, and your work practices appropriate. Unlike cervical spondylosis, however, in rheumatoid arthritis the bones around the joints can be very thin indeed. This is of immense importance in the neck because it means that it becomes even easier to damage the neck. In particularly bad cases it may be necessary to wear a cervical collar (a neck brace of sorts) to prevent the neck and head being moved around too much and certainly any sufferer from severe rheumatoid arthritis should *always* have a head restraint in the car to avoid the worst effects of a whiplash accident. In really severe cases of rheumatoid arthritis in the neck it is absolutely vital to wear an orthopaedic collar (which provides support for the neck) in the car. Any sudden jerk may be enough to fracture the remaining brittle bone on the odontoid peg, dislocate the neck, and paralyse the patient. Don't forget that most road accidents occur within three miles of the victim's home and you are probably much more likely to have a collision in a built-up area than when travelling quickly on a motorway.

Granted, a high-speed collision is much more dramatic and potentially more dangerous, but it is amazing how much force you experience when decelerating suddenly from three miles an hour – for example, when running into a bollard while parking – or suddenly stamping on the brakes. So, if you've been given an orthopaedic (cervical) collar to wear in the car, wear it. It may save your life.

Other self-help mechanisms include taking your tablets regularly to reduce the level of inflammation. If the joint isn't inflamed then it is much harder to injure it during the normal hurly-burly of the day; but if the joint is red raw inside, then little movements can do a lot of damage.

Complementary treatment

Complementary treatment abounds for rheumatoid arthritis, probably in response to the fact that at best orthodox medicine can only alleviate, it cannot cure. All sorts of alternative techniques have been tried – copper bracelets, and special diets in which food items are either omitted, or else added in profusion. Because rheumatoid arthritis is an inflammatory disease it is probably wise to make sure that your intake of Vitamin C is adequate (about 60 mg per day is the current RDA).

As for diets – some cases of rheumatoid arthritis may well have a big food-allergy factor in them and an exclusion and provocation test will help to find out which foods may be the culprits . Do note that in rheumatoid arthritis the time scale of a food sensitivity tends to be elongated – it takes a great deal longer for the symptoms to clear, and equally when the provocation test is performed and the food being tested is put back into the diet, it may be several days before any symptoms recur. Therefore, if you are doing food sensitivity testing you would be wise to exclude the foods to be tested for two to three weeks and put them in not more often than one food every three days, adding the food at each meal, to ensure that there really is a good loading dose.

It is not easy to do exclusion tests under these circumstances. While it's easy to go on virtually a total exclusion diet for five days, trying the same thing for twenty-one days is asking for trouble, nutritionally speaking. Therefore, a modified diet needs to be undertaken in which the main culprit foods are excluded, leaving a wider range of foods to be eaten during the exclusion time. Note, too, that the foods which cause trouble in rheumatoid arthritis are often not the same as the ones that cause the biggest problems in migraines. In the case of migraines, dairy products, wine and chocolate must be high on the list of suspect foods; in rheumatoid arthritis it is the grains (wheat, rye, oats, barley) that often cause the biggest problems. In assessing symptoms from the various diets, often stiffness of the joints is the most sensitive indicator.

All these comments apply equally, whether you're doing a classic exclusion/provocation food-allergy challenge test, or one of the alternative diets that abound. There are all sorts of diets that have been recommended for rheumatoid arthritis – the Dr Dong diet, diets excluding red meat, diets high in fish, vegan diets, vegetarian diets; diets high in celery, garlic, onions, kelp and apples have all been suggested as well. Try it and see. *If one particular diet seems to suit you and seems to alleviate your symptoms, then fine. Do remember, however, that rheumatoid arthritis is an episodic disease and you have to make sure that your change of diet hasn't coincidentally aligned itself with one of the good or bad episodes. Repeat the tests on a number of occasions to make sure that you are observing a genuine effect.*

Also ensure that the diet you go on is a balanced one. The advice of your doctor, your health visitor, or a dietitian may be appropriate; you need to make sure that the diet you choose is both well-rounded, providing you with all the proteins, minerals, fats, vitamins and carbohydrates you need. It should go without saying that any dieting or allergy testing when you are pregnant should first be discussed with your doctor; similarly, if you suffer from asthma, or have swelling of the lips or tongue.

Once there is inflammation within the joint the neck reacts in much the same way, irrespective of what is causing the inflammation. Therefore, most of the treatments for cervical spondylosis also apply to rheumatism. Gentle and appropriate exercise, massage (not manipulation), physiotherapy, are all helpful; and do be careful when doing exercises to pick those that are not likely to jar the neck. Even large or boisterous dogs while on a leash can provide sudden and dangerous jerks to the head and neck . If you have a dog it might be a good idea to invest in a sprung leash, which absorbs some of the blow.

If you decide to visit a chiropractor or an osteopath, remember that some of their massage and physiotherapy-like techniques are very acceptable and helpful, but manipulation is absolutely contra-indicated *in rheumatoid arthritis of the neck.*

Acupuncture may be helpful in relaxing some of those muscles that are in spasm, and can control the pain. Acupressure has a similar effect. Moxibustion, where the acupuncture needles are heated by putting small burning wicks on top of them, is frequently used.

The Alexander technique may help in the rehabilitation stage of the disease; and with those migraines which occur as a result of neck problems .

A homoeopath might suggest apis, arnica, ledum and rhus tox, and there are literally dozens of herbal remedies. Many sufferers say copper is extraordinarily successful in preventing attacks. Helpful herbs include bogbean, celery seed, meadowsweet and white willow. A poultice from cayenne and slippery elm should help during an attack.

Pantothenic acid, taken regularly, might help, as will Omega-3 oils. Feverfew is excellent. The leaves of the feverfew plant have anti-inflammatory properties which may help migraine and arthritis sufferers. Tinctures of burdock root are said to neutralise and remove poisons from the body, and act as a mild diuretic. Dandelion root (in the forms of tea, coffee or tablets) may help.

Capsaicin (in the form of capsicums, or hot, red peppers) have the ability to block something called substance P, which is involved in inflammation and pain. It should, however, be avoided if you have a bleeding problem, or are taking anything to thin your blood, as it has an anti-clotting effect.

Aromatherapists would offer oils of cypress, fennel, juniper and lemon to detoxify, and to reduce inflammation. Benzoin, camomile and rosemary can relieve pain. Hot compresses, alternated with cold, will offer considerable relief. Massage should be given to stimulate local circulation.

Garlic, taken internally in the form of teas, in cooking, eaten raw, or in capsule form, or rubbed into the joints, is an ancient and valuable remedy.

Inflammation in the joints can be reduced by the natural production of cortisone in the adrenal glands. When too much supplementary cortisone is taken to control the arthritis, the adrenals shut down. Reflexologists say that they can stimulate those adrenals, not only to reduce cortisone dependency, but to increase the natural ability of the adrenals to produce it.

All forms of relaxation therapy will help reduce the muscle spasm that accompanies neck injury or inflammation.

NECK INJURIES

Any injury to the neck can cause headaches, both at the time of the injury and later and it's worth remembering that any injury bad enough to damage the skull may also damage the neck at the same time. There are too many different types of injury to go into detail about each one, but it's enough to say that any direct or indirect injury to the neck can cause problems. This includes blows at work or during sport (rugby, in particular, but any of the contact sports can cause problems). Any occupation where the hands are frequently held above the head, and especially where the neck is bent back (such as in plastering) can cause neck injuries. Sometimes the accident isn't obvious – such as a sudden jerk on the arms when out walking the dog, a fall on the out-stretched hand, or turning over in bed when asleep. Even a severe blow to the *bottom* of the spine can cause trouble at the *top* – for example, falling downstairs, banging your buttocks.

Sometimes injury can occur while under general anaesthetic in an operation. Because the patient can feel nothing (and because one or other arm may be held out at an awkward angle for the insertion of drips, etc.), it is possible for the neck to be tugged inappropriately, or put into the wrong position for some considerable time.

Poor posture can also cause neck injuries, but over a long period of time. It is surprising how holding a joint at slightly the wrong angle can cause difficulties. For example, those who wear bifocals may end up straining the joint between the fourth and fifth cervical (neck) vertebrae, because when looking at the top of a piece of paper, the vision is often obscured by the junction between the lower and the upper lens of the bifocals. The reaction of the reader is to tilt his head back slightly, to bring the top of the paper into view through the lower lens. Five years of this can be enough to strain the joint slightly, causing headaches!

Other 'small' habits like this that can cause neck problems when repeated over a long time, include driving with your arms too straight: adopting the 'ten-to-two' wheel position is *not* good if you've got short arms. You can also irritate your neck joints by using computers when sitting with your chin jutting forwards, which is easy to do, if the computer has been incorrectly set up, ergonomically speaking.

Wearing headgear that is too tight can also cause headaches, and heavy headgear that is not well-balanced may do the same, by causing too much stress on the muscles and joints of the neck as they seek to hold the head in the correct position against the pull of gravity from the headgear.

Treatment for a neck injury depends very much upon the nature of the injury, and will probably need the advice of your doctor for anything other than the mildest sprain or strain. You should find relevant much of the advice in the section below, on whiplash injuries.

Whiplash injury

Unfortunately, a whiplash injury is all too common an occurrence today. This happens to the occupant of a car when it is shunted, usually from behind. The essence of the injury is that the head is forced too far backwards, often coupled with an earlier or subsequent over-bending of the head forward. If there is no head restraint then, as the car is shunted, all of the driver except his head is moved suddenly forwards; the head accordingly rotates backwards, and the neck over-arches backwards. Then, as the head is pulled forwards by the rest of the body, it swings forward and suddenly bends over on to the chest. It may even rebound up again.

In a head-on collision the reverse happens. The body decelerates quickly because it is strapped in, but the head, being free, doesn't stop as quickly and bends forward on to the neck – often far too far. Then, as the body stops, the head is flung backwards, again arching the neck over the back of the seat.

Accidents like this are very common, though the increasing use of head restraints has considerably reduced their severity. A whiplash accident like this (and it's called a whiplash because the head whizzes backwards and forwards rather like the end of a whip being cracked) causes quite specific damage to the neck. If you've been hit from behind it's usually the fourth and fifth joints of the neck that are damaged. If you're hit from the front, the fifth and sixth joints are usually affected. There is no bone injury, but the ligaments and muscles are stretched, bruised and torn, and the joints may be jammed together, just as a drawer in a desk jams if it is rammed in firmly when slightly at an angle.

Typically, there is little pain immediately after the crash, though the neck may feel sore, but the neck stiffens up and becomes severely painful in the next few hours. Surprisingly, however, the pain is often perceived at a point slightly higher up the neck than the place at which the injury has occurred.

In a whiplash accident, the ligaments around the joints can be severely stretched. Unlike muscles, ligaments are not very resilient. When stretched a little, they behave like crêpe paper. If you stretch crêpe paper slightly, then let go, it returns to its original crinkled form. However, over-stretch it – perhaps pressing your thumb into it – and it won't go back to its original shape when you take your thumb away. Ligaments around joints are very much like this – resilient to a point, but beyond that they become torn and bruised; and then they stiffen up.

Immediately after the incident there is little pain, but the neck progressively becomes stiff and sore over the next few hours. The vicious circle of 'joint pain causing muscle spasm, which causes joint pain which causes spasm' sets itself up again as a result of the muscle spasm following the soft-tissue injury. The result is a stiff, tender neck with pain radiating into the back of the head, and knotted-up muscles in spasm at or above the level of injury.

The whiplash accident is potentially a very nasty injury. Fortunately, it's not life-threatening, but its effects can be life-long and I always counsel patients with a whiplash injury to expect a degree of pain for a very long time. In addition, the joints that have been injured remain vulnerable to further injury for the rest of your life, in just the same way that you can get a 'weak ankle' after twisting it once.

Diagnosis

Diagnosis is pretty easy – the condition comes on shortly after a whiplash-type injury sustained in a car crash or similar accident. Note that the injury is not usually perceived immediately. If there is *immediate* pain in the neck then there is always the possibility that the neck may have been broken, and immediate and careful transportation to casualty is necessary, followed by an X-ray. Don't try to get to casualty yourself; get someone to ring for the ambulance, and let the ambulancemen strap the neck appropriately before anyone attempts to move you.

Diagnosing the longer-term effects of a whiplash injury is not always so easy, but victims nearly always remember the fact that they once had a whiplash injury to the neck, even though it was many years ago. It is useful to remember that the effects of a whiplash injury never really go away and may be responsible for triggering other problems, such as tension headaches. An old whiplash injury can also multiply the effects of cervical spondylosis or osteo-arthritis in the same joints.

What else could it be?

Apart from their manner of onset, tension headaches, cervical spondylosis, osteo-arthritis of the neck, and whiplash injury can all look and behave in much the same way. In addition, they can add to one another and multiply each others' effects, and it may be difficult to sort out which is the main problem. The mode of onset, the history of injury, and the existence or otherwise of cracks from the neck are the main differences. Clicks and cracks usually indicate osteo-arthritis; numbness or tingling in the hand or arm indicate cervical spondylosis (a disc injury), but in practice there is a lot of overlap between the two.

Orthodox treatment

Painkillers are essential, to remove pain and to reduce the chances of developing the pain/spasm/pain/spasm syndrome. So, too, are anti-inflammatory drugs, which reduce the tissue reaction to the bruising and stretching of the whiplash injury. Use of an appropriate anti-inflammatory drug such as ibuprofen (trade names Brufen and Nurofen) during the ten days immediately after the accident may enable the joint to settle down more easily, but you must be sure you take the drugs *after* meals, and stop taking them if you start to develop stomach discomfort.

Initially, it may help to apply icepacks. Wrap a bag of frozen peas taken from the freezer in a piece of cloth – to reduce the chance of 'cold burn' – and apply it to the damaged muscles for fifteen minutes at a time, four times a day for the next two days. Local application of heat will make matters *worse* if applied in the early stages of an injury. Later on, after the initial phase has passed, warmth can be immensely helpful in reducing muscle spasm, but applying warmth at the time of the injury just causes more rather than less soft-tissue swelling.

In the days after the accident, the use of rubefacient creams may help. These are medicines that make the skin feel hot when they are rubbed or massaged in. They act partially by providing counter-irritation, which reduces other forms of pain. The massage the neck gets when the cream is rubbed in also helps. Rubefacients such as Aspellin Linament, Algipan, etc., feel comforting and relaxing; the local skin irritation produced by the cream brings more blood into the area (which is why it feels warmer).

Many casualty departments routinely put their patients with whiplash injuries in a cervical collar (an orthopaedic neck brace). Personally, I don't like these for anything but the most severe injuries. The real problem with the whiplash injury is that after the original trauma, the soft tissues become bruised, and then fixed, and then the neck won't move properly at the affected joints. It seems much better to let the joints move rather than immobilising the neck in a collar. The orthodox medical theory (with which I disagree) says that fixing the neck in a collar stops any further damage to the joint, and minimises further stretching and bruising to the ligaments. This is true, but really this is secondary to keeping the neck moving – not moving violently (no neck-rolling exercises) – but allowing the normal gentle movements of day-to-day living to keep the neck loose, and thus prevent the neck stiffening up.

Self-help

Prevention is certainly easier than cure for a whiplash injury. So, drive safely!

You're much less likely to get a whiplash injury in a car fitted with head restraints. Don't forget that in a collision, rear passengers are subjected to just the same forces as the driver. This is short-sighted. If your car hasn't got head restraints, fit them – to all seats, if possible. If your children aren't tall enough for their heads to protrude over the back of the seat then they won't need head restraints yet; the seat itself will act as one, even though it's bouncy rather than just supportive. Do make sure, however, that the children are buckled in with seat belts that cross over the right bits of their anatomy; otherwise, in a crash they will either bend forward too far (with a strap that's too low and doesn't restrain the shoulder) or get garotted (with an adult strap that's at the level of the neck). A well fitting lap- and crossbelt is essential for all children travelling.

As far as treatment of the whiplash injury is concerned, there isn't much that you can do yourself. Professional advice will be necessary, and continue to take any prescribed tablets (see above). However, *after* you've been checked out by the doctor, it may help to apply cold compresses in the early stages (as mentioned above).

Complementary treatment

Acupuncture and acupressure, physiotherapy and sometimes manipulative medicine may be appropriate; however, we must be cautious about advising manipulative medicine in neck injuries. It is vital not to manipulate someone who has the slightest chance of having a fractured vertebrae and it may be necessary to exclude a fracture by performing X-ray before even attempting manipulation. Soft-tissue work by an osteopath or physiotherapist will probably help; and if the joints in the neck have been jammed together by the accident then manipulation may be appropriate.

Reflexology for solar plexus/chest/spine and breast/chest may help.

In an emergency situation, 30c arnica, every five minutes, up to about ten doses, is helpful. To reduce bruising, try rhus tox, ruta, hypericum or bryonia.

For pain relief, try a tea made from the spray and flowers of the catnip plant (also called catmint); one teaspoon of the tea before meals should soothe the pain. A cold balm of melissa, and a very light massage of lavender oil will help. Olbas oil (or lotion) may help relieve muscle spasm, and again try a peppermint mash. Where there is inflammation, a compress dipped in strong marigold tea (calendula) and cider vinegar may give relief.

Essential oils of ginger, juniper, lavender, marjoram and rosemary, inhaled, gently massaged or added to your bath, may relieve pain and inflammation. Try one or a blend of the oils, with a light base oil.

Following your recovery period, Alexander technique and Eldenkrais method can help you to regain body confidence and posture, which will encourage your natural reflexes to start moving again, relieving pain and allowing unrestricted movement.

Although it's right to be cautious about the use of manipulation in the immediate post-accident phase, manipulative medicine can help later on. At this point the joint is often solidifying into a fixed, immovable state as the bruised ligaments heal by forming scar tissue. Manipulation at this time may help to keep the joint mobile. An injured joint throws strain upon other joints because these have to do the work that it once did; manipulation and soft-tissue treatment can often keep the other joints working where they are in danger of giving up through being progressively over-stressed. Loosening the related muscle spasm stops the other joints from seizing up.

The object of all of this treatment is to keep the movements of the neck as free and easy as possible, and to reduce the chances of the neck stiffening up with muscle spasm or scar tissue. To this end, all techniques can be useful – painkillers and anti-inflammatories to reduce the pain and spasm; manipulation to keep the joints moving; acupuncture to reduce pain and spasm; and massage to help the muscles relax.

ANNE

Anne is a twenty-seven-year-old professional dancer, so the ability to move her body gracefully and accurately is of greatest

importance to her. Unfortunately, she had been in the driving
seat of her stationary car when another car ran into her from
behind. The collision wasn't a bad one – she'd had head
restraints fitted to the front seats, so the resulting damage to
her had been minimal, but even with an accident at a speed low
enough to cause little damage to the cars, she had still
sustained a minor whiplash injury and had now developed neck
pain.

Typically, for a soft-tissue neck injury, the pain came on some
time after the injury – a few hours afterwards to be precise. On
examination, her doctor noted that there was spasm of the
muscles in the middle of the neck, especially on the left side,
with pain radiating down over the shoulder and into her back.
She also had a headache at the back of the head.

She could still move her neck quite well, considering what had
happened, but the range of movement was much less than she
would have liked it to be. Normally she can move her neck
around as if it were made of elastic, and she needs to be very
lithe for her dancing. To have a neck that may seize up (either
now or in the future) is not going to help her.

So, despite the fact that she had had a very small accident,
and had been saved from the worst of it by neck restraints, she
was still suffering from a lot of pain. In her own words, 'It felt
as though a good pull on the neck would help.' While
manipulation was a possibility for the future, her doctor decided
it was better to start off by giving her painkillers, muscle
relaxants, and an anti-inflammatory drug, to try to reduce
bruising in the soft tissue of the neck. Because muscle relaxants
can often make patients sleepy, her doctor warned Anne not to
drive or use machinery if she were affected.

To a dancer, a whiplash accident, even a minor one like this, is
actually something of an emergency. Swift treatment may make
all the difference between a neck that becomes pain-free
quickly, with minimal bruising and few long-term effects, and a
neck that persistently causes trouble, especially when jarred, or
irritated by being put into odd positions – which is precisely
what a dancer does. Treating Anne's neck quickly and
aggressively was important for her long-term professional
activity.

Gratifyingly, she responded well. Although she soon didn't
need the combined pain-killer/muscle-relaxant tablets, her
doctor encouraged her to continue the anti-inflammatory drugs
for some time, to make sure that the strained and bruised
ligaments were adequately treated, and to minimise internal
bruising and scarring.

What else could it be?

Because there are many different causes of anatomical problems in the neck, there are a wide variety of possible diagnoses, but in this chapter we are really concerned with the question *Is this headache basically caused by a structural problem?*. It can be a difficult question to answer, because often an underlying physical abnormality has overlying spasm and muscular tension which may be of much greater intensity than the structural abnormality itself.

A tension headache alone will cause the same type of headache as cervical spondylosis or osteo-arthritis, but cervical spondylosis with nerve entrapment will also produce pain radiating down the arm or over the top of the shoulder. In *osteo-arthritis* there are likely to be grating and clicking sensations issuing from within the neck, and the neck is sore, and much stiffer on sideways bending and twisting than in tension headache.

Straight tension headaches give a similar sort of pain, except that there isn't the same degree of grating in the neck, and simple tension headaches normally don't cause pain radiating out into the fingers or arm, though they commonly produce pain in the top of the shoulder and the top of the back.

Self-help

Using the neck properly by correct posture and working positions will bring great benefits to the neck. It's important to remember that each joint in our body has a 'natural' way of working. Use it excessively (more than it is intended to be used), or use it inappropriately (perhaps always bent at an awkward angle, or over-loaded by over-frequent use) and the joint will become worn and injured more easily. Jerking the joints doesn't help either! On the other hand, if you respect that joint you'll use it in a more effective and natural way, reducing the strain upon it and in turn reducing the wear the cartilage receives.

It is obvious that excessive use of a particular joint is likely to cause problems and it is relatively easy to spot the occasions when this may be a problem. If your job involves a frequent movement of a joint – especially when under a lot of muscular tension – then this may cause problems for the future. This is easiest to spot in the limbs; quite often a person whose job involves repetitive movements tends to have problems with just those joints that are involved.

Unfortunately, it is all too easy to get into a way of moving in which most of the movement occurs at just one joint in the spine, leaving this joint worn out, while the other joints have very little to do (often being stiff through lack of action). This happens more often in those with a poor posture. Instead of a neck which can bend a little at each joint, bad posture means that one or more of the joints is always working at or near the limits of what it can do. Then, when you try to bend a little more in the same direction, other joints have to do more than they would normally like to do – or else the original joint itself has to do too much, and promptly seizes up.

Defects of posture and poor positioning at work often take a long time to produce symptoms. It may be many months or even years before the most stressed of the joints finally gives up and starts producing pain. Once it's in pain, muscle spasm reflexively occurs around it, fixing it and stopping it from bending. Because the joint is fixed by spasm, even more work is given to other joints, which in turn tend to get over-stressed.

Don't forget either that the neck is just one part of the spinal column and that injuries to one part of the spine have knock-on effects elsewhere. The old osteopathic principle of injuries being reflected up the spine at roughly every third joint has particular relevance here – look after your back and you'll minimise neck problems, and vice versa. Back care is essential. We spend a third of our lives asleep, so it pays to have the right type of bed, the right type of pillow, good seats in the car, and appropriate easy chairs.

For those who lift and carry, it is important to make sure that loads are balanced evenly, that there is a good lifting position with a straight – not a bent – back, lifting by bending and straightening the legs and thighs, rather than by bending and straightening the back. Try not to carry out repetitive movements in the same way all the time, so that you spread the activity and the load among more muscles and joints. For example, if you are carrying bales of straw, don't carry them just on one shoulder – alternate. Not only will you strain the joints in a lopsided fashion, you'll build up lopsided, unbalanced muscles, so that they pull on the joints unevenly and cause even more joint misalignment and stress. Therefore, get into the habit of putting the object you're lifting on the right shoulder the first time, the left shoulder the next time, and so on.

Once you've started to develop anatomical neck problems you'll need to think about lifting, moving and posture in a completely different way. Although some of the neck joints may be damaged already, it's not too late to re-learn good posture and good lifting practices, because at the very least these will minimise any further damage to your neck.

TERESA

Teresa is a forty-year-old woman who works in telephone sales. She came in complaining of pain in the neck, a headache, and pain going down the right arm; she seemed quite terrified by it all. (She was worried that she might be developing a brain tumour.) On examining her it was obvious that the muscles at the junction of the neck and shoulder had gone into spasm – the slightest touch on them gave immense pain both into the neck and down the arm and she couldn't bend her neck sideways without causing more pain.

The interesting part was yet to come. She had two other problems, both of which contributed to the neck spasm: she was deaf in the left ear, and very dominantly right-handed. Being involved in telephone sales, she spent a lot of the day writing down customer details, so she needed her right hand free. However, as she was deaf in her left ear she couldn't use her left hand to hold the telephone, and instead had got into the habit of holding the earpiece between her right ear and the point of her shoulder, pulling her neck up in the process. This left both hands free to write with – the left hand to hold the paper, the right to hold the pen. She spent much of her day like this, with her right ear holding the phone against her right shoulder.

Teresa's doctor pointed out that she was putting her neck into exactly the wrong position and was getting recurrent spasm of the neck muscles as a result. Could she use the telephone any other way? Not easily. She had to write at the same time: holding the telephone to the right ear with her left hand was going to be very difficult. Teresa's doctor suggested that her employers might like to buy her a lightweight telephone headpiece so she could use the phone easily, keeping both hands free, and not bending her neck awkwardly.

To help matters along, her doctor suggested she buy some Syndol, which is a combination painkiller and anti-spasm agent available over the counter. This can make patients drowsy so she was warned of the importance of not using machinery or driving until she knew what its effects would be.

As she got up to go out her doctor noticed she had a large and heavy bag with a shoulder strap, which she immediately put over her right shoulder. He recommended that she alternate the shoulders on which carried her bag, as she was making the muscles of her right shoulder work twice as hard. In this way she would even up the load on her neck and make sure that one set of muscles didn't become over-developed (and hence become likely to go into even more painful spasm) leaving the other side of the neck under-developed (and unable to oppose the spasm if it did develop).

Ten days later she came bouncing in, pain gone, to tell her doctor delightedly that as soon as her employers found out what was causing the problem they immediately volunteered to fit her telephone with a headset, which was installed at very small cost. Now, as a result of the medication, the alteration of her working position, and the change in habit holding her bag, she was now pain-free; the headaches had gone, and so had the neck spasm.

It's important to emphasise keeping the neck pain-free. If there's no pain, then no reflex spasm can be set up. Many people prefer to do without painkillers, but regular painkillers can help a great deal in staving off the beginnings of that syndrome. In degenerative neck disease and other forms of backache, taking painkillers regularly may make all the difference.

The bottom line is that by giving yourself adequate pain relief (and in some cases, anti-inflammatory drugs as well) you will reduce the amount of discomfort you experience, and even more importantly, reduce the chances of further damage to the neck joints.

Complementary treatment
Massage, acupuncture and reflexology are all likely to help. You might think that osteopathy and chiropractic would be of value – and they are, but only to a point. Manipulative techniques are most useful where there is no anatomical change to the joints or muscles. The more anatomical changes in the joints, the less likely is manipulative medicine to help, over and above simple physiotherapy, or osteopathy using soft-tissue techniques without manipulation.

There is a great deal on offer from other therapies; in particular, aromatherapy and herbalism. Any pain that is the result of muscle spasm, or muscle or bone compressing the nerves, may benefit from gentle massage with a vegetable oil and mustard or pepper oils. Try eucalyptus, niaouli and rosemary in a vapouriser. Warm baths with aspic, juniper, nutmeg, and a very tiny quantity of black pepper oil will reduce inflammation and relieve pain.

A poultice of pine, rosemary or lavender oils, or herbs, may help relieve pain. Four products with analgesic properties commonly used with for pain and neuralgia include cajuput oil, camphor, menthol, and clove oil. Tiger balm contains all four ingredients. Rosemary is excellent for muscular pain – taken internally, or pressed on the painful areas as a poultice. Tea tree and eucalyptus have similar external benefits.

The Alexander technique is enormously beneficial. By adjusting your carriage and means of sitting, working, etc., you learn how to move and, indeed live day to day, in a manner that best benefits your body. You also learn how to prevent the distortion that comes from the misuse of the body, relaxing tightened muscles that are the result of pulling yourself out of shape.

Reflexology and acupuncture can help with the pain, and will relieve spasm and stiffness in the neck, easing the accompanying headaches. Dance therapy encourages freedom of movement, which helps to loosen what are often self- or sub-consciously tensed neck muscles. Learning to move properly – altering your carriage appropriately – is essential for living without pain.

Associated problems
Any neck or back injury will be made worse by poor posture, bad lifting practices and poor ergonomics both at work and at home.

Chapter Five

MENINGITIS AND ENCEPHALITIS

MENINGITIS

Of all the causes of headaches, meningitis must surely be the one that is most feared – and justifiably so. Within the space of forty-eight hours, meningitis can turn a previously normal, healthy child or adult into a corpse; those that survive may be deaf or mentally impaired.

This is meningitis at its worst; but the good news is that only a small percentage of cases end up with such an appalling outcome; the rest recover, often with little or nothing to show for their ordeal. Fortunately, meningitis is *rare* – which is surprising because the bacteria that cause it are quite common.

The brain floats in a bath of cerebro-spinal fluid (CSF), which supports and protects it from unnecessary shocks. Because the brain is floating, its supporting tissues don't have to pull on the brain too hard. All they have to do is moor it, like a boat! The brain and spinal cord are wrapped in a set of loose coverings, called the *meninges*.

Normally the spinal fluid and the meninges are completely sterile and totally closed off from the outside world, so there is little chance of infection getting into the delicate tissues of the brain or the spinal cord.

However, just occasionally this barrier is breached and infection gets in. When this happens, the coverings of the brain (the meninges) become infected, and, like any other infected area in the body, start producing pus. This pus, full of bacteria and viruses, goes directly into the spinal fluid which bathes the brain. Unfortunately, this only serves as a quick way to spread the infection; any infection in the meninges quickly develops into infection over the whole of the outside of the brain and spinal cord. And this is meningitis.

Two groups of organisms can cause meningitis – bacteria and viruses. *Bacteria* are tiny self-contained organisms; typical bacterial infections include boils on the skin, urinary tract infections, sinusitis, and some types of pneumonia. Bacteria are usually susceptible to one or more antibiotics.

On the other hand, *viruses* are much smaller than bacteria; they don't have a complete set of cellular 'organs' (organelles) and can only reproduce by burrowing into body cells, hijacking the cell's own organelles, and using them to recreate more viruses. Then the cell dies, bursting open to release hundreds more virus particles. Viral infections include the common cold, influenza, and many childhood ailments such as German measles, chicken pox, and mumps. Unlike bacteria, viruses aren't susceptible to antibiotics. Viral infections are frequently impossible to kill off artificially. Instead, we have to wait until our bodies develop a natural immunity to the diseases, and once this happens the immune system starts to fight the viral invaders and destroy them. Unfortunately, in the more virulent illnesses, the viruses do a lot of damage to the body before it can get round to mounting a proper immune response.

The reason why it's been easier to find antibiotics to kill bacteria, but not many to stop viruses, is because of the different nature of the two infections. Because viruses burrow *into* the cells of the body it's difficult to kill them off without killing the cells. There *are* various agents which now can stop viral infections, but these are often toxic, don't always work very well, and are usually extremely expensive.

In summary, the two forms of meningitis are bacterial and viral. You might think that viral meningitis, being difficult to treat, was likely to be the bigger killer – but as we mentioned earlier this isn't the case. It's bacterial meningitis, often caused by small round bacteria called *meningococci*, that causes the greatest damage; another type of bacteria that often causes meningitis is *haemophilus influenzae*.

Many of us actually carry the meningitis bacteria in our noses. Surprisingly, they don't cause us problems. Why not and why do only certain people get meningitis?

There are two theories. The first is that, although the brain is usually tightly sealed off from the outside world, this barrier isn't always as complete as it could be. There are a number of places where structures have to enter or leave the brain cavity; for example, where nerves pass in and out to the face; where arteries bring in fresh blood; and where veins take away the used blood. Normally these potential channels are well sealed off. However, there is always the possibility that the seal may not be complete, and that bacteria or viruses could squeeze through.

One place in particular seems to be a most likely candidate. The nerves responsible for our sense of smell pass directly into the base of the brain from the nose, through a sheet of bone called the *cribriform plate*. We now think that in some people these nerve channels aren't sealed off properly, and therefore connect the outside (dirty) world with the inside (sterile) world of the brain. This would explain neatly why certain individuals get meningitis and others never do.

On the other hand, if there's some form of gap, you might expect the same individual to go down with different forms of meningitis on separate occasions, which in practice doesn't seem to happen. Enter the second theory, which says that it is a hiccup in our immune system which gives entry to the infection in susceptible people.

What has to be said – and said very loudly – is that meningitis is an *uncommon* disease. It is, unfortunately, appallingly vicious when it strikes, but for all that it is uncommon. There are about 3000 cases a year in the UK, which is about one per 18,000 people. In the last fifteen years I've seen *just one case*, which is about average.

Although meningitis is rare, it isn't completely random. Predominantly it attacks children and young adults, but people of all ages can get it. At times certain areas of a country have higher rates of meningitis than the rest; Stroud in Gloucestershire is a recent example; so too are Norway and Nepal.

The classic symptoms of meningitis are seen in a child or a young person who has suddenly become ill with fever, headache, neck stiffness and vomiting. The light hurts the eyes. The patient may soon become drowsy or even unconscious, and in certain cases has a livid, patchy, purplish rash shaped like a little group of dots or blotches which is spread sparsely over the trunk and limbs and doesn't go away when you press it. These dots rapidly develop into large purplish bruises.

The speed of the onset of the disease can be frighteningly quick. A child that is fit and well at lunchtime may be near death by the evening.

Not all these symptoms and signs may appear. The prime symptom is a stiff neck, and *anyone* with a stiff neck (where they cannot bend their neck *forwards*, on to their chest) should be considered to have meningitis until proved otherwise, especially if they also have a temperature.

However, *children under the age of eighteen months often don't get a stiff neck.* Instead, they may often have a bulging fontanelle (the soft bit on the top of the head where the skull bones haven't yet fused). The skin of the fontanelle lies directly over the meninges and the brain. In meningitis, pressure rises in the spinal fluid, which is why the fontanelle bulges. (Note that the fontanelle also bulges in a child that is crying, so you have to check it when the child is quiet.) Other than a bulging fontanelle, a child under eighteen months may have little specific to show for the illness. They may be vomiting, and will probably look really ill; they may be uttering a shrill, moaning cry, and be very fretful, or else have convulsions. They may be irritable, or conversely drowsy or unnaturally still; and may suddenly develop a squint.

If you suspect that you or your child has meningitis then you must act *immediately*. Quite literally, every minute counts. You need a doctor there and then. If, when you ring, she's out on her rounds, don't wait. Dial for the ambulance and say you think the patient has meningitis. Even if your amateur diagnosis is wrong it doesn't matter: the ambulance service would rather turn out unnecessarily to six cases that aren't meningitis than miss one that was. Many doctors will give an injection of penicillin before sending the patient off to hospital. That extra twenty minutes of penicillin (while the patient is still getting to the hospital in an ambulance) may make all the difference between life and death.

NICOLA

Nicola was a twenty-three-year-old secretary who called out her doctor one morning complaining of a severe headache and vomiting. At first there didn't seem to be much the matter with her. She had a mild temperature, and the light seemed to hurt her eyes, but when the doctor tried to bend her chin on to her chest, her neck was extremely stiff.

She obviously had meningitis. Her doctor immediately gave her an injection of penicillin, and then arranged for an ambulance to come urgently to take her to hospital.

On admission she had a lumbar puncture. The fluid dripping out of the lumbar puncture needle was clear, which meant that Nicola probably had a viral meningitis (cloudy fluid contains pus, which usually means a bacterial infection). In addition, there was no blood – so her symptoms weren't due to a sub-arachnoid haemorrhage.

The first results soon came back from the lab – Nicola had viral meningitis. This was confirmed two days later when the results of culturing the cerebro-spinal fluid (CSF) showed that there were no bacteria in it. Virus infections don't respond to antibiotics, so there wasn't much to do except to give Nicola painkillers and wait while she got over the infection.

Nicola was soon on her way to recovery but was still easily exhausted, very lethargic and typically post-viral. However, over the next few weeks she made an excellent recovery and after about a month went back to work, none the worse for wear.

Orthodox treatment

There is only one place for a person with suspected meningitis, and that is the hospital, and very quickly, too. After a quick examination, the hospital doctor will perform a lumbar puncture, in which a needle is put in the small of the back so that it reaches the fluid surrounding the spinal cord. This is the safest place to tap cerebro-spinal fluid (CSF) without damaging the spinal nerves.

The doctor will then check if the CSF is cloudy. If it is, the patient has meningitis, probably bacterial. If it is clear, the patient may still have meningitis (more likely viral in this case). Analysis of the CSF in the lab, in particular culturing it for bacteria, will not only tell the doctor what type of infection the patient has, but also show the antibiotics to which the bacteria is sensitive.

The treatment for *bacterial* meningitis is antibiotics. Often a cocktail of several antibiotics is used, in case the bacteria are resistant to one of them. Often these antibiotics are initially given by injection, sometimes into muscle, sometimes into a drip which is inserted directly into a vein, which takes them directly into the bloodstream. In some cases, the doctor will inject antibiotics into the spine at the time of the lumbar puncture, so that the antibiotics go directly into the spinal fluid surrounding the infected meninges.

From then on it is a matter of waiting and hoping. Despite the fact that in lab tests the bacteria causing meningitis are often sensitive to antibiotics, in the patient the same antibiotics do not necessarily work as quickly nor as effectively as we would like. Even with full doses of antibiotics it is still quite possible for the patient to die, or be brain damaged, by the infection. One reason for this is that some types of bacteria release toxins, so that even if the bacteria have been killed the toxins are still in the system, doing damage and causing toxic shock.

After the initial infection is over, rest and recuperation are the order of the day, and it may be many weeks before the patient is fit enough to resume their usual duties.

What about *viral* meningitis? Here is a different problem. While bacterial meningitis is sensitive to antibiotics, viral meningitis isn't. There are one or two anti-viral agents that can sometimes be used, but by and large, viral meningitis has to resolve of its own accord rather than by anything the doctor can do. After a time the immune system of the body works out how to respond to the invading viruses, and starts destroying them. Thankfully, viral meningitis doesn't do anything like the same amount of damage as bacterial meningitis, though it can still be lethal.

Type of headache

The headache of meningitis is pretty phenomenal, but often the patient doesn't know much about it because they are delirious or unconscious. The headache may be over the whole head; alternatively, it can be located at the front, or the pain can extend into the neck and back. As the disease progresses, the headache becomes more and more severe.

Headaches *after* meningitis are also quite common and it will be some time before the pains go away completely.

What else could it be?

Meningitis is characterised by a stiff neck, a temperature, sensitivity to light which hurts the eyes, and vomiting. In some *flu-like viral infections* it's possible to get a condition called *meningism*, in which there is spasm of the muscles in the neck but without the same degree of neck stiffness. In meningism the neck can be bent, but the chin won't always reach the chest. However, the difference between meningitis and meningism is far too subtle for lay people to diagnose with confidence. Even as a doctor I'm reluctant to diagnose meningism, just in case in doing so I miss its far deadlier cousin. Any feverish condition where there is a stiff neck should be considered to be meningitis until proved otherwise.

Sub-arachnoid haemorrhage can give a stiff neck and altered consciousness, but without the temperature; *tension headache* can produce a neck which is stiff on side bending and twisting, but not usually on bending forwards, and there won't be a temperature; and ordinary viral infections such as gastric flu can produce headaches, vomiting, and a rise in temperature *without* causing neck stiffness.

In children, *febrile convulsions* can be mistaken for the convulsions of meningitis. Some children get convulsions when they get a fever. Once you know your child has a tendency to febrile convulsions, then there's not the same fear that the convulsion may be meningitis. However, when it's the *first* convulsion, you don't know whether it's meningitis, or a susceptibility to febrile convulsions, so hospital admission is necessary, for a lumbar puncture to exclude meningitis.

Finally, *flu-like infections* can produce vomiting and photophobia (where the light hurts the eyes), but without a stiff neck; and *migraines* can produce vomiting, headache and photophobia, but with neither a stiff neck nor a temperature.

Prevention

We can now immunise against two of the bacterial types of meningitis. There's been a vaccine against the A and C strains of *meningococcal meningitis* (one of the bacterial forms) for some years, but there isn't one against the B strain yet, which is unfortunate, because that's the one that mainly does the damage.

Immunisation against meningococcal meningitis may be useful in a persistent local outbreak, and there are some countries (notably Nepal, Kenya and Norway) where meningitis is currently prevalent. Travellers to these countries may be offered meningitis vaccination before they go. Travel vaccination requirements change from month to month – check the current requirement with your doctor or practice nurse at least six weeks before you are due to travel.

Secondly, immunisation against Haemophilus Influenzae is now available, called the Hib vaccine. It's presently being offered to children under age of four in the UK. Haemophilus Influenzae more commonly produces severe respiratory infections, especially in children. Despite its name, it doesn't cause influenza.

A full course of immunisation consists of three injections at intervals of about six weeks. Older children will require fewer injections, and adults don't need it because they will have developed a natural immunity.

Treatment of contacts

In *bacterial* meningitis, it is usual to give special antibiotics such as Rifampicin to those people who are close contacts of the patient; in practice, this usually means just those who are living in the same house. These antibiotics hopefully will kill off any of the organisms in these exposed people. It is not usually thought necessary to treat the more occasional contacts, as meningitis is not that infectious, and in practice only close contacts are likely to be vulnerable.

Self-help

The only self-help of relevance is to be on the look-out for a stiff neck (on bending forward) whenever you get a fever or a headache. This applies especially if you live in a community which seems to have a large number of meningitis cases. Watch for that stiff neck, without getting paranoid about it. Always check for a stiff neck whenever you or someone in your family gets a headache or a temperature then if it is meningitis you'll spot it early.

Testing a young child for a stiff neck isn't easy; they don't like having their neck forcibly bent. Instead, make a game of it. Ask the child if she can touch her knee with her nose. If she can, she's very unlikely to have a stiff neck. And don't forget that children under eighteen months don't always get a stiff neck. Instead, where it's still present, the fontanelle bulges.

Complementary treatment

There are no complementary treatments for meningitis. Orthodox medicine is what you need – and very quickly, too. In meningitis, delay might be fatal. Dial 999 immediately, and while waiting (and only if the patient is conscious) you might try giving him or her arnica or aconite every ten minutes until help arrives. Alternatively, sipping valerian tea while waiting will ease the pain and shock, and provide a distraction.

Try rubbing Rescue Remedy (a Bach Flower remedy) into the pulse points and behind the ears of the patient, while waiting for help. Lavender and camomile oils can be soaked in a handkerchief and pressed to the nostrils, or as a compress to the forehead. All of these therapies provide some relief from the symptoms of meningitis while you wait. Orthodox medical attention must be sought immediately.

Severe headaches following meningitis can be treated with lavender oil, in any of the popular aromatherapy forms. Lavender tea with a pinch of rosemary, or as a tincture, acts as a stimulant, and strengthens the system. Some therapists recommend Royal jelly as a supplementary nutrient source.

If you suffer from anxiety following meningitis, try camomile or orange blossom tea, or vervain. Aconite, ignatia and phosphorous would be recommended by the homoeopath. Geranium lavender, melissa, neroli and rose oils can be used in a vapouriser, in the bath, or, mixed with a carrier oil, lightly massaged into the temples, shoulders and neck.

Depression may be treated with Bach flower remedies, various herbal preparations, homoeopathic medicine and many other forms of treatment, in particular art and music therapies . It is essential that you consult a registered practitioner following any severe illness, and certainly when suffering from depression of any kind.

Associated Problems

After an attack of meningitis, the brain may take some time to recover, and it is common for headaches to persist for some time.

ENCEPHALITIS

Meningitis is an infection of the *coverings* of the brain, whereas encephalitis is an infection of the brain tissue itself usually as a result of a viral infection. Often a small amount of encephalitis occurs as part of a viral illness, such as mumps or measles. Mostly the inflammation is minimal and spontaneously disappears without trace once the infection is over. In the moderately severe viral infections such as influenza it is probably a mild degree of encephalitis which is responsible for the transient disordered dreams, drowsiness, and slight irritability that sometimes accompanies these conditions.

More rarely, a more severe form of encephalitis from mumps, measles, etc., can cause permanent brain damage such as deafness or mental handicap. Sometimes infection is primarily in the brain itself, and in the really bad cases, encephalitis can be life-threatening. In cases like this there may be fits, gross alterations in the level of consciousness with extreme drowsiness or even coma. Severe cases of encephalitis look more or less exactly like meningitis, with vomiting, a stiff neck, and a severe headache.

The approach to treatment is the same, too. Clinically it is often impossible to tell meningitis and encephalitis apart without doing a lumbar puncture and other special tests. *Urgent* hospital admission is necessary, exactly as in the case of meningitis.

Patients with severe encephalitis are obviously ill; but because most cases are due to viral infections, often little can be done; unlike bacteria, viruses don't respond to antibiotics. However, the herpes virus group does respond to the anti-viral agent acyclovir and in severe cases acyclovir given by injection may help to *limit* (not remove) an encephalitis thought to be caused by this type of virus.

Fortunately, severe encephalitis is rare; treatment is entirely in the hands of orthodox medicine and no self-help nor alternative therapies are appropriate. Mild cases of encephalitis (where the encephalitis is really just part of an overall infection, such as flu or mumps) usually resolve spontaneously; the headache and other symptoms they produce are best treated symptomatically.

TIMOTHY

Timothy is a thirty-seven-year-old planning officer in his local council. Over the course of several days he developed a severe headache in both temples, and a slight temperature. Then his memory became poor, he felt nauseous, and he had great difficulty 'finding words' and doing calculations. Things came to a head when eventually he blacked out with the pain.

He was admitted to hospital where he had to undergo a large number of tests. He was given blood tests, followed by a CAT scan and a lumbar puncture to sample the cerebro-spinal fluid (CSF). Analysis of this indicated that he might have a viral encephalitis. Finally he had an electro-encephalogram (EEG) which showed that the whole of the electrical functioning of the brain was markedly disturbed.

Timothy had a severe viral encephalitis, disrupting the whole of his brain in a non-specific way. Because of the severity of his symptoms he was given the anti-viral agent acyclovir by intravenous drip, for ten days, and slowly his mental functions started to return. His EEG improved, as did all the tests of his mental functioning. His headaches started to disappear too.

Eventually he become well enough to go back home. He still had intermittent headaches which moved from temple to temple; and although to the outside observer he seemed to be back to normal, Timothy still felt 'woozy' at times and still couldn't calculate quite as quickly as he'd been able to in the past. Also, in keeping with the after-effects of a severe viral infection, he felt exceptionally tired.

Over the next few weeks he gradually returned to normal. The headaches disappeared, and his mental functions returned to what they were before he contracted the illness.

Chapter Six

OTHER INFECTIONS

We've looked specifically at meningitis, but as a general rule, *most* infections (especially viral ones) can cause headaches. These are usually accompanied by a general feeling of malaise, and sometimes a sore throat; contrary to what many people think, however, you don't have to have a running nose.

Infections fall into two main groups – those caused by bacteria, and those caused by viruses. *Bacteria* are relatively large organisms, existing outside the body cells, while *viruses* are much smaller, and need to get inside the body's cells in order to multiply. Viruses are responsible for many of the major infective illnesses that still trouble us in the West – the common cold, influenza, chickenpox, measles, German measles, hepatitis, and, of course, AIDS.

Unfortunately, the only way to stop most viral infections is by preventing them from occurring in the first place through immunisation. Immunisation, however, has to be carried out disease by disease – a separate immunisation is required for polio, influenza, German measles, and so on, even though sometimes the inoculations can be mixed in one injection. The point of immunisation is to expose the body to each type of virus, but in a safe, inactive form. This activates the immune system, which remembers the chemical shape of the outside coat of the virus. Then, if any of the 'real' viruses invade in the future, the body quickly recognises them and mobilises the immune system to destroy them before they can do any damage.

Bacterial infections include most of the infections that produce pus or boils; in addition, such infections as typhoid, gonorrhoea, diphtheria and whooping cough are all bacterial infections. The body's immune system will fight bacteria, but nowadays bacteria can also be killed off by antibiotics – at least, in most cases. Bacteria are usually quick to succumb once a suitable antibiotic has been given, but sometimes an infection gets too tenacious a hold for antibiotics to do any good, and on other occasions bacteria can develop resistance to particular antibiotics.

As well as bacteria and viruses there are other groups of infective agents, such as *spirochaetes* (which in this country cause syphilis and the water-borne Weil's disease). In tropical climates, infections by worms and other parasites can be common; these include malaria, which is a small parasitic organism that lives in the red blood cells and the liver, and is transmitted by the bite of an infected mosquito.

The characteristic sign of an infection (other than very minor ones) is a raised temperature. The temperature rise varies according to your age, and the disease itself; as a rough rule of thumb, anything above 101°F is likely to be a viral infection (with the exception of urinary infection, malaria and septicaemia, commonly known as blood poisoning). Smaller rises in temperature are usually associated with bacterial infections.

The age of the patient has an important bearing on the temperature, too. By comparison with adults, children produce much higher temperatures: in an adult, a minor infection which causes a temperature of 99.5°F may produce a raging temperature of 102°F in a child. In the same way, the temperature rise is usually much smaller in the elderly, in comparison to the middle-aged adult.

Often children don't complain of headaches when they have infections, but perceive the pain to be in their abdomens. 'I've got a tummyache, Mummy' is the childhood equivalent of the adult's 'I've got a headache'.

It's generally true that any illness that produces a fever can produce a headache; the headache is worse in the earliest and middle parts of the infection, and usually dies down as the fever starts to wane.

In the specifically childhood diseases – chickenpox, measles, and so on – it is often only when the rash comes out that the parents realise their child is suffering from something other than a heavy cold or a dose of flu, as intrinsically, there is little difference between the infection caused by influenza and that caused by chicken pox. It really doesn't matter, anyway, because once a viral infection has taken hold there's very little we can do except treat the symptoms as they arise, using extra fluids, paracetamol for the temperature (aspirin can be used for adults) and bed rest. For uncomplicated viral infections, ordinary antibiotics are useless and there is no point in prescribing them.

Sometimes a simple viral infection becomes more complex: perhaps a secondary infection such as a bacterial chest infection develops in a patient who started off with flu. Often it's obvious what has happened – such as when the patient starts coughing up coloured sputum. In children, a viral infection of the nose and throat can sometimes be followed by an ear infection. Most secondary infections are caused by bacteria, so in these cases the doctor will want to prescribe an antibiotic. Although the primary cause of the illness (the virus) won't respond to an antibiotic, the secondary (bacterial) infection will.

In a bacterial infection, a headache usually comes on only if there is quite extensive infection. The two bacterial infections most likely to do this are a urinary tract infection, and a chest infection.

However, infections in the face, head and neck areas can produce headaches directly. Sinus infections produce headaches through pressure on the facial bones, dental infections can also produce headaches, and viral infections which affect the lymphatic glands in the neck can cause muscle spasm of the neck muscles.

Type of headache

The headache accompanying an infection is usually generalised and pounding, at its worst in the early stages of the illness, often pounding in time with the pulse, and made worse by straining. The intensity of the pain is often (but not always) related to the height of the temperature.

What else could it be?

The chief pointer to an infection is that the temperature rises; so a headache accompanied by a temperature is almost certainly infectious in nature.

There are two dangerous varieties of infection. The first is *meningitis* – so check that the patient can bend their neck far enough for the chin to touch the chest. If they can't, contact your doctor *immediately*. In a toddler, an alternative way to check for neck stiffness is to ask them to touch their nose to their knee. If they can do this, they haven't got neck stiffness. Do remember, by the way, that neck stiffness doesn't always occur in babies with meningitis; instead, the fontanelle bulges (the fontanelle is the soft area on the top of the head). There may be a high-pitched cry, convulsions and irritability, or – conversely – drowsiness, apathy and stupor.

The other unpleasant cause of headache plus temperature is malaria (rare in Great Britain and much of the Western world). The patient will have been abroad recently, or else have had malaria in the past. Any severe headache and high temperature that comes on within six weeks of travelling to or through a region where malaria is common should immediately be reported to the doctor. This applies even more if the patient has failed to take anti-malarial tablets regularly and routinely. In malaria, there is a swinging temperature, with rigors (violent shaking and teeth chattering); but you can also get rigors like this in both flu and urinary-tract infections.

Finally, there's a trap that catches not just patients, but also doctors. A high temperature and a headache (normally a sign of a virus infection) can also occur with a bacterial *water infection*, especially in a child. Often there's stinging or burning on passing water. The urine may be smelly, you may need to go to the toilet more frequently than normal and once you sense you want to go to the toilet, you may need to go *urgently*. But these symptoms don't always occur, and it's easy to overlook a urinary-tract infection, *particularly in the young child* who can't talk about their symptoms. Treatment is simple – an antibiotic usually clears things up quickly. The danger is in *not* giving an antibiotic, because long-standing, unrecognised water infections can damage the kidneys (see below for further information about water infections).

Orthodox treatment

The most important thing is to be sure that you're not dealing with meningitis or malaria. The next question is to ask whether or not it is a bacterial infection. If there are symptoms of a water infection, earache, coloured sputum, or a severe sore throat, then you will need to contact your doctor, because an antibiotic will probably be required.

If it's none of these, then probably you're dealing with a virus infection, in which case little else remains to be done except to treat the symptoms. Paracetamol, fluids and bed rest (if necessary) are usually all that is needed. Regular paracetamol (according to the dose on the bottle) will bring down your temperature and ease the aches and pains. In infections aspirin is not appropriate for anyone under the age of twelve, because it has been known in rare instances to cause Reye's Syndrome, which is a disorder which can lead to severe brain and liver damage, and sometimes death. In adults, however, aspirin often brings down the temperature more effectively than paracetamol, though aspirin can upset the stomach in certain sensitive individuals, and is not suggested for anyone suffering from bleeding disorders such as haemophilia, patients on steroids, and those with ulcers or gastritis. Nor should you take aspirin if you are pregnant.

Although safe in normal doses, paracetamol is actually quite toxic to the liver and can be *very* dangerous in overdose, especially if taken with excess alcohol. As few as twenty tablets taken in twenty-four hours has been enough to kill. So *don't be tempted to double the dose of paracetamol* if your headache hasn't gone away – you may damage or even kill yourself.

If you're still having problems dealing with the headache or bringing down the temperature, despite full doses of paracetamol, and you're an adult who is able to take aspirin, then try alternating full doses of paracetamol and aspirin every three hours. Start off with two paracetamol, then three hours later have two aspirin, then three hours later have two paracetamol, and so on. In this way, neither paracetamol nor aspirin is being taken to excess, but the effects of each continue the anti-temperature and anti-headache effect of the other. A regime like this can be very effective, especially in settling the unpleasant symptoms of flu, which is often quite resistant to treatment.

Antibiotics are not required for a simple viral infection, unless there's a secondary infection – such as a chest infection, or an earache. However, in anyone with an underlying illness (such as asthma or diabetes), antibiotics may be required more quickly, or even straight away, to try to prevent secondary infections starting.

Opinions vary about whether bringing the temperature down is all that important. Aspirin and paracetamol work by re-setting the body's internal thermostat, and after a dose the temperature drops, or at least stabilises.

Some doctors recommend tepid sponging as well, at the beginning of a fever, purely to bring down the temperature. It's certainly useful when the fever is subsiding; the body is trying to lose heat, which is why we sweat at this time. In providing more fluid to take away the heat of the skin by evaporation, tepid sponging helps cool the body without fluid loss and debilitation of heavy sweating.

Tepid sponging is always useful in those children who are prone to febrile convulsions, in whom it helps to bring the temperature down as quickly as possible to terminate or prevent fits. In children with febrile convulsions, it isn't the height of the temperature that gives the convulsion, but the speed with which the temperature rises. So a child may throw a fit if she reaches a body temperature of 99.5°F in twenty minutes, while that same child may tolerate a temperature of 103°F with no problems at all, *provided she goes up to that temperature slowly*. In really severe cases, a dose of phenobarbitone prescribed by the doctor may help to reduce the tendency to have fits.

Only certain children seem susceptible to febrile convulsions: febrile convulsions disappear by the age of seven, and *never* lead to epilepsy. There is one common trap: in a child who's never had a febrile convulsion before, a convulsion with a temperature could be meningitis, so you need to contact your doctor straightaway.

Self-help

For most febrile illnesses, paracetamol and/or aspirin, fluids, and bed rest are all that is needed. Don't worry if the patient doesn't eat for a few days; it doesn't matter. Even in small children a period of up to a week without food is unlikely to cause any problems; after all, that's what fat stores are for! Just make sure there's an adequate intake of fluid, which is simply enough fluids to ensure that the patient is passing water regularly.

Uncomplicated viral infections don't need a doctor. On the other hand, you *should* call the doctor if other symptoms occur, such as: earache, coloured sputum, or jaundice; if the patient seems particularly ill or is getting much worse; if there is pre-existing disease such as diabetes, chest disease or heart trouble. If the sufferer is very old or young you will probably want to call the doctor earlier, too. It's also worth contacting the doctor if they don't seem to improve after three or four days.

Most febrile illnesses start to resolve themselves after a few days, and there is normally little that the doctor can do, other than advise treatment of the symptoms with paracetamol and fluids. It's only the *complications* of viral infections that the doctor can treat.

ROBERT

Robert is twenty-four, and was confined to bed with a temperature of 103°F, a severe headache, aching muscles and a slight sore throat, but nothing else, and he didn't have any of the symptoms of the common cold. However, his doctor was very alarmed at the high temperature.

*Robert felt **dreadful.** However, he could bend his chin on to his chest, so he didn't have meningitis; and he didn't have a cough or any trouble passing water, nor any diarrhoea, so he didn't have a chest, a urinary-tract, or a bowel infection.*

In fact, Robert had simple flu – but as he'd never really had a dose of flu before he was taken aback by the severity of the symptoms. His doctor remarked that those who say they've 'had a dose of flu, but worked through it' never actually have flu in the first place, just a heavy cold. Robert nodded enthusiastically in agreement, then winced with the extra pain that moving his head produced.

The treatment was simple: regular paracetamol and extra fluids to cope with the fluid loss caused by sweating. As he was feeling so terrible he used the trick of two paracetamol alternating every three hours with two aspirins.

Gradually he got better. The combination of paracetamol and aspirin brought his temperature down – making him sweat in the process – and curbed the headache at the same time. Even so, it took him two weeks before he felt able to go back to his job as a carpenter.

Robert didn't feel completely back to normal for about six weeks, illustrating what is so commonly not appreciated – that viral infections such as flu take six or more weeks to go. Robert asked about using extra vitamins but his doctor doesn't usually advise extra vitamins during the recovery stage some doctors do, but most feel they are not usually needed unless the patient is a child who is off his food, or an old person who doesn't eat much at the best of times.

Complementary treatment

Children who are coming down with any one of the childhood diseases are usually pale, listless, tired and irritable. Recognising these signs, and increasing fluids and making sure the child is well-rested, will decrease the severity of the illness. Homoeopathy is effective at all stages of the illness, and is perfectly safe for children. Individual consultation will be necessary, but some of the suggested remedies are: morbillinium for measles, phytolacca for mumps, pertussin, aconite and bryonia for whooping cough, and rhus tox, sulphur and belladonna for German measles.

Herbal remedies abound for both the treatment of the illness and for dealing with the temperature and headaches that are the symptoms of the illness. Yarrow as a tea can be taken in measles, as well as poke root. Echinacea tablets or tincture may help clear rashes, and catmint (catnip) can be infused to bring down fever. Poke root in tincture or tablet form are helpful for mumps, as well as taking senna for fever, and freshly chopped ginger as a poultice on the skin.

German measles might respond to chicory and cherry plum Bach flower remedies, and for whooping cough you might try coltsfoot, elecampane, and black root. Wild cherry can help the cough itself.

Children who are suffering from fever can be gently sponged with a few drops of camomile or bergamot oils in tepid water; alternatively, use tea tree and eucalyptus dropped on a hanky and tied to the end of the bed or cot. Hornbeam, chicory and holly Bach flower remedies might help, and acupuncture can bring down fever.

There are many alternative therapies for febrile convulsions. In terms of prevention, anything that prevents a fever from climbing is helpful, like belladonna or merc sol. Use Rescue remedy in a crisis.

The relief of adult infection and fever is somewhat similar, but there are plenty more options. Aromatherapy is useful in many cases. Basil, camomile, *rose and tea tree will induce sweating, while eucalyptus, lemongrass, tea tree and rosemary can bring down fever. You could massage your temples and the back of your neck with camomile in a base oil, and baths of any of the above oils should help. Try a tepid bath when suffering fever. Cooling oils are bergamot and lavender, and oils used in viral infections include tea tree, eucalyptus and bergamot.*

Camomile, eucalyptus, rosemary and thyme can be mixed or taken separately as a tea, to relieve fever. Where there is infection of the urinary tract, diuretic herbal teas might help. Try pine, parsley or celery. Chlorophyll tablets and barley water can ease out infection. Drink plenty of water and camomile tea, when suffering infection of any kind, and try eating fresh garlic.

The same homoeopathic remedies for children will bring down high temperatures in adults, and specific illnesses will require specific doses and dilutions. The symptoms of malaria, for example, can be eased with china, china sulph and arsenicum, though othodox medical advice must be taken as well. (It was while trying to find a cure for malaria, and observing the effects of quinine, that Samuel Hahnemann discovered the principles of homoeopathic medicine.)

The clinical nutritionist would recommend black cohash, devil's claw and quinine for malaria. There is some evidence that other viruses can be controlled by increased intake of zinc and Vitamin C. Extracts of licorice and St John's wort may have anti-viral properties.Acupuncture, acupressure and Bach flower remedies may all help deal with the pain of headaches caused by infection, and help ease other symptoms. Some claim to go to the root of the pain, and deal with the diseases themselves, by stimulating the body's own resources. See what works for you.

HERPES ZOSTER (SHINGLES)

Chickenpox is an almost universal childhood disease characterised by blistery spots scattered all over the body. These are often exceptionally uncomfortable, especially where they occur in the throat, ears and other orifices. Other than this, chicken pox is usually a relatively benign illness, with few side-effects. However, after the infection is over, the chickenpox virus lodges in the ends of the nerves near the skin. Many years later these viruses can re-activate and when they do they form the condition called shingles.

Shingles produces much the same sort of crusty abrasions as chicken pox, except that whereas chickenpox occurs over the whole body, shingles occurs only along the distribution of one single spinal nerve. So, typically, the little marks of shingles will appear in a band or a patch round the trunk; or down the arm; or over the buttock; or down the leg. Occasionally, the nerve affected is the one which supplies the forehead region, or alternatively the eye itself. Shingles here can cause severe head pain.

Although chickenpox and shingles are essentially the same virus, the infections themselves couldn't be more different. Whereas chickenpox is usually a mild infection leaving no after-effects, shingles can be a very nasty infection indeed. For a start, it's painful; and what's more the pain of shingles can continue for *years* in the area of skin supplied by the nerve that has been affected. Secondly, although chickenpox is a disease of the young, shingles generally affects those who are older, and those whose immune system isn't working properly (the 'immunocompromised'). This included sufferers from AIDS, and those who are on certain types of medication such as for cancer.

Shingles has been very aptly described as 'a belt of roses from Hell'. The pain of shingles doesn't have to persist afterwards, but in a good proportion of cases it does. Shingles can be very unpleasant, but fortunately we have a number of drugs that can counteract it. The secret of good treatment is to use these drugs as soon as the condition is diagnosed, and to make sure that the treatment is fully carried out. The less that the virus in the nerve endings is allowed to proliferate, the less pain will occur in the future.

One of the classic places for shingles to occur is over the forehead and around the eye. It starts with an odd sensation in the skin over one side of the forehead and scalp, which then gradually turns into pain, but at this stage there is nothing to be seen and both doctor and patient may wonder what is happening, or where the severe pain is coming from. Then the skin lesions begin to come out – typically, little cyst-like blebs which soon crust over. The blebs can be few in number, but in severe cases they can cover the whole area supplied by the affected nerve, and so one side of the forehead can become a mass of ulcerated abrasions. Typically, new crops of blebs appear each day while the older ones start to crust over. Eventually, no more new vesicles are formed, and the crusts finally drop off, often leaving skin which is red, peeling and very tender to the touch. The skin symptoms of pain and sensitivity may persist some time after its colour and consistency have gone back to normal.

Even if you don't get post-infection pain, shingles is a *very* debilitating disease and it may take three months before you feel back to normal.

Orthodox treatment

The secret is to nip the disease in the bud. As soon as the diagnosis is made your doctor will probably prescribe some anti-viral ointments to put on new lesions as they form, and anti-viral tablets to take by mouth. Only small quantities of ointments will be prescribed because they are *immensely* expensive to manufacture.

There are a number of drugs available – these include idoxuridine, which is applied as paint, and amantidine, which is taken as in tablet form, though others are available. Make sure you tell our doctor if you think you are pregnant as some anti-viral agents shouldn't be used in pregnancy. Where there is a lot of pain a prescribed painkiller will also be useful.

Herpes zoster infection doesn't give a true headache as much as severe localised superficial pain. However, in some cases the after-pains may last for a very long time indeed (of the order of years, if not for life) and can be very difficult to treat adequately.

Self-help

If you suspect you've got shingles then go to your doctor straight away. The sooner you can start using the drugs she prescribes, the greater your chance of escaping without too much after-pain.

Complementary treatment

According to some complementary therapists, shingles often indicates an inadequate supply of B vitamins, the major role of which is ensuring a healthy nervous system. A clinical nutritionist might suggest thiamine by supplement or injection. Adenosine may help the disease – relieving the symptoms of eight-eight per cent of those tested, none of whom had a recurrence. Adenosine is taken in the form of adenosine monophosphate (AMP) injections.

Infusions of lady's slipper, oats, skullcap and St John's wort (which is also an anti-depressant) might help. Tinctures of marigold (calendula) can be used to bathe the affected area. Topical creams which contain capsicum help to cool the pain of nerve disorders affecting the skin, like shingles. It can also provide substantial relief of the pain that develops in the wake of the illness. Try to include hot red peppers in your diet, if you are suffering from this. Glycyrhizin is an extract of licorice root and has been reported as being beneficial in the treatment of shingles, showing anti-viral activity.

A reflexologist would massage the following reflex areas: solar plexus/diaphragm, chest/lung, shoulder/arm, and neck/thyroid. The second stage would be breast/chest, lymph, neck/chest, shoulder/arm, thymus, neck/throat, spine, lymph/groin.

A homoeopath might suggest arsen alb, kali phos and rhus tox, but all chosen remedies would, of course, be dependent on a full consultation.

Acupuncture can help deal with the pain, and facilitiate faster healing, as well as stimulating the immune system.

Aromatherapy can soothe painful symptoms of shingles, but contact a registered aromatherapist for a suitable blend of oils that will not irritate the skin condition, particularly if you plan gently to massage the body. Light massage with camomile, bergamot, eucalyptus, geranium and tea tree can soothe the painful blisters, or try applying a poultice with essential oil of rose. Bergamot is an anti-depressant and can be applied to the blisters, or in a bath at night. All of the above oils can be vapourised to relieve the symptoms of shingles.

Chapter Seven

SINUSITIS

The sinuses are large hollowed-out areas in the bones at the front of the skull. We need them for two reasons. Without sinuses the bones would be solid and heavy, so that our heads would tend to drop forward, especially as the bones concerned are at the front of the face, well away from the centre of gravity of the head, so the extra leverage the bone would create would be very great. The sinuses are small in children, and grow in size from the age of about six upwards, as the face enlarges towards the adult shape. The second reason why we need our sinuses is to give richness and reverberation to the voice.

There are four groups of sinuses – the *frontal* sinuses are in the bones of the forehead over the eyebrows; the *maxillary* sinus is underneath the eye, to each side of the nose; the *ethmoid* sinus is deeper in the facial bones, at the level of the eye, and the *sphenoidal* sinus is deep within the nasal cavity.

The sinuses are not closed spaces within the bones, but open – like little sacks, whose mouths open into the nasal cavity. This opening is called the *antrum, which is* very important in sinusitis, as we'll soon see.

The sinuses are lined with mucus-producing cells, together with cells with a covering of little hairs on top. These hairs are called cilia; they all move in unison and under the microscope the surface of the cells looks like waving fields of corn. As the cilia move, they propel any mucus that's collected in the sinus out towards the antrum, from where the mucus enters the main nasal cavity, and thereafter can get to the outside world, blown out on to the handkerchief or swallowed down the back of the throat. The mucus traps any dust, dirt or bacteria, and the cilia propel the accumulated rubbish out through the opening.

The weak point of the system is the small size of the antrum, which can all too easily become blocked. The cells lining the antrum can swell with inflammation (both allergic and infective), and the sinuses themselves can get infected, changing the thin mucus into thick infected pus, which is much harder for the cilia to waft out.

Once the antrum is blocked there's a quick rise in pressure inside the sinuses as more and more pus is produced. This pus is a mixture of bacteria, mucus, extra fluid from the inflamed cells lining the sinus, and white cells from the blood, which have migrated in to fight the infection.

Because the sinuses are carved out of bone, there is nowhere for this excess fluid to go, and consequently the pressure inside the sinuses rises very quickly. (It's exactly the same as with a pimple on your nose. These are unbearably painful, simply because there is the same rise in pressure: when the pimple erupts to the outside surface and bursts there is an immediate reduction in pressure, and a corresponding immediate reduction in the amount of pain – even though the amount of pus released from that small spot may be little more than a pinhead.) It's not the amount of pus that causes the pain, it's the *pressure* it creates that causes the discomfort.

Sinusitis often follows a cold. The pain can be fiendish, with constant pain in the face or head, which gets worse on bending down, a stuffed-up sensation in the nose, and (often) infected green mucus coming down the nose. You may have a temperature. The sense of smell usually goes away (the sensitive organs of smell in the nose get liberally covered with sticky green pus, which delicate smells can't penetrate), though sometimes when the infection is more or less localised to the sinus itself the patient can smell the pus.

You might think that infection in a small bony hole would be insignificant as far as the rest of the body is concerned – don't you believe it. Sinusitis can make you feel *dreadful*, not just because it's painful, but because a *lot* of pus is produced. The toxins that this pus liberates can enter the bloodstream and make you feel very rough.

An important diagnostic feature of sinusitis is that the pain is much worse when putting your head down. Often, there is local tenderness of the bone over the sinuses, and your doctor will press over these areas to see if this increases the pain (pressing on the bone increases the pressure inside the sinuses even more, and it's basically pressure that causes sinus pain).

In more difficult cases, or where there is long-continued sinus infection and inflammation, it may be helpful for the doctor to arrange X-rays of the face and skull. It is easy to see when the sinus is infected – normally sinuses have air inside them, which shows up as dark shadows in the bone (X-rays penetrate air more easily than bone). If these air-filled sinuses get filled with pus or fluid, under X-ray they look more like the shading of the adjacent bone, so the radiologist can quickly spot which sinus is infected.

Type of headache

Typically, the pain is in the front of the face, around one or both eyes, though as there are four different sets of sinuses, the site of pain coming from each is slightly different. Pressure over the affected sinus causes an instant increase in pain; and the pain also worsens when the head is bent down towards the knees (because the pressure of the blood pooling in the veins adds to the pressure inside the sinuses). Anything that increases the pressure or the amount of fluid in the sinuses will increase the pain, so often sinus pain is worse on lying down. You may wake with a headache, which will go after being upright for a time as the blood-vessel congestion reduces slightly. However, pain from the frontal sinus can sometimes start an hour or two after getting up, and then get better in the afternoon.

What else could it be?

Pain centred around an eye could be *migraine* (but in migraine there are usually changes in the vision, together with vomiting). The pain of *glaucoma* settles round one eye, but the eye is usually inflamed and the vision will be blurred; pain radiating from the back of the neck in a *tension headache* or in *cervical spondylosis* can be sensed in one eye, but there won't be a raised temperature, and the pain won't increase much if you bend or lie down.

Toothache and sinus pain can often be very difficult to tell apart, particularly as some of the upper front teeth, especially the upper canines (the 'eye teeth', slightly pointed ones just to the side of the front of the mouth) have their roots embedded in the bottom wall of the bone that forms one of the sinuses. A *root abscess* in a tooth here (that's an abscess at the very end of the root of the tooth) can be excruciatingly painful and, just like sinusitis, can also give more pain if you put your head down. However, the offending tooth is often very tender when touched or banged, and the pain doesn't normally increase when pressure is put on the bone overlying the sinuses (though pressure on the bone under the gum certainly increases the pain).

In addition, a nasal-sounding voice, a history of nasal allergies, or pus dripping down the nose are usually pretty obvious indicators that the pain is sinus rather than dental. However, in difficult cases you may need to see both doctor and dentist – sinus and dental X-rays may be necessary before the diagnosis can be made with certainty.

Just occasionally sinus pain which doesn't go away with treatment can indicate a *cancer of the sinuses*, so if your pain doesn't get better, be sure to check with your doctor – though in most cases, it will be simply because the bacteria responsible for the infection are resistant to the antibiotics that are being used.

Finally, *high blood pressure* can give the same pattern of headaches – worse on rising – but there won't be facial tenderness, and, obviously, your blood pressure will be high.

Orthodox treatment

There are three aspects to orthodox medical treatment. The first is to stop any infection with an *antibiotic*; the second is to reduce the swelling of the lining of the nose with a *decongestant*, such as pseudoephedrine, thus enlarging the opening to the sinus; and thirdly, to *reduce any allergic response*.

Why is the allergic response so important? Simply because it causes the cells round the hole leading to the sinus to become inflamed, swollen and produce even more mucus. All this reduces the diameter of the hole of the antrum even further. In fact, a large number of people get sinusitis mainly because they have nasal allergies to inhaled pollen, dust, tobacco smoke, or other substances. The more allergic we are, the more the cells lining the nose are likely to swell, and the more the antrum will get blocked.

Because the allergic response is so important, often your doctor will prescribe anti-allergic medication – an antihistamine; sodium cromoglycate as drops or spray; or a steroid nasal spray. Sometimes it's convenient to use an over-the-counter decongestive cough remedy for a short time – these typically contain a decongestant to dry up the production of mucus, and an antihistamine to reduce the local inflammation.

Some people are more prone to sinusitis than others. In some, the antrum is anatomically on the small side; in others, allergies to pollen, dust, or foods may cause the cells lining it to swell, blocking it, or reducing its size enough to cause problems whenever an infection strikes – a cold, for example. Anyone with frequent attacks of sinusitis is usually well advised to try to keep under control any allergies he has.

Food allergies may also have a part to play. Some patients find that they are sensitive to a particular food, which makes them sneeze, and gives them a blocked-up, running nose. However, the role of food allergy in sinusitis is not fully accepted by all doctors, and while all agree that pollen and dust can cause problems in sensitive individuals, many doctors are hesitant about the role that food sensitivities play.

However, all doctors agree that once an allergy has been identified the substance causing it should be avoided where possible. Often this is easier said than done; for example, although it is possible to reduce your exposure to household dust, it's impossible to get rid of it altogether, because even the best-kept house has dust floating in the air. Nor is it easy to avoid pollen; you can stay indoors on days with a high pollen count, wear dark glasses, avoid parks, gardens, fields and the countryside in general, and walk on the shady side of the street, but all you'll do is minimise your exposure rather than remove it altogether.

Unfortunately, minimising your exposure in this way may not be enough. Because allergies tend to work in an all-or-nothing fashion, exposure to even small quantities may trigger off almost a maximum response.

On the other hand, it is quite possible, if sometimes a little awkward, to avoid foods to which you are sensitive. And, if there are other substances you're allergic to, like chemicals, paint, and so on, you may be able to adapt your lifestyle to avoid them.

If it's impossible to avoid those things to which you are allergic, then you'll need a second or third line of defence. Calming down the inflammatory reaction in the nose with antihistamines, anti-allergy drops and sprays (such as sodium cromoglycate) and local steroid preparations (such as beclomethasone) can often be very helpful. Drops of dilute salt solution can also help by liquefying mucus.

One thing the chronic sinusitis sufferer should *not* use for any length of time are decongestant sprays, pills or linctuses. While these are very useful in the short term – say, up to ten days – using them for a longer period lets the mucous cells lining the nose get accustomed to the medication. Then, when the spray is stopped, there is rebound extra production of mucus. So the patient starts using the spray again, What he doesn't realise is that the spray itself is making matters worse – the more he uses his decongestant spray the more rebound secretion will occur.

The really long-term sinus sufferer may need to see an ear, nose and throat (ENT) surgeon. Doing an operation to wash out the sinuses may help clear out accumulated debris and infection. This is important because the presence of foreign material, old pus, etc, can often act as a source of further and continuing infection.

Sometimes, where the hole into the sinus is small, or there's gross obstruction from allergy or infection, and particularly where the sinuses never drain properly and keep on re-infecting themselves, the ENT surgeon can perform an operation called an *antrostomy* to widen the antrum, the hole which leads from the sinus into the nose. Because the sinuses are formed inside bone, the surgeon has to drill bone away in order to enlarge this hole.

Sometimes just a small increase in the aperture of the drainage hole is sufficient to allow the infected secretions inside to get out properly. An antrostomy is often combined with a sinus washout. Operations like these are done quite frequently, and are often very successful.

I mentioned earlier that the cells lining the sinus are covered with microscopic hairs, called cilia, which waft debris out of the sinus. These cells are very important. The antrum is actually up at the top of the sinus, so gravity won't drain away debris. The cilia must be intact and working properly in order to pull the debris up the incline to the antrum.

Unfortunately, tobacco smoke poisons the cilia and stops them working, which is one reason why sinusitis sufferers should *stop smoking*. Without the cilia working properly, it's much easier for debris to remain within the sinus – a prime source for infection.

The second reason why smoking is bad for your sinuses is that both by the direct effects of the smoke particles and through the allergic reaction of the lining of the nose to tobacco smoke, smoking inflames the cells lining the sinuses and closes off the antrum, making infection more likely.

Self-help
If you're a regular sinusitis sufferer then there are a number of things that you can do. Firstly, go to your doctor at the first sign of a sinus infection – you may nip it in the bud. Secondly, when an infection begins, a *short* course of decongestants may open up the antrum and allow proper and adequate drainage of the sinuses. But beware, decongestants should only be used for a maximum of ten days without seeking further advice from your doctor, as otherwise rebound congestion can occur to make matters much worse.

A word of caution here. If you're on anti-depressant drugs called *monoamine-oxidas inhibitors* (MAOIs for short) you can get a severe reaction if you use decongestants, either by mouth or as nasal drops. You should know if you're on an MAOI because you will already have been warned not to eat cheese. These drugs are not in common use now, but because the blood pressure is sent sky high, the interaction is potentially fatal.

If you're an allergic person, then try to avoid the things that you're allergic to; not always easy, but worthwhile if you can do it. Hay fever and dust-mite allergy are significant causes of nasal allergies. What we call *hayfever* is actually a reaction to a large number of different types of airborne pollens, and not just to those produced by grasses.

These pollens are released at specific times of the year, for example, silver birch in April to May; plane (a common tree in London) in May; grasses from May to August; and nettle from June to September. After this, in the autumn come the spores from moulds and fungi.

Many hayfever sufferers are allergic to only one or two types of pollens and spores, and the timing of their worst symptoms coincides with the release of pollen from those particular species. Pollen is so small that it needs a microscope to be seen, and being small and very light it remains suspended in the air for considerable periods of time. When it lands on the lining of the nasal passages the allergic reaction it provokes causes inflammation and swelling of the cells lining the nose, together with increased mucus production. Both these processes cause the nasal passages to become blocked.

Hayfever is worst when there is the most pollen in the air. This depends upon a large number of factors, whether the plants you are allergic to grow in your area (or up-wind), whether they are sporing at the time, and the weather conditions (which can either encourage sporing and also keep spores in, or wash them out of the air). In general, dry sunny weather encourages plants to produce spores. The amount of pollen in the air increases during the morning when the pollen is released. This pollen rises, sometimes into the upper atmosphere. The pollen count also goes up again in late afternoon when this pollen starts to descend. Rainy conditions tend to wash the pollen out of the atmosphere, but on the other hand, wet conditions before the pollen season encourage plants to produce even more pollen when eventually they pollinate.

· The chief self-help principle for hayfever sufferers is to avoid the pollen to which you are allergic. Try to avoid parks, gardens, and the countryside in general; watch the weather reports, which often include a pollen count, and on days that are likely to be bad try to stay indoors with the windows shut. When driving in the countryside keep the windows closed, and when out walking use sunglasses.

If you are severely affected it may help to take a short holiday during the worst of your own hayfever season – because there is relatively less pollen in cities you may have less trouble there. The seaside also tends to have less pollen – if for no other reason than if there is an on-shore breeze it will be coming from over the water and thus blowing pollen-free air towards you. High mountain areas are also a good place to go to; up in the mountains the grasses tend to produce less pollen.

Going abroad may help. For a start the same plants may pollinate at slightly different times because the seasons may be earlier (if you go south) or later (if you go north). In addition, the plants that are common to the new area may be ones to which you're not allergic. Often hayfever sufferers find that their symptoms go almost completely when they go on a foreign holiday.

Allergy to dust mite is like hayfever, except that it occurs all year round. House dust consists largely of old skin flakes that have been shed by people living in the house, and dust mites are microscopically small insects that live off these flakes of skin. Both of these substances can prove highly allergic to certain sensitive people, and are often responsible for the symptoms of a continual running nose, made worse by exposure to dusty rooms.

Self-help is not easy because it is impossible to remove dust completely from your home. However, a reduction in soft furnishings will help. Polished wooden floors, linoleum or cork tiling may be better than a deep-pile carpet; Venetian blinds better than curtains, and duvets better than blankets.

You can cut down the amount of dust by frequent damp dusting (dry dusting merely serves to push more dust into the air again). Regular vacuuming of the carpets helps (especially in the bedroom and under the beds), and of the curtains, and from time to time the mattress and the blankets.

Wash your curtains, and of course your blankets, regularly; sunlight kills off the dust mite so drying blankets in the sunshine will help considerably. Put clothes away in wardrobes rather than leaving them hanging on chairs or on the back of a door; and, finally, remember that the dust mite tends to inhabit wool in preference to man-made fibres. Therefore, if you choose mainly man-made fibres for your clothes, your bedding and your soft furnishings, you may reduce your long-term problems.

Passive smoking can cause a lot of problems for those who are sensitive or allergic to tobacco smoke, and is yet another good reason for banning smoking – or, at least, providing smoke-free zones in offices, restaurants, public transport and other public places. Even a brief exposure to tobacco smoke can block you up for the next twenty-four hours, if you are sensitive to it.

A filtered air purifier may be a useful and inexpensive option; one look at the used filter gives you an idea of the kind of dust and dirt that exists in the air of our day-to-day environment.

Many sufferers from sinusitis find that they are worse in the artificial atmosphere of the air-conditioned office. Poor quality air-conditioning produces air that is too dry, which irritates the lining of the nose. Air-conditioning produces air that is high in positive ions, and there is some evidence that these also irritate the nasal passages.

Poorly maintained air-conditioning can often recycle fumes and solvents round the office, causing problems in those who are sensitive to these substances; both air-conditioning and (especially) domestic warm-air central-heating systems, if poorly maintained, can encourage moulds and fungi to grow in the warm, dark and sometimes moist conditions in the pipes. These produce millions of spores, and when the air-conditioning/central heating is switched on, these spores are blown out into the room air, causing further problems in those who are allergic to them.

It's not always easy to get round problems caused by office air-conditioning. Often the windows are fixed shut; but, if you are able to open them, you may find your symptoms are alleviated by breathing in fresh outside air. Alternatively, you may be able to counter the effects of positive ions by using an ioniser. And, finally, if you always get sinus and nasal troubles when the hot-air central heating is switched on, get someone competent to check it.

If you do get a cold, resist the temptation to blow your nose hard – you may well blow infected material from the centre of the nose into the sinuses. Sucking it out again is nothing like as easy as it was to blow it in there! Do resist the temptation to blow your nose too vigorously. Just wiping it is usually quite sufficient.

Anything which causes pressure inside the nose should also be avoided. So, if you go swimming, you would do well to avoid diving or duck-diving because the pressure that is generated inside the nose can easily push material into the sinuses. Similarly, it's inadvisable to go scuba-diving when an attack of sinusitis is brewing.

Complementary treatment

Anything which reduces inflammation of the lining of the nose is going to help sinusitis sufferers. The less the inflammation, the wider the diameter of the antrum and the better the sinuses will drain. Herbal decongestants may be helpful, as are all anti-allergy measures; don't forget this includes checking for food allergies.

In the acute attack of sinusitis, inhalations of steam can be helpful. As children, we were often given what seemed to be a cross between a stone hot water bottle, a teapot, and a hookah, filled with boiling water to which a little drop of Friar's Balsam was added. The resultant piping-hot aromatic steam was inhaled through a glass mouthpiece. I remember distinctly that it seemed to have a particularly soothing effect – though it probably had its greatest effect on the lungs rather than the nose.

Inhalations of benzoin, cajuput, eucalyptus, niaouli or tea tree can be inhaled to clear the sinuses. Any of the above oils can be added to a carrier, or base, vegetable oil (or soya) and then rubbed on the outside and inside of the nose. Lavender and eucalyptus can be similarly used over the sinus regions (externally, of course), and on the temples, to open up the passages. Peppermint oil can be inhaled to reduce stuffiness, and thyme and lavender are beneficial in reducing pain.

Acupuncture and acupressure are alternative ways of reducing nasal congestion. The Hegu point is used to control pain and sinusitis – find it in the web between the thumb and the index finger, about a thumb's width from the edge of the web. The direction of massage is towards the wrist.

Other remedies, particularly for catarrh, include fenugreek tea which can be drunk or sniffed up the nostrils, and red rose petal and rosehip tea. Two common herbal remedies involve a tea made from meadowsweet (among other herbs). As meadowsweet is an unprocessed form of aspirin, perhaps this is why it works to reduce inflammation. In the past, powdered bark of white willow would also have been prescribed; this, too, is a source of aspirin.

Lemon juice, diluted in warm water, may be sniffed up the nose; some people even use it neat! Alternatively, steep the peel and juice of a lemon in boiling water and inhale it. Garlic decongests, detoxifies and disinfects, relieving a build-up of catarrh. Echinacea is supposed to fight infections; elderflower, eyebright and peppermint are anti-catarrhals; golden rod acts as an anti-inflammatory; lemon and horseradish are said to stimulate the immune system, and reduce fluid in the sinuses. Two or three drops of eucalyptus with a teaspoonful of honey can be taken two or three times a day. Honey and lemon is a traditional soothing remedy, which may also fight infection. A peppermint poultice to the sinus area helps, as does the inhalation of onion (if you can bear it!). Eating onion reduces mucus production. Elecampane and hyssop help clear nasal passages. Homoeopathic remedies include teucrium marum verum, aconitum and pulsatilla nigricans.

Hayfever sufferers may find help from this tip: eat the local honey. Because this contains minute quantities of the very pollen that you are exposed to locally, it is actually acting as a homoeopathic/desensitising preparation.

Many alternative practitioners are convinced that extra Vitamin C will treat and ward off colds; there is no concrete evidence but as Vitamin C is unlikely to cause any damage there's no harm in trying it. Paradoxically, using large doses regularly for long periods may actually make you more liable to get a rebound scurvy when you go back to your normal Vitamin C intake.

Ensure that you are getting enough Vitamin A in your diet. Natural sources of Vitamin A include fish-liver oils, meats (especially liver), carrots, broccoli, spinach, canteloupe melon and tomatoes. Remember that Vitamin A is toxic in large doses, and can cause birth defects in pregnancy, even if supplementation occurred before conception. Vitamin C, up to one gram daily, may help prevent some symptoms of allergies; Vitamin B12 may help with the prevention and treatment of sinusitis.

MICHAEL

Michael is a twenty-three-year-old student who developed severe pain in the right side of his face. He hadn't had a cold, but had recently been doing a lot of duck-diving in the local swimming pool.

The pain in his face was intense and constricting. When he tried to lie down the pain just got worse, and by morning it was unbearable. Putting his head between his knees increased the pain greatly, and he was very tender over the bone just underneath the right eye.

Michael obviously had sinusitis and his doctor prescribed an antibiotic to get rid of the infection, a decongestant to help the sinus to drain more easily and some painkillers. These soon began to work and within three days the pain gone completely.

Although he hadn't had a cold, Michael had done a lot of swimming and diving. Probably the increased water pressure during duck-diving drove infected material from his nasal passages into the sinuses where it started to cause an infection.

Chapter Eight

STROKES

Cells in the body get their energy by slowly burning energy-rich sugars. This is very much like the burning process that goes on when we light a bonfire or a candle, except that it takes place at a much lower temperature. The net result is the same, however; oxygen combines with complex carbon-containing molecules, which break down to release energy. In a flame, the energy is released as heat, but in the body the energy is captured and used to drive its processes and actions.

Most cells in the body contain stores of a substance called *glycogen*, which is, effectively, stored glucose. Glycogen provides the constant supply of energy the cell needs on those occasions when its blood supply is inadequate, or cut off.

In the temporary absence of oxygen, most cells can go over to a form of energy production called *anaerobic metabolism*, which doesn't need oxygen, but they can only maintain this type of energy production for a short time. So, if the blood supply to a muscle cell is temporarily unable to support the oxygen or energy requirements of the cell – during a sprint, for example – the cell lives on happily, burning glycogen as an energy source and, if necessary, going over to anaerobic metabolism. When the sprint is over and the demands on the cell drop, it returns to its normal method of getting energy.

Nerve cells are unique in the body in that they have no in-built store of glycogen to keep them going; nor can they go over to anaerobic metabolism if they haven't got enough oxygen. Nervous tissue is therefore excessively vulnerable to losing its blood supply. A nerve cell deprived of its blood supply stops functioning within seconds, and will die if its blood supply isn't restored within minutes. This is why a heart attack can cause death even if the heart can be re-started. If the blood supply to the brain has been cut off for more than about three minutes then damage and eventually death occurs, even though the rest of the body may be alive, with the heart once again beating spontaneously.

Overall brain death like this occurs when the supply of oxygen-containing blood to the whole of the brain has been interfered with – such as when the heart stops, in drowning, or in strangulation. In comparison, a *stroke* occurs when the blood supply to *part* of the brain is cut off. This happens in one of three main ways.

• *A small clot* (known as an *embolus*) finds its way into one of the arteries supplying the brain, and lodges there, blocking the artery and cutting off the blood supply to the part of the brain that the artery supplies. Deprived of its blood supply the brain tissue, in the area supplied by the artery, dies. *Transient Ischaemic Attacks* (TIAs) are clot-type strokes, except that the clot quickly disperses. TIAs cause a stroke-like episode which then spontaneously recovers, leaving no residual problems. We'll be looking at these separately, later on in the chapter.

• *Plaques of arteriosclerosis* (thick fatty deposits on the inside of arteries) can slowly increase in size and eventually block the whole of the channel inside the arteries in the brain. Often the final event is a slowing down of the blood through the furred-up artery until a clot forms in what remains of the central hole, blocking it completely.

• *A bleed*. If an artery *inside* the brain substance ruptures, blood is pushed into the brain itself. This blood acts exactly like a bruise (after all, a bruise is simply blood in the wrong place) and the effect is to put stale, old, stationary blood between the nerve cells and the active blood supply.

Clinically speaking, it can be very hard to distinguish between the three types of stroke.

Permanent interruption of the blood supply in one of these ways is called a stroke. What happens next depends on several things: where the blockage/bleed is situated, how big an area of the brain has had its blood supply cut off, and whether the area of brain tissue normally supplied by the affected artery is able to get its blood supply from another source (called collateral circulation).

The anatomy of the brain is important here. The blood supply to the brain itself comes via three arteries, which ascend through the neck, and then join together into a ring of arteries called the circle of Willis, inside the skull at the base of the brain. From here, further arteries lead the fresh blood into the brain, supplying all parts of it with oxygen and nutrients. The blood then takes away carbon dioxide and other waste products in the veins. For some reason, one of the weak points in the system is in the artery that supplies the part of the brain that controls movement – the *motor cortex*. A stroke here affects *movements*. Interestingly, because the motor fibres cross over, the muscles affected by a stroke are on the opposite side of the body to the side the stroke has occurred in the brain, so a stroke in the left side of the brain affects movements on the *right* side of the body, and vice versa.

Although to the naked eye the brain is symmetrical, it certainly isn't, as far as function is concerned. In particular, the control of speech is located only on one side of the brain; in general, on the opposite side of the brain to the handedness of the patient. For example, a right-handed man usually has his speech centre on the left side of his brain, and vice versa.

The speech centre is situated near the motor cortex, so it is often affected by strokes. Therefore, a right-handed man who has a stroke in the left side of the brain will be paralysed in some muscles in the right side of his body – arm, leg, or both – and *may also lose his ability to speak*. If he were to have an exactly similar stroke on the right side of his brain he would lose power in the left side of the body, but his speech and understanding would be unaffected.

Typically, a stroke occurs very quickly, which is why it is called a stroke. It appears that the sufferer really has been struck down. In a bad stroke the patient may become unconscious, but more often he will remain awake, though suddenly aware that he cannot use an arm or a leg (or both), or that he has lost his power of speech. He may have a headache. Often the headache of a stroke is sudden, violent, and painful; but, equally, strokes can occur with little or no headache at all. Some strokes can make the sufferer feel exceedingly unwell, whilst other people notice only that they can't move one of their limbs or hands quite as well as they used to. Sometimes all that happens is that the patient loses his ability to speak, or his ability to understand words; or, perhaps, he undergoes a slight personality change, becoming more vague and less able to think swiftly.

What happens during a stroke depends on which part of the brain is deprived of its blood supply. For some reason one of the most frequent blood vessels to be affected is the artery supplying the part of the brain which controls movements of the arm and leg, though it's possible to get strokes in all areas of the brain.

You might be tempted to think that if an area of the brain were destroyed then it would be final – no further recovery of function would be possible. Surprisingly, it doesn't work like this at all. Immediately after the brain has been damaged by stroke it tries to re-route messages, to bypass the obstruction of the dead and dying brain cells. Often this re-routing can be extremely successful and it is not uncommon to find that a patient with a severe stroke has, three months later, recovered all or nearly all power in the affected limbs.

Type of headache

The headache associated with stroke usually comes on suddenly, at the time of the paralysis. The pain can be really severe and is often bursting in nature. Headaches can also occur after a stroke, because of the generalised damage to the brain. Usually these disappear with the passage of time.

What else could it be?

A stroke is typified by one-sided paralysis with or without loss of speech. A true stroke implies permanent damage to the brain, but there are two processes that can cause temporary interruption to the normal workings of the brain in a similar sort of way. The first is a Transient Ischaemic Attack (TIA), which is discussed later in this chapter. However, TIAs and strokes can only be distinguished because one goes away and the other doesn't; at first they are indistinguishable.

The second process that can cause temporary paralysis is *hemiplegic migraine*. This is a moderately uncommon, but particularly alarming type of migraine, especially the first time you experience it. Not only do you get the normal symptoms of migraine – but also weakness or even paralysis of one or more limbs on one side of the body. Fortunately, hemiplegic migraine resolves spontaneously, and although dramatic and frightening, seldom causes permanent damage.

However, there is a sort of halfway house between a stroke and hemiplegic migraine, and this is the type of migraine that sometimes comes on as a side-effect of the contraceptive pill. In this it is possible to have a hemiplegic migraine that actually progresses to a stroke. If you have your first ever attack of migraine on the contraceptive pill, you should stop taking it *immediately*. Migraines *caused* by the Pill (rather than just *exacerbated* by it) may well go on to cause a stroke.

Orthodox treatment

Once a stroke has occurred there is often little that can be done, at least as far as the stroke itself is concerned. The doctor will want to check to see if a part of the body is throwing off little clots – such as a damaged heart valve. If a source of clots is found it may be appropriate to thin the blood to prevent these clots forming, and later becoming lodged in the brain. In some cases, it may even be necessary to surgically remove the offending area.

At the moment, most stroke victims have to wait for the body to recover naturally, by itself. On the horizon, however, are some interesting clot-dissolving drugs, and in the future it may well be that stroke victims immediately get sent to hospital for clot-busting injections given directly into the veins, as is often done now with heart attacks.

Good post-stroke treatment can make a lot of difference to the patient's quality of life. Much of the treatment centres around physiotherapy, teaching people to re-learn movements; speech therapy; and so on.

MARGARET

Without warning, at the early age of sixty-one, Margaret had a series of strokes which affected the left side of her body. On the first occasion she woke up with a severe headache and found she couldn't use her left arm properly. Over the next few days she started to recover; she could move the arm more, but she still had a lot of headaches.

Three months later she had two further strokes, which made it impossible for her to walk. She couldn't get her balance for a start, but in any case her left leg wasn't strong enough to keep her upright.

Then her problems really started. She began to get painful spasms in her back, shoulder and arm muscles. Some of this was because the paralysis stopped her stretching properly, but many of the spasms were in the muscles affected by the paralysis. (The muscles themselves aren't affected in a stroke. It's the connection to the brain that's been destroyed, so now the muscles can seize up of their own accord.) In turn these spasms caused her to have further severe headaches.

Muscle relaxant drugs did help a bit, by reducing the reflex spasms from muscles that were now out of her conscious control. But even these didn't do very much, and eventually she had to be admitted for two weeks of intensive physiotherapy. This, by contrast, helped a lot, and since then she has had intermittent physiotherapy as necessary. She's also had a long course of reflexology, which she says has helped her considerably.

Now, at the age of sixty-nine, she is confined to a wheelchair. Her spasms are under control for much of the time using a combination of physiotherapy, reflexology and anti-spasmodic drugs, and as a result her headaches have lessened as well.

Because most stroke victims are elderly, all other types of headache affecting the elderly can combine to multiply their effects and cause greater headaches. For example, a patient with a stroke may also have a considerable degree of osteoarthritis of the neck, which irritates the neck further, causing even more headaches from muscular tension. As well as muscular imbalance, which aggravates the neck problem, there may also be anxiety, tension or depression as a result of worrying about the illness itself. This further knots up the neck muscles and causes yet more headaches.

Prevention of stroke is important. You're more likely to have a stroke if you've had high blood pressure for a long time, – and by that I mean *many* years. We now know that bringing the blood pressure down, and keeping it down, reduces the chance that you'll suffer a stroke. This is why doctors are so keen to discover those who've got high blood pressure. Treating a thirty-year-old's high blood pressure may prolong his life by *years*.

Self-help
The key to self-help is avoidance. Make sure that you have your blood pressure measured from time to time. This is especially important if you have a family history of high blood pressure, or if your own blood pressure is known to be a little higher than normal. (In this case, more regular checks are likely to be needed.)

If your doctor is giving you tablets for blood pressure make sure you take them regularly, even if you get some side-effects. Do, by the way, tell your doctor about any side-effects. There are many different ways of treating high blood pressure and it may be that the drug you're using at the moment doesn't suit you as well as some of the others might.

If you've already had a stroke, then do attend to what your doctor and physiotherapist are telling you. In particular, if your physiotherapist is suggesting some exercises, take time to do them. It will help considerably to keep your remaining muscles trim and get the very best out of muscles that have been partially paralysed. By exercising properly you will be minimising the after-effects of your stroke to a degree you might not think possible at the moment.

Finally, if you are getting pains in your head, neck, or back following a stroke, don't suffer in silence – tell your doctor.

Complementary treatment
The prevention of stroke, and rehabilitation after suffering a stroke, are the main focuses for several complementary therapies. The circulatory system is the centre of attention in terms of prevention, and the control of cholesterol, high blood pressure and cardio-vascular disease are most important. Try hawthorn (berries and leaves) and lime blossom in tea or dry form. Massage with juniper and lemon are said to help break down fatty deposits in the bloodstream.

Aromatherapy is a good way to prevent circulatory problems, and strokes in particular. Oils pass quickly into the bloodstream, when used in massage, and there are a number that you should find helpful. Black pepper, juniper and marjoram will stimulate the circulatory system locally, while cypress, neroli, lemon and rose will improve circulation generally.

Royal jelly is thought to lower blood pressure. Vitamins C and E aid the whole circulatory system, acting as anti-oxidants. In America and Finland, studies have indicated that low levels of selenium in the blood are linked to strokes and to heart and circulatory diseases. However, selenium is potentially toxic, so do consult a registered practitioner before using it. Selenium is often used with Vitamin E. Do note, however, that the effects of selenium are blocked when Vitamin C is ingested at the same time.

Niacin (Vitamin B3) also lowers blood cholesterol, and protects against cardio-vascular disease. Niacin may actually be capable of reversing some arteriosclerosis, in many cases a forerunner to strokes. Niacin is, however, toxic in high doses; a niacin flush – hot, reddened skin, a tingling and burning sensation in the face, neck, arms and chest area – indicates toxicity. Consult your GP or clinical nutritionist for a sensible dose.

The Feldenkrais method, which is a new kind of learning system that uses movement as a means to change and develop a more healthful way of using your body, helps those who have suffered strokes.

Stress-reduction techniques are essential to help prevent strokes, and gentle exercises – like those involved in T'ai Chi or yoga – keep the circulatory system in good order. Acupressure, acupuncture, chiropractic and osteopathy can help deal with the pain of headaches, and the anxiety that can exist following stroke. The muscle spasm in the neck and shoulder areas that is common in stroke victims benefits from physiotherapy or soft-tissue manipulation (osteopathy) and the headaches and psychological effects that often follow a stroke may react well to cranial osteopathy. Music, dance and art therapy can teach the patient to use weakened limbs and reflexes, and provide distraction from the pain, fear and depression that may ensue after the illness.

Reflexology may assist the muscles to relax, and relaxation therapy will be beneficial if you are tense. As post-stroke therapy, reflexology can help patients recover more quickly and return to regular living. Strokes can make the patient less in control of his emotions, which can well up in a childlike fashion. Relaxation techniques and perhaps psychotherapy might be appropriate here.

TRANSIENT ISCHAEMIC ATTACKS

As we discussed earlier, there is a second type of stroke-like event: *Transient Ischaemic Attacks* (TIAs). These are exactly what they seem. *Transient,* meaning they don't last long; *ischaemic,* meaning the blood supply has been cut off; *attacks,* meaning episodes. In other words, TIAs are like repeated strokes, which then go away after a matter of minutes or hours.

In a TIA, a tiny clump of cells forms in the blood, then jams in one of the smaller arteries in the brain. This temporarily interrupts the blood supply to a small area of the brain, which immediately ceases to function properly. However, the clump quickly disperses and the blood supply is restored. During the short time the clump is in place the patient experiences the symptoms of a stroke, which then go away again. The difference between a TIA and a stroke is that a TIA spontaneously resolves – usually within twenty-four hours, and often within a few minutes.

We think now that TIAs are caused by little clumps of platelets; these are tiny cells in the blood that initiate blood clotting. Under some circumstances platelets stick together too easily, forming little clumps which are small enough to pass round the general circulation, but can get jammed in the smaller arteries.

Most cells in the body can function for a short time without a blood supply, so platelet clumps like this can block blood vessels in the muscles, the bones, or the skin without causing symptoms; by the time they are likely to cause symptoms they will have dispersed. However, because nervous tissue cannot function for even a few minutes without an intact blood supply, even a small clot interrupts the workings of the brain. As the clot disperses, the blood supply returns, and that area of the brain starts working properly again.

TIAs are exactly like small strokes which come and go. A patient suddenly finds he has lost the use of an arm or a leg; he can't speak properly or understand what someone else is saying; shortly afterwards the power returns to the muscles, the speech comes back, and comprehension returns.

PETER

Peter is a sprightly seventy-eight-year-old man who woke up one morning with weakness on the right side of his body and a throbbing headache. He could understand what was said to him, but couldn't speak, and could only communicate by nodding or shaking his head. Within a few minutes he started to improve, and could walk normally. Soon his speech started to return.

In view of the rapid improvement, his doctor diagnosed a Transient Ischaemic Attack (TIA), and prescribed a small dose of aspirin, to be taken regularly each day.

Six months later he had a further episode. Again his right side was weak, and again there was loss of speech (obviously his speech centre is on the left side of the brain, the side which was affected when there is paralysis down the right side of the body). Again, his speech became thick and garbled, though as

before he appeared to understand everything that was said to
him. He recovered completely during the next twenty-four
hours.

   This pattern is typical of Transient Ischaemic Attacks, which
at first appear to be a stroke, but which recover speedily to
leave no trace twenty-four hours later.

   Peter continues to be well. The TIAs are under control,
providing that he takes his regular dose of aspirin.

Type of headache
Just as a stroke can sometime cause a headache, so TIAs can also be associated with a headache, exactly like the headache of a full-blown stroke.

What else could it be?
At first a TIA is just like a stroke; you only know it's a TIA because it goes away again after a time. Any TIA that *doesn't* go away isn't a true TIA. It must have been caused by a clot which didn't disperse, and which blocked the artery long enough to kill off some of the surrounding nerve cells.

Just occasionally what looks like TIAs can actually be the tip of the iceberg for a rather more sinister event, such as a *brain tumour*. It can be remarkably difficult to spot these, but unexplained, recent weight loss, increasing or continuous headaches, no response to treatment, and abnormalities in blood tests are all features that point towards this diagnosis; but it often needs some very specialised tests such as MRI (Magnetic Resonance Imaging) scanning to be sure of what is going on.

Orthodox treatment
Although TIAs are like mini-strokes, unlike strokes TIAs are eminently treatable. The aim is to reduce the stickiness of the platelets and stop them clumping together. A tiny dose of aspirin is sufficient – just a child's dose (75-150 mg) once a day is all that is required to make the platelets a little less sticky (the normal adult dose of aspirin is 600 mg every four hours). Alternatively, your doctor may use a drug called dipyridamole (Persantin) which has the same effect.

Self-help
Firstly, don't panic. Although at first it looks just like a stroke, a TIA goes away completely after a short time. Once you've had one TIA, you may be prone to others; be sure to consult your doctor to be sure of the diagnosis. And do remember that TIAs don't necessarily lead to full-blown strokes.

Complementary treatment
A regular infusion of white willow bark or meadowsweet tea might help, as both of these contain aspirin in natural form. However, it may be best just to use a tablet of the pure drug, in a proper controlled dose. Taken regularly, aspirin will reduce the stickiness of the latelets help prevent clots.

Associated problems

Strokes are often associated with *high blood pressure* ; imbalances in the muscles of the neck can lead to muscular spasms and *tension headaches. Physiotherapy,* or some of the other *manipulative medicines* may be helpful in dealing with this. Strokes mainly occur in older people, many of whom have a degree of *cervical spondylosis* or *osteo-arthritis* in the neck. *Depression* may follow a severe stroke and make muscle tension, and tension headaches, worse.

Chapter Nine

SUB-ARACHNOID HAEMORRHAGE

The arachnoid is one of three layers of tissue which cover the brain in much the same way that a loaf of bread is wrapped in thin cellophane. The main blood vessels supplying the brain itself run between the arachnoid and the next layer of covering. In a sub-arachnoid haemorrhage, one of these blood vessels bursts, releasing blood into the gap between the arachnoid and the brain. In essence, it's a burst blood vessel on the outside surface of the brain. Blood squirts out from the artery under high pressure, and because the skull is a closed cavity with soft tissue inside, as the blood cannot expand outwards, instead it pushes on the delicate brain substance, raising the pressure inside the head. The brain is squeezed in the process and the pressure inside the brain rises progressively until it stops functioning properly.

Genetically, certain people are prone to having little balloon-like blebs, called *berry aneurysms*, on the arteries supplying the brain, and because these blebs have thinner walls than the arteries, they are more prone to rupture. Arteries supply blood, so the blebs are under high pressure, making them more likely to rupture, especially in someone who has high blood pressure. When an aneurysm ruptures, the blood spurts out with some force into the surrounding space overlying the brain tissue itself. Often the haemorrhage occurs at a time of straining; for example, on trying to open the bowels; during exercise; or during intercourse. On these occasions the blood pressure has (naturally) risen slightly, but this extra rise in pressure is the proverbial straw that breaks the camel's back: an already weakened and thinned artery wall finally gives way under the strain, and the high-pressure blood inside forces its way out.

The results can be dramatic. A sub-arachnoid haemorrhage can strike down a previously healthy man or woman in seconds: typically, the patient feels as though she has been hit on the back of the head with a lump of wood. Exactly what happens after this depends on where the leakage has occurred, and how big it is. A sudden big leak can produce an explosive headache, then render the victim unconscious within seconds; she collapses as though pole-axed. In less dramatic bleeds, the patient may well not lose consciousness completely, but may be drowsy and irritable, with altered consciousness – and a massive headache. Others, who have just a tiny tear with a continuous but small leak of blood, may feel unwell in a vague sort of way, without any obvious pointers to what is going on, except for the feeling that they have had a knock on the back of the head, and, of course, a headache.

Often the patient develops a stiff neck, just as in meningitis, but unlike meningitis, the stiff neck will have come on very quickly (within minutes) and the patient won't have a temperature or any other signs of infection. On the other hand, a small leak from an aneurysm may produce little in the way of a stiff neck – or, indeed, any other symptoms, other than a headache.

Sometimes the amount of bleeding can be very small, and in a number of cases there are several small 'warning' bleeds before the big one strikes. It's only on looking back that these warning bleeds can be recognised for what they are, rather than being dismissed as minor headaches from viral infection or stress.

Type of headache

The headache starts very suddenly, without any warning at all, and feels as if you've been hit hard on the back of the head or neck or, alternatively, that there's been an explosion inside the head. The pain is extreme.

What else could it be?

Four conditions can mimic or be mimicked by a sub-arachnoid haemorrhage:

Meningitis gives the same type of stiff neck, in which the patient is unable to bend his chin to his chest (remember that a true stiff neck is one that cannot be bent *forwards*). Like a sub-arachnoid haemorrhage, meningitis can also come on quite quickly (but in a matter of hours, not minutes) and soon produces altered consciousness, irritability and drowsiness. But patients with meningitis almost always have a temperature, even if it's only a small one,.

In practice, for the lay person the difference is unimportant. In both cases you need a doctor and you need one now. Don't wait for the morning; don't wait even five minutes – it could be the difference between life and death.

A *stroke* can cause sudden headache, collapse and unconsciousness, within a few minutes. However, paralysis is usually one-sided, with one arm or leg obviously more floppy and paralysed than on the other side.

Headaches coming on during intercourse can mimic a sub-arachnoid haemorrhage, because they come on very quickly, and sometimes almost explosively; and, of course, a sub-arachnoid haemorrhage can be precipitated by the excitement and stress of intercourse. In fact, if a headache of this type and magnitude occurs during intercourse, it may be wise to do a full medical investigation, just to be sure. Once a sub-arachnoid haemorrhage has been eliminated, then it is fair to assume that any further headaches during intercourse are not likely to be sub-arachnoid bleeds.

A very severe *tension headache* can actually be quite difficult to distinguish from a sub-arachnoid haemorrhage, particularly if it has a sudden onset – such as a sudden tensing of the muscles as a result of a fright; or in a minor injury to the head which reflexively results in all the neck muscles going into spasm (for example, bringing your head up underneath a cupboard, hitting it hard and finding that the resultant reflex pulling of the head downwards by the neck muscles has sent all of them into spasm).

Orthodox treatment

A sub-arachnoid haemorrhage is a medical emergency of the first order. *Immediate* admission to hospital is necessary. Recovery from a sub-arachnoid haemorrhage can take a long time and may not be complete. The degree of recovery depends very much on how big the bleed was, and how quickly the patient was operated on. Untreated, sub-arachnoid haemorrhage is usually lethal; even after operation, in severe cases, there may be permanent brain damage; but a gratifyingly high proportion of patients make an excellent and complete recovery.

Sub-arachnoid haemorrhage leaves scars, both physical and mental. The external scars of the operation are unimportant; operations inside the brain are surprisingly easy to disguise because mostly they are hidden by hair.

The real scars are internal. There may be the after-effects of brain damage – stroke-like symptoms, where there is weakness or paralysis of the hands or feet; impediments in the speech; reduction in concentration; reduced quality of mental functions; and, of course, persistent headaches.

Often the biggest scar is psychological. There is frequently a feeling of terror that the same thing is going to happen again; after all, berry aneurysms are often multiple, and at first any headache (even from flu) is likely to set the patient telephoning the doctor in a panic. It can often take a long time for the patient to recover their confidence after such a near-death experience.

In actual fact, the prognosis for the future is bright. There's often a slow, but steady return of physical and mental functions, with few set-backs. Second haemorrhages are very rare (though this doesn't stop the patient feeling frightened, especially when doing anything that requires exertion or straining). In fact, the only thing that needs observation and control is blood pressure; sub-arachnoid haemorrhage tends to occur more frequently in patients with high blood pressure.

The bad news, however, is that persistent headaches may follow the haemorrhage, even after the patient has recovered from the bleed itself. Undoubtedly, some of this is due to anxiety and tension; but it would be amazing if there were no ill-effects after the bashing the brain has received from the massive bleed, the subsequent extra pressure, and the ensuing operation. These headaches are controllable, though, and usually subside with the passage of time.

ELIZABETH

Elizabeth was in her late forties, and was fit and well when, suddenly one morning, she had a severe pain in the back of the head. She felt as if something had hit her on the back of the neck, and immediately began to vomit. The severe headache continued, her legs became weak and she had double vision.

Even before the doctor could get there she had lapsed into semi-consciousness, and was only partly aware of what was going on. Her neck was stiff when the doctor tried to bend it forwards, and on scraping the soles of the feet, both of the big toes moved upwards, which indicated that whatever had happened, it had affected both sides of the brain, not just one, as a stroke would.

The sudden onset of the condition, severe pain in the back of the head, loss of consciousness, stiff neck and the fact that both sides were affected all indicated that Elizabeth had had a classic sub-arachnoid haemorrhage.

Elizabeth was transferred to hospital as soon as possible and immediately had a lumbar puncture. A needle was inserted into the spinal column to draw off some of the cerebro-spinal fluid (CSF). Straightaway the doctor saw that it was heavily bloodstained, confirming that Elizabeth had indeed had a sub-arachnoid haemorrhage. She was then transferred to another hospital where she had an angiogram. This showed the site of the leaking artery and soon Elizabeth was taken to the operating theatre to have the leaking aneurysm clipped off.

After the operation she made a slow but steady recovery, though for some time she was unable to speak. However, this passed and eventually she was able to go home.

Since then she has made a complete physical recovery. Her mental recovery wasn't quite so smooth, because for the next two years, every time she had a headache she became terrified that it was the beginning of another attack; in fact, she often gave herself a tension headache just worrying about the situation. And she was still getting headaches from the after-effects of the original attack.

Gradually she regained her confidence, though it took time; there was a period when she was frightened to go to sleep because she had aching in the back of the neck; and, at one point, she needed anti-depressants. At the time of the attack, Elizabeth had been the nearest to death that she'd ever been, and she knew it.

Now, however, she's well, relaxed, and has finally got over her anxieties. It's good to see her smiling again.

Self-help
The only self-help measure is to call a doctor *very* quickly.

Complementary treatment
There are no complementary therapies that will deal with sub-arachnoid haemorrhage during the attack. You need a doctor, a hospital and a neuro-

surgeon, and the quicker the better. Call for emergency services as soon as you suspect sub-arachnoid haemorrhage. While you are waiting, you can offer the sufferer arnica (30c every five minutes until medical attention arrives), and rub Rescue Remedy (a Bach flower remedy) into pulse points to prevent shock. However, don't attempt to give anything by mouth if the patient is unconscious.

After emergency help has been sought, and after the haemorrhage has been controlled, there are a number of things that can be done to help the patient rehabilitate. Paralysis of any kind can be helped by reflexology, chiropractic and osteopathy. Dance and music therapy, as well as yoga and T'ai Chi offer an enormous psychological boost, as well as gentle physical exercise to help ensure a speedy recovery. It is essential that all exercise is gentle, and that you consult your GP before beginning any exercise programme.

Acupuncture and acupressure, as well as cranial osteopathy, can help you to deal with headaches following the illness; persistent headaches can be controlled with lavender oil. Relaxation methods can be undertaken, if discussed first with your doctor. Certainly there is a great deal of fear and anxiety following such a frightening attack, and psychotherapy may help you deal with that. Bach flower remedies are good for this sort of problem.

Chapter Ten

HEAD INJURIES AND CONCUSSION

Injuries to the head sometimes cause physical damage. In general, the harder the blow, the worse the damage, but the site and *direction* of the blow are both very important. There is a long list of different types of injury that can occur after a blow to the head. These are:
- Concussion
- Undisplaced fracture of the skull
- Depressed fracture of the skull
- Fractured skull with underlying bleed
- Sub-dural haemorrhage
- Post-traumatic problems

Note that this is *not* a progressive list – you don't have to have the first four items on the list before you get number five. The common factor is that all the items in the list can produce headaches of one sort or another.

CONCUSSION

Concussion is a severe, non-specific upset in the functioning of the brain following a blow; to cause concussion, the blow usually has to be severe enough to knock the patient out.

The brain is soft and delicate, and needs protecting from direct blows by the solid walls of the skull, which completely enclose it. Even though these bones are quite thin, they protect the brain very effectively from all but the heaviest blows. The part of the skull which surrounds the brain is shaped like the shell of an egg – thin, but amazingly strong. Like the egg, the skull derives its strength from its smooth, ovoid shape, which distributes the force of incoming blows in such a way as to disperse their energy evenly. There are very few discontinuities, which act as weak points where stress might build up, so it usually takes a very hard blow to crack the skull and an even harder blow to stove it in.

Although the brain is well protected against direct injury, no amount of external protection can ever prevent the disruption that occurs from a twisting, rotating force suddenly applied to the head – such as a sideways punch to the jaw. When this occurs, the skull spins round rapidly, but the brain doesn't follow quite so fast, being semi-solid (rather like blancmange). In just the same way that you can split a plate of blancmange by suddenly twisting it, so the shearing forces from a blow pull and stretch the nerve fibres as they travel across the brain. In minor cases, this stretching merely causes a temporary disruption of brain activity (being 'knocked out', or made unconscious). In more severe cases there is permanent brain damage, as the fibres are stretched until they snap, or small blood vessels rupture and bleed.

It doesn't need a single, severe injury to cause brain damage. Repeated blows can have the same effect, even if they're not strong enough to knock you out. The 'punch-drunk' fighter is a classic example – a boxer who over the years has sustained many blows to his head. As a result of these frequent minor injuries his brain functions slowly deteriorate, his IQ drops, his speech is slurred and his movements are uncoordinated.

FRACTURED SKULL

The importance of a head injury is not whether the patient has been knocked out, nor even whether the skull has been fractured in the process, *but whether or not the injury has caused damage to, or pressure on the brain*. This pressure can come from a number of sources, such as bleeding – either into the brain or underneath the skull – which presses on the brain, or else from a depressed fracture where the bones themselves are pressing directly on the brain.

All other considerations are secondary. To be honest, after a head injury, it really doesn't matter if the patient *has* sustained a fractured skull – the bones of the skull are just like other bones of the body, and will heal. A hairline crack or fracture is really of little importance (other than that it causes pain), *as long as there is no bleeding underneath, or swelling of the brain substance*.

This can't be emphasised enough. All too often, people imagine that it's the concussion that we should look out for, or the fractured skull that is so important. That isn't the case. The only reason for admitting a patient to hospital after concussion or a fractured skull is that a blow big enough to cause concussion is hard enough to rip nerves and blood vessels within the brain or cause swelling of the brain itself; and where there is a fractured skull there may also be treacherous and unseen underlying bleeding. So the patient is admitted, and observed carefully for the next twenty-four hours, to spot any signs of progressive internal injury.

Most head injuries result in simple *superficial* bruising; a small proportion concuss the patient. Harder blows may cause a skull fracture, though the position and angle of the blow often determines whether or not the skull will fracture. One part of the head is particularly prone to direct fracture – the temple (at the side of the head, between the eye and ear) is the most vulnerable area for fractures that are the result of a direct blow from a small object, such as a golf ball.

A simple undisplaced fracture of the skull (where the bones haven't moved) is usually relatively unimportant. Provided there is little bleeding from the broken edges of the bone, then a crack in the skull bones can be treated much like a crack in any other bone, such as at the wrist. In fact, because the skull is such a solid, well-constructed egg shape, even if there is a crack, the edges of the bone are usually held closely together and will soon heal without needing bandaging or plaster to hold the ends of the broken bones opposite one another.

DEPRESSED SKULL FRACTURE

On the other hand, sometimes a blow is sufficient to dish in the skull, in which case the broken bones are now pressing on the brain and preventing its proper functioning. When this happens, many of the same symptoms occur as with bleeding underneath a fracture. Briefly, pressure on the brain causes a stroke-like effect, the patient becomes drowsy or loses consciousness, has a dreadful headache, may lose control of his vision so that he sees double, and the automatically controlled irises in the eye may go awry, so that one pupil becomes large and won't react to light.

If these things occur, then the patient urgently needs an operation to lift the depressed pieces of bone. Once the pressure on the brain is relieved, it starts to work normally again. And provided the head injury has not irreparably damaged the brain tissue underlying the fracture, full recovery should follow.

How do you know if you have a fractured skull? A useful rule of thumb is that if you've been knocked out, or if you've had a blow from a blunt object which was hard enough to rupture the skin, you need to be seen in Casualty straightaway.

If you've been knocked out, or if the X-ray shows that you have fractured your skull, you'll need to be admitted to hospital for observation for twenty-four hours, to make sure that internal bleeding isn't developing.

One small event causes a lot of confusion and is worth mentioning. A relatively minor blow to a child's forehead often brings up the most mountainous bruise, which usually frightens the life out of his parents! The child falls, bashing his head on the edge of a table and within minutes, there's the bruise – rising a quarter of an inch above the normal level of the skin.

I call this the 'Korky the cat' phenomenon! If you remember back to the days when you read the 'Dandy', you'll remember that every time one of the characters received a bang on the head, immediately he was pictured as having a mountainous bruise. This is really only a reflection of what happens to so many small children in the same circumstances. Although the bruise often *looks* awful, it seldom means anything important. So long as there is no cut in the skin, a cold compress will help to reduce the swelling, as will a hanky dipped in witchhazel, pressed to the bruise. And it usually goes down quite quickly, too. However, if the blow caused a cut in the skin; if the child was knocked out or can't remember the incident; if he seems drowsy, is seeing double, or is vomiting, or in any way seems to be behaving unusually, then it is time to take him to Casualty.

FRACTURED SKULL WITH UNDERLYING BLEED

At certain places, the bones of the skull have arteries running through them. And, if the skull bone fractures across the artery, it ruptures; blood forces its way out, getting underneath the inner lining of the skull. Arteries are under high pressure, and this bleeding produces symptoms by pressing on the brain, giving a headache, drowsiness and sometimes symptoms like a stroke; often the eyes don't work properly, causing double vision; in particular, the pupils don't react properly, often reacting to light differently on each side of the body.

The sudden development of a widened pupil that won't react to light indicates that something has gone very wrong within the skull, and usually means that the patient needs an urgent operation to suck out the blood clot pressing on the brain.

SUB-DURAL HAEMORRHAGE

After passing through the brain, used blood is collected in large veins lying directly on the inside of the skull. Sometimes, as a result of a minor head injury, these veins can snap or tear. When this happens, blood slowly leaks out between the two outermost coverings of the brain (the dura). This is called a sub-dural haemorrhage. Because veins work at a much lower pressure than arteries do, blood leaks out only slowly, so the effects of a sub-dural haemorrhage are much slower in onset than with bleeding from an artery. With a sub-arachnoid haemorrhage (which occurs in the next layer of the brain covering), the ruptured vessel is an *artery* under high pressure and blood leaks out very quickly indeed. With a sub-dural haemorrhage it is more of an ooze.

The large veins draining the brain can be stretched and broken, particularly by blows to either the front or the back of the head. It doesn't need a particularly violent bang to do it, either – even a blow which isn't enough to cause concussion or loss of consciousness is still capable of causing a sub-dural haemorrhage. In older age the brain sometimes shrinks, and a sub-dural haemorrhage is more likely to happen simply because the brain can move around more inside the skull: hence sub-dural haemorrhages are more common in older people.

Bleeding inside the skull compresses the brain, causing it to function less well; the higher the pressure inside the brain, the more it cuts off the normal flow of blood through brain arteries, and so the less oxygen can pass into the nerve cells – which therefore don't function as well as they used to. Patients with a sub-dural haemorrhage gradually think more slowly, become less alert, and eventually become drowsy: they may go into coma. Typically, the degree of drowsiness comes and goes. In the worst cases the patient can develop a stroke-like condition. If untreated, a sub-dural haemorrhage may end in death.

Pressure like this is likely to cause a severe, continuous headache. A slow bleed into the inside of the skull is ultimately just as devastating as a fast one but is far less dramatic, and the symptoms come on more slowly. In the older person, where the brain has already shrunk slightly, the extra blood may create very little extra pressure at first, because there's more space available within the skull. However, in younger people, excess pressure can develop to a much greater degree.

WINNIE

Winnie is a seventy-five-year-old widow who lives in a small cottage. One morning she miscounted the steps and fell down the last step of her stairs. Although she hit her head, she didn't knock herself out and her main trouble was a severely bruised right hip. After a few days she seemed to be recovering well, but gradually she became less alert, slightly more befuddled, and her memory wasn't quite as good as it used to be. At first, her friends and relatives thought that it was merely the onset of older age, but soon she couldn't remember what she had been doing the day before, when three weeks previously she'd had a clear, agile mind. Her son got worried and rang the doctor.

When the doctor examined her she found very little – other than the fact that Winnie thought today was Thursday when it was Tuesday, couldn't name the current prime minister, and seemed generally vague and slightly drowsy. The doctor found that Winnie's left big toe moved upwards when her feet were tickled on the soles, which indicated that there had been a stroke-like event on the opposite side of the brain.

Because of the recent fall, her headache, and the slow onset of the symptoms, her doctor wondered whether Winnie had had a sub-dural haemorrhage and arranged for her to be admitted to hospital. There, scans of the brain proved that this was exactly what had happened. Winnie was taken to the operating theatre, anaesthetised,and a small hole was made in the skull. Through this the surgeon sucked out the blood and blood clot that had escaped from the punctured vein and was pressing on the brain.

A week after the operation, Winnie was back to her old self, alert, interested and well on the way to recovery.

Type of headache

The headache of a sub-dural bleed is severe and may last for a long time. Typically, it will come on *slowly*. The degree of drowsiness fluctuates.

Orthodox treatment

Treatment is simple, but requires an operation. The surgeon drills a hole in the bone of the skull overlying the point where the blood clot has formed, and sucks out the excess blood. This immediately reduces the pressure on the brain. The blood flow inside the brain returns to normal, and full recovery usually occurs.

However, sometimes the situation may have progressed too far and permanent brain damage or even death can occur.

Self-help

There are no self-help measures.

Complementary treatment

As always in the case of any medical emergency, you must not waste time by trying to find suitable complementary treatments. You need to get orthodox medical attention immediately. *Complementary medicine comes into its own in the recovery stages of illness, and that is where it is used to best effect.*

Homoeopathy does provide emergency treatment suggestions, but these are to be undertaken only while waiting for medical attention and never if the patient is unconscious. Belladonna, nux or aconite can be given every fifteen minutes, while waiting for help, in the case of sub-dural haemorrhage. Homeopathic Opium could be tried, if the face has turned blue or congested. During recovery, try baryta, gelsemium and lachesis, with ledum for pain. Do, of course, consult a registered homoeopath for individual diagnosis and prescription.

Infusions of balm, camomile, peppermint or skullcap can be sipped by the victim, while waiting for attention. These deal quite effectively with shock.

Lavender, melissa and neroli can be inhaled to prevent shock, and Rescue Remedy (a Bach flower remedy) can be taken internally (a few drops), or rubbed in at pulse points.

In the recovery stage of head injuries, many many therapies can be used. You might try the Feldenkrais Method, acupuncture, osteopathy (cranial, as well), psychotherapy, medical herbalism, biofeedback and kinesiology, to name but a few.

DEALING WITH A HEAD INJURY

Three important questions need to be answered following any head injury.

- Has there been concussion or any other form of brain damage?
- Is there any bleeding in or around the brain?
- Is there a neck injury as well?

As far as the direct head injury is concerned, the following facts are important to take into consideration.

1. If the victim has been knocked out, or cannot remember the exact incident or the few seconds leading up to it, then he needs to be admitted to hospital for at least twenty-four hours observation. .

2. An injury from a *blunt* object (either one that hits you or one that you fall on) that has caused a cut in the skin may have been sufficient to break the skull as well. You will need an X-ray to show whether there is a skull fracture underneath the cut.

3. If any of the following occur in the first twenty-four hours after a head injury, the injury to the brain may be more severe than previously thought, or there may be internal bleeding. The symptoms are: *severe, increasing* headache; vomiting; double vision; incoordination; drowsiness. (There's a great difference between drowsiness and sleepiness: when you feel sleepy you want to sleep, but can be roused to full consciousness. When you're drowsy, you can't be roused properly.)

If any of these occur; if there is any odd behaviour; if there is a general deterioration of the patient's condition; or if there is anything else that is causing concern, you should go to Casualty *immediately.*

Usually the above symptoms occur within the first twenty-four hours, but in some cases they can occur much later, perhaps over ten days. This is particularly the case with sub-dural haemorrhages in older people. Even when the injury is several days old, if the patient starts showing some of these symptoms, they should see a doctor *immediately*.

The only reason why patients are admitted to hospital following a head injury is to be certain that they do not have any hidden bleeding inside the skull causing pressure on the brain, or else swelling of the brain substance itself. Any extra pressure needs to be relieved as soon as possible, whether caused by stoved-in bones in the skull; from high-pressure bleeding; or from slow low-pressure bleeding, as in a sub-dural haemorrhage. An urgent operation may be necessary to elevate stoved-in bones and suck out any blood clots: swelling of the brain substance itself can be treated with steroids.

Orthodox treatment

Even where there is concussion and/or an undisplaced skull fracture, most cases of head injury resolve spontaneously with no need for any special medical involvement. However, it is good medical practice to observe the patient for twenty-four hours, because just occasionally the damage to the brain is greater than was first thought, or else there is internal bleeding. Increased pressure in the brain may cause an increasing headache, the patient's mental functions may drop, his ability to move may be impaired, and his blood pressure often rises progressively. Putting the patient under observation allows the doctors to spot any sudden deterioration quickly. At regular intervals throughout the night a nurse shines a light in his eyes to see if their pupil reflexes are working properly, and asks him to move his feet and hands to make sure that all his movements are intact. The nurse will also check that the patient can be roused fully, because changes in the level of consciousness indicate a worsening of the situation. He will also measure the blood pressure and take the pulse, as certain changes in these can indicate that complications are starting.

Self-help

The prevention of head injury and brain haemorrhage is simple, but often neglected. If you are given head protection in your job, or for driving a motorcycle or pushbike, then *use it* – it's not macho to do without.

Motorbike helmets are deceptive – they are very effective in reducing head injury, but they rapidly lose their strength if previously dropped or banged, even if the blow wasn't particularly hard.

Helmets don't respond well to being painted, either. The solvent in some paints dissolves the plastic of the helmet, weakening it considerably.

Increasingly, cyclists are being recommended to wear helmets; the neuro-surgical units are spearheading campaigns to encourage their use.

Repeated violent head movements can result in torn nerve fibres, small bleeds in the brain, and in some cases more serious bleeds from ruptured blood vessels. 'Headbanging', a dance popular more in the Seventies and Eighties, in which the head is repeatedly jerked violently up and down, can cause severe brain damage and even death as a result of rupturing blood vessels inside the head.

The second dangerous activity is boxing. You can suffer *brain damage even when wearing headguards*. Although a headguard may protect against direct blows to the face, there is virtually no protection against the twisting force of a sideways blow to the chin, and it is these twisting, rotating forces on the brain that probably do the greatest damage in producing a punch-drunk fighter.

Contrary to the impression given in the movies, keeping the patient awake after a head injury doesn't help. In any case, the stress of the circumstances surrounding the head injury usually makes him want to sleep – especially if the patient is a child.

Self-help after a head injury is largely a matter of common sense. If you've been knocked out, or show any of the symptoms described above, then you will need to get to hospital as soon as possible. On the other hand, if the injury is minor, you haven't been knocked out, and you haven't got any of the other symptoms, then a couple of paracetamol (or in adults, aspirin, if you're able to take it) may be all that you need to get rid of the headache. If you've jarred your neck as well as banging your head, then an anti-inflammatory drug such as ibuprofen can often be more effective than simple analgesics. (This is available over the counter as Nurofen; don't take it if you have stomach ulcers.)

If there is a lot of spasm in the neck muscles then a cold compress and massage may be helpful. However, *don't* apply *heat* to the site of a recent soft-tissue injury; it will make the swelling worse. Instead, cold compresses will reduce the swelling, the inflammation, and the pain. Warmth is for a few days later, after the initial injury has started to settle down.

One very important word of warning: where there has been a head injury, there may also be a neck injury. If the patient is complaining of severe neck pain, or if you think the neck may have been damaged, then *do not move them*. If the neck has been broken, moving the head or body may rupture the delicate spinal cord inside the neck. There have been instances where patients have been damaged more by the actions of their first-aid 'helpers' than they were by the original injury. There is one horrific case of a motorcyclist who came off his machine and was found lying on the ground with his neck broken but his spinal cord intact. Somebody took his helmet off, and in doing so bent his neck, and severed his spinal cord, paralysing him permanently. So, if there is a neck injury of any severity (which usually means the patient is in severe pain, and perhaps unable to move without experiencing agonising pain), or else is unconscious, then *do not move them*. Wait for the ambulance to arrive: ambulancemen and paramedics have specialised equipment to allow them to move patients without causing further movement to the head and neck.

Complementary treatment

There is no alternative to proper hospital care for those who have had a head injury severe enough either to knock them unconscious, or give any of the symptoms described earlier. If you've been knocked out, you will need twenty-four hours' observation. On the other hand, minor degrees of head injury and superficial bruising can be successfully treated with all sorts of therapies.

Acupuncture can help when there is local muscle spasm, and soft-tissue injury. It is especially effective for pain, and can be helpful for bones that are slow to heal.

After an accident, Bach flower remedies can be applied to pulse points, and again, a good herbal treatment for shock is an infusion of balm, camomile, peppermint and skullcap, which can be sipped, or applied as a compress to the head area. Arnica can be taken while awaiting medical attention.

Biofeedback and kinesiology can be useful in the recuperative stages of injury, as can therapies like colour therapy (to help with persistent headaches), flotation therapy, relaxation and psychotherapy. The latter can be especially good, since anxiety can play a part in injury-related headaches. Reflexology to treat the head and neck area could be helpful; therapists say this revitalises the body so that it can better heal itself. It should also relieve some of the pain and tension. Osteopathy and cranial osteopathy may help, after the initial injury has begun to settle down.

Comfrey root (in small doses) can be taken internally to encourage bone healing in the case of fracture. (The old name for comfrey is 'knitbone'.) Valerian tea combined with skullcap may help with spasm-caused headaches. Bumps and bruises can be swabbed with witch hazel, which will prevent swelling. A poultice of mustard seed stimulates circulation and relieves muscular and skeletal pain. Anti-inflammatory herbs include comfrey, marigold and yarrow. Apply as a compress.

An aromatherapist could suggest lavender, marjoram and thyme to sooth aching and promote healing. Essential oil of fennel will ease muscular pain. Rose in the bath can help headaches, and try essential oil of lemon on the bandage to arrest bleeding. Anti-inflammatory oils include bergamot, marigold (calendula), lavender and myrrh. Black pepper is rubefacient and can be used in massage after healing has begun. Analgesic oils are bergamot, camomile and lavender.

The homoeopathic remedies of nat sulph, china and camomile can be taken after a head injury, and bryonia can relieve discomfort, along with arnica, hypericum and symphytum. But do see a registered homoeopath who will assess your particular needs.

PAIN AFTER A HEAD INJURY

Firstly, there is the immediate post-injury headache, occurring during the first week after the accident. Secondly, there can be post-concussion headaches – which may be a concussion headache that doesn't go away, or else a headache which comes on even as late as six months after the original injury.

Pain immediately after a head injury

A lot of things can happen from a blow to the head. Firstly, there's local bruising to the skin, fat and muscles overlying the skull, each of which will cause pain. The bones of the skull may be bruised or broken, which is another source of pain. The brain may undergo a shearing force, pulling and stretching its nerve fibres;

surprisingly, the brain hasn't got any sensory pain fibres in it, so it can't feel pain directly from this, but headaches often occur after concussion for other reasons. Bleeding into the skull raises the pressure inside the head, and this can cause an intense headache.

Any injury to the skull is likely also to injure the neck to some extent, and there may be pain from muscles and ligaments which have been over-stretched, joints that have been moved into abnormal positions, and bones that have been broken.

Obviously, not all of this happens in every head injury, but it does give an idea of the large number of different sources of pain that can follow after a single blow.

One of the most potent sources of pain after a head injury comes from the neck muscles. Often a simple head injury traumatises the neck sufficiently to cause all the muscles to go into spasm. This can occur after relatively minor blows; for example, on banging your head under a shelf.

TREVOR

While on holiday, Trevor went on a tour of a tin mine. He was told to put on a protective helmet, which he thought was a bit over the top. Surely, he thought, they wouldn't be taking visitors anywhere where the roof might fall in?

He soon discovered the hard way why visitors were given helmets. Going along a low passage he misjudged the height of the roof and banged his head firmly on a projecting piece of rock. The helmet took the force of the blow, but almost immediately Trevor felt his neck seizing up and becoming sore at the very top. Within five minutes he developed a sickening headache, together with a tight feeling at the top of his neck, where it met the skull. Every time he tilted his head back, the pain in the nape of his neck became worse, and probing gingerly with his fingers he became aware that the muscles in that area were very sore.

Realising that the blow was too soft to have done much damage, he made a point of massaging the muscles and gently stretching the neck by bending his head forwards and putting his chin on his chest. This relieved the spasm that had reflexively occurred in his muscles as a result of the bang on the head, and soon he was more or less pain-free. However, the pain didn't really settle until the next morning – wisely, he took a couple of paracetamol just before going to bed and that, plus the normal muscle relaxation of sleep, stopped the spasm of the upper neck muscles that was causing the problem.

Trevor's case is a typical example of how a small bump to the head can cause the muscles in the neck automatically to contract to protect the spine from further injury, and how this spasm can cause more pain and problems than the direct blow.

Type of headache

The headache immediately after a head injury is usually throbbing, with tenderness locally at the site of the injury; it is frequently accompanied by a generalised headache, from spasm in the neck muscles.

Treatment

Treatment following head injury depends on exactly what injuries have been sustained; see the relevant section above for each type of injury.

Long-term headaches after injury

As well as damage from concussion, the brain can also be injured without receiving a blow. Internal damage can occur through pressure; for example, from a sub-arachnoid haemorrhage, from a stroke, from hydrocephalus, and tumours. The non-specific injury the brain receives from these can also cause *post-traumatic headaches,* a term which includes headaches both from direct concussion and from other forms of brain injury.

Assessing post-trauma headaches is not easy, if for no other reason than the fact that any blow to the skull almost certainly strains the neck as well. For example, a car crash which knocks out the driver will probably cause a whiplash accident as well. So is the post-trauma headache due to the head injury or the neck injury? Other than neck problems, true post-concussion headache is by far the most common *continuing* symptom after a severe head injury. Interestingly, the degree of headache depends on what the patient was doing when they had their injury – head injuries sustained during recreation seem to cause far fewer post-concussion headaches than do injuries sustained at work. Obviously there must be some psychological element in the degree of pain experienced.

One interesting aspect of post-traumatic headaches is that they sometimes don't start until six months after the original injury. These 'late acquired' headaches may be related to depression, especially if the patient has lost their job as a result of their injuries.

Type of headache

Most post-traumatic headaches are over the whole of the head, and are usually accompanied by poor concentration and dizziness. Just occasionally a head injury can start off migraine-type headaches, but this is very rare.

What else could it be?

It's not always easy to disentangle headaches caused by direct brain damage (concussion), and those arising from *injury to the neck.*

Don't forget that it's quite possible for other types of headaches to occur coincidentally, unrelated to the injury. Unfortunately, the idea that the two things are unrelated is often very difficult for the patient to comprehend. After all, he thinks, *I injured my head and then six months later I start getting migraines.* Surely the two are related? They may be, but then again, they may not.

Orthodox treatment

Post-concussion headache sometimes responds to mild analgesics, including the non-steroidal anti-inflammatory drugs (NSAIDs). These are drugs that are commonly used for rheumatism; for example, ibuprofen (also known as Brufen or Nurofen), diclofenac (Voltarol), and indomethacin (Indocid). There are *many* others. In addition, a small dose of the beta-blocker propranolol may help. This drug is principally used in treating blood pressure and angina, though it can also be useful in cases of migraine. It relaxes the muscle lining of blood vessels in the brain, which may be the way that its anti-headache effects occur.

Complementary treatment

Acupuncture lessens healing time and trauma associated with concussion and head injury. Cranial osteopathy may help some sufferers, as can reflexology (for calming down muscle injuries and broken bones). Where there is a coincidental neck injury any of the manipulative medicines may be appropriate.

An aromatherapist might suggest the anti-depressant oils bergamot, clary sage, camomile, geranium, jasmine, melissa, neroli and ylang ylang, used in any of the usual aromatherapy forms (baths, vapourisers, massage, etc). You might also try some of the anti-inflammatory oils in the same way – marigold, camomile or myrrh.

Basil leaves can be steeped in boiling water and drunk as a tea. Basil oil can be massaged into the temples. Bach flower remedies (especially the Rescue Remedy) can help with emotional problems that might follow, and lead to further headaches. A homoeopath would have to prescribe according to very specific symptoms, but cicuta or nat sulph are two possible remedies.

According to complementary practitioners calcium and magnesium are nature's tranquillisers, and supplementation may help some sufferers. Music and dance therapy is useful, following healing of the injury. Relaxation therapies and the Alexander Technique both claim to help post-accident suffering, by facilitating quicker recovery and dealing with tensions and stress. Obviously, any of the post-operative or post-illness suggestions offered in Chapter Nine will be useful.

Associated problems

Injuries to the neck often occur at the same time as head injuries: *whiplash injury* and *cervical spondylosis* may all create further problems. In addition, if the head injury has resulted in severe brain damage with *paralysis of some groups of muscles*, the effects can be similar to those caused by strokes, in that an imbalance in the pull of opposing muscle groups may cause stress on the neck and spine.. *Depression* is a real cause of headaches, and may well occur if the patient has received a permanent injury.

Chapter Eleven

HIGH BLOOD PRESSURE

One of the biggest misconceptions about headaches is that they're commonly due to high blood pressure. Certainly, patients with *severe* hypertension get headaches, and those with moderate blood pressure seem to be more prone to headaches *from other sources*, but there is no hard and fast relationship between blood pressure and headaches. In fact, high blood pressure is renowned for producing no symptoms at all in the majority of sufferers.

Very high blood pressure does cause headaches, though. They are characteristically severe, and typically worse on waking up, rather than later in the day – which is interesting because you'd expect it to be the other way round. Blood pressure falls during sleep, and on waking your blood pressure is likely to be lower; yet, it's at this time that the headaches occur!

'Blood pressure headaches' like these only occur if the hypertension is severe and untreated. However, those with a moderate rise in blood pressure do tend to suffer more frequently from headaches *from other causes*. In other words, *severe* blood pressure can trigger early-morning headaches by itself; lower levels of blood pressure seem to multiply headaches due to other causes.

Headaches caused by high blood pressure are probably related to the direct effects of pressure on the arteries of the brain, and the number and frequency of headaches largely depends upon the extra pressure. Reduce the blood pressure and the headaches go away.

Sometimes blood pressure can rise as a side-effect of the contraceptive pill. It can also rise in pregnancy. However, the rise of pressure is small by comparison with 'ordinary' blood pressure. Small increases in blood pressure are potentially much more serious if you're on the Pill or pregnant. Changing to a different pill, or even stopping entirely may be necessary: in pregnancy, rest and sedation may be required. You will need to consult your doctor about both these situations.

Type of headache

The headache of severe blood pressure is typically worst on waking. It's also worse if you sleep in, so headaches from high blood pressure are often worse at the weekend because of this. The headache is on both sides, and can be at the front or the back of the head, severe, bursting or throbbing, and sometimes accompanied by blurred vision, dizziness and in extreme cases, vagueness. Headaches like these are entirely related to the level of excess blood pressure: reduce the pressure and the headaches reduce also.

What else could it be?
As we just discussed, the headache of high blood pressure is typically worse on waking up, and often made worse by lying in. This is also typical of *migraine* where sleeping in late can trigger off an attack. But from there on the symptoms diverge. There are no visual changes such as flashing lights accompanying the headache of high blood pressure and a migraine is usually one-sided. In any case, it's easy for the doctor to distinguish between migraine and hypertension headaches just by measuring your blood pressure.

Tension headaches can also be worse on sleeping in; but in this case the muscles in the back of the neck will be sore and tender, and, of course, the blood pressure will be normal. Don't forget that worrying about your blood pressure can give you a tension headache!

Orthodox treatment
The treatment of blood pressure almost needs a book on its own, because there are so many methods, and so many ways in which the doctor, patient and complementary therapist can join forces to help.

In a few cases, high blood pressure has a basic cause, and in these cases removing the underlying problem may bring the blood pressure down to normal. Underlying problems like this include obstruction of the arteries to the kidney; certain rare types of kidney disease; and various tumours (some benign, a few malignant) that secrete excess hormones which raise the blood pressure.

One of these hormone-producing tumours is called a *phaechromocytoma* and it's a non-malignant growth of a type of tissue that normally forms part of the adrenal glands. It produces excess, uncontrolled quantities of adrenalin-like substances which can raise the blood pressure to very high levels. Finding and cutting out offending cells brings the blood pressure back to normal.

Other hormonal causes for raised blood pressure include tumours of the pituitary gland (a gland at the base of the brain) which secrete too much growth hormone and *diabetes* is associated with higher blood pressure. However, with the exception of diabetes, all these conditions are rare: most doctors are unlikely to meet even a single case in their whole lifetime.

Once we've eliminated these conditions, we're left with what is called 'essential' hypertension, and this forms the majority of cases of high blood pressure. Many cases of essential hypertension are probably genetic, and at the moment there is very little that we can do to cure it. Just keep taking the tablets! On the other hand, there are many things that can make blood pressure worse, chief of which is being too fat. For every extra pound of fat you put on, your blood has to go through an extra mile of capillaries; the fatter you are the harder the heart has to work. Mild to moderate blood pressure frequently rises in those who are overweight, and often returns to normal if the patient goes on a diet and returns to normal size.

Exercise also helps, making the body more efficient in how it uses biochemical raw materials, and regular exercise reduces blood pressure in the long run.

Stress, too, is associated with blood pressure, though the relationship is far from precise. Undoubtedly, extra levels of stress put up the blood pressure over a short period of time; for example, frantically rushing to get to work on time puts up the blood pressure *transiently*. Some people seem to get high blood pressure when stress is maintained for a long time, yet others don't get a raised blood pressure in these situations.

There are many things that the orthodox practitioner can do to treat high blood pressure. These fall into four main sections: dealing with obesity; encouraging exercise; reducing stress; and, prescribing medicines. However, we shouldn't look at these four groups independently; they all interact one with the other. A little less stress, a few extra pounds off, a little more exercise and a mild diuretic may together bring the blood pressure down to normal levels, but it might require a far higher dose of medicines if the first three procedures aren't undertaken.

Let's look at each of these in turn:

• Obesity. Without doubt, being fat causes your blood pressure to rise, and shedding those extra few pounds may make all the difference to your overall health and wellbeing.

• Exercise. Firstly, exercise uses up the excess adrenalin that swills round the system when we are in a state of alertness as a result of a fright or stress. Secondly, the fit person who exercises is less likely to become obese. Thirdly, the body systems of fit people work in a slightly different way to those who are unfit.

Exercise promotes a greater sense of well-being, a sense of relaxation, and causes some significant but subtle changes to occur in the body, particularly in the way in which the cells of the body handle sugar.

• Stress. Our bodies are good at responding to external stress; they do so by putting up the blood pressure transiently, which is useful if we need to run away quickly in the face of danger. However, if stress is applied for days and weeks on end, or if we don't get any opportunity to relieve the stress, then our bodies become constantly over-stimulated, with adrenalin swimming around the system; no wonder the blood pressure goes up!

Anti-stress measures can be simple, but very effective in reducing the levels of stress within the body; and by reducing stress we may reduce blood pressure fairly quickly.

However, stress *on its own* is unlikely to be the entire cause of high blood pressure; it probably has an effect mainly on those with an underlying predisposition to high blood pressure.

• Medication. There are five main groups of drugs to treat high blood pressure.

1. *The thiazide diuretics*. These are drugs which are often used to produce extra urine and dry out the body.

2. *Beta-blockers* are drugs which block the effects of adrenalin and nor-adrenalin, and so reduce the contraction of the arteriolar muscles, reducing blood pressure. They also stop the heart over-exerting itself, in much the same way that putting a wooden block under the car's accelerator pedal prevents you over-revving the engine.

3. *Calcium channel blockers* such as nifedipine (Adalat, Verapamil, Diltiazem, etc) block the movement of calcium ions across the outer membrane of muscle cells and, in doing so, reduce the force with which the involuntary muscles can act. As all the muscles controlling blood pressure are involuntary, these medicines are excellent for reducing blood pressure.

4. Drugs which act to *block the transmission of nerve impulses, e.g.* Alpha-methyldopa. After being absorbed in the body this is changed into an imitation transmitter chemical – one that doesn't stimulate the nerves – so, effectively, the nerve starts firing blanks! As a result the nervous system can't force the muscles to contract as strongly, so the blood pressure drops.

5. The group of blood pressure reducers called *ACE-inhibitors* (which stands for Angiotension Converting Enzyme Inhibitor). These block the effects of a hormone called angiotensin which when converted into its active form normally acts to constrict the muscle cells in the arterioles. Blocking the conversion reduces the stimulus on the muscle cells.

PRESIDENT ROOSEVELT

It's interesting to remember that until the Fifties we hardly had any medicines to control high blood pressure. Had we had them earlier, the fate of Europe might have been quite different, because President Roosevelt suffered from extremely high blood pressure. In the last few months of the Second World War, his blood pressure was uncontrollably high, a condition called malignant hypertension (it's not related to cancer, by the way).

This severe blood pressure had profound effects upon the President, giving him severe headaches, making him feel 'woolly headed', and making it difficult for him to think carefully and properly. This had unfortunate consequences, for at that time he was meeting Stalin and Churchill at the Yalta Conference. In fact, the effect of his extreme high blood pressure was to make him unable to exert his usual political and diplomatic power, and the result was that Stalin got his own way over the plans for the post-war control and division of Europe. It is a salutory thought that had we been able to control blood pressure twenty years earlier, the face of Europe might have changed in the process.

In controlling your blood pressure your doctor may use one drug on its own, or several of them together. Often the control of blood pressure is easier using two different drugs that work in different ways. Diuretics and beta-blockers are often used together; but, in fact, most anti-hypertensive drugs can be combined usefully with one another. Some combinations of drug even come together in one capsule, for convenience and ease of administration.

Once your blood pressure is under control you'll probably only need to see the doctor once every six months for a routine blood-pressure check.

Once drug treatment has started, it is usually for life. While it is often possible to bring down minor degrees of raised blood pressure by curbing obesity, instituting relaxation therapy, etc., if hypertension remains despite these measures, then permanent drug treatment is likely to be needed. High blood pressure like this doesn't often come down of its own accord, and although the drugs currently used reduce the blood pressure directly, they don't affect what causes the alteration in blood-pressure control. So, in effect, they are just ameliorating the effects of high blood pressure, rather than curing it so that it goes away.

Just occasionally the blood pressure does come down again, but this is either after some years have passed, or else after a major event such as a heart attack or a stroke. In these circumstances it may be possible to reduce the medication.

A problem with taking drugs is that occasionally they can give side-effects – dizziness, weakness, coughs, difficulty with erections, etc. As they are being given for a condition which is largely symptomless it's often difficult to persuade the patient to continue taking the medication, because as far as he is concerned, he feels fine when he's off the medication, and worse when he's on it. It is *vital* to keep taking your blood pressure pills; if you don't you run the risk of an earlier stroke, which may reduce your life expectancy by several years, or paralyse you.

Self-help

Two of the most important things you can do to get rid of high blood pressure are to *keep slim* and *exercise*. The results of dieting can be quite dramatic. An obese person with moderately high blood pressure can have their blood pressure brought down to normal simply by getting rid of their excess fat.

It may also help to limit your alcohol intake to four units a week (one unit equals half a pint of beer, one measure of spirits, or one glass of wine).

Some doctors feel that limiting salt intake can help. The evidence for this is a bit mixed, but some patients with high blood pressure may be helped by reducing excess salt in their food. Don't use too much in cooking, and *certainly* don't add salt at the table.

Relaxation therapy (particularly biofeedback) is also thought to benefit the reduction of high blood pressure. However, relaxation therapy by itself will probably not bring down established high blood pressure. On the other hand, it will join together with other forms of treatment to reduce high blood pressure without requiring such heavy doses of drugs.

Complementary treatment

Most of the complementary therapies offer advice for sufferers of high blood pressure. Stress reduction is an obvious target for the therapies, but there are many that are more specific in their aims.

Royal jelly is reputed to lower high blood pressure, and can be taken in many forms on a daily basis. Garlic and onions reduce cholesterol, which has been linked to high blood pressure, and hawthorn berries and rosemary can help to lessen oedema. Yellow dock can be taken as a tea to stimulate kidney function. Uva ursi and corn silk are good natural diuretics, aiding kidney function. Passionflowers calm, and dandelion leaves provide calcium and potassium which therapists say vitalise the kidneys and reduce oedema. Raspberry leaf has a similar effect.

Acupuncture can help, as can acupressure and reflexology, to cause the body to relax, and to stimulate the body's ability to work efficiently. In pregnancy, acupuncture can help with pre-eclampsia but only in conjunction with orthodox medicine. Homoeopathy has remedies too numerous to mention; because high blood pressure can be caused by any number of things, it is best to consult a homoeopath who can diagnose and treat your specific causes.

A clinical nutritionist is likely to suggest you reduce sugar, animal fats, and red meats; the reduction of salt, as previously mentioned, has been recognised as having some effect in the fight against high blood pressure. Tea, coffee and alcohol should be kept to a minimum, while grains, fibre and fresh fruit and vegetables should be increased in your diet. Vitamin B3 (Niacin) can control blood pressure, but only under the supervision of your GP. Omega-3 oils and calcium can also be supplemented.

Massage with oils thought to decrease blood pressure is an option; try soothing oils like lavender, marjoram, melissa or neroli. Vapourisation and bathing with a few drops of the oils in your bath water are also useful. Camomile, bergamot, rose and frankincense can invigorate and rejuvenate, and some have anti-depressant qualities. Fennel and lemon cleanse and detoxify.

Bach flower remedies are directed not towards the blood pressure, but at the irritability which may be causing the underlying stress. Vervain is used for strain; impatiens for impatience and irritability; agrimony for those who hide worries behind a brave face. Oak and elm are for anyone who feels overwhelmed.

A good exercise programme can keep you fit, which helps to reduce high blood pressure. As well as being an exercise T'ai Chi is also a mechanism for relaxation: relaxation therapies themselves can also help in high blood pressure. Reflexology reduces stress, and stimulates the circulatory system.

Associated problems

Strokes and *sub-arachnoid haemorrhages* can both be caused by high blood pressure. *Stress* can both increase blood pressure and cause *tension headaches*. Certain *hormone problems* cause high blood pressure as a side-effect.

Chapter Twelve

TUMOURS

Probably the most common fear of patients with prolonged or severe headaches is that they have a tumour. Thankfully, the answer they hardly ever do, although rarely headaches can be a symptom of a growth in the brain or skull.

However, it is *very* uncommon for a headache to be the first indication of a brain tumour; paralysis, stroke-like attacks or fits, yes. Headache, no. On the other hand, headaches are common symptoms of brain tumours, *but only as a late event*, long after the diagnosis has been made.

Tumours form when cells don't know how to stop dividing; essentially, a tumour is an overgrowth of cells. There are two main types of tumours – *benign* and *malignant*. In benign tumours the cells overgrow, but don't invade the tissue surrounding them, and there is often a layer of squashed normal tissue around the tumour. Often a benign tumour can be shelled out of the tissue it's buried in, almost as one would shell the kernel out of a nut.

Benign tumours cause problems because they press on other tissues and organs in the body; and because benign tumours are very similar to the tissues they are derived from, they can produce the same chemicals – so it is quite possible for a benign tumour at a hormone-producing site (like the thyroid gland) to produce an uncontrolled excess of hormone.

Basically, these are the only two ways that benign tumours can exert any unpleasant effects; simply by their physical presence, and sometimes by secreting excess hormones. Benign tumours never spread to distant parts of the body, and they seldom change into malignant ones.

What sort of tumours are commonly benign? Often breast lumps are found to be harmless; those little skin tags that often come round the neck are small benign tumours; and, as mentioned above, deeper in the body the thyroid can have benign tumours that may secrete extra thyroid hormone. The gut may have small benign growths in it.

Malignant tumours are a different kettle of fish altogether. These are cells which have *really* got out of control. As well as not knowing when to stop dividing, they also infiltrate the tissues surrounding them. Whereas a benign tumour frequently has a cyst-like shell around it, a malignant tumour doesn't – which is why it is frequently difficult to remove, because there is no clear borderline between normal and abnormal tissue.

As well as spreading locally malignant tumours also spread to distant sites. A primary tumour (i.e., the tumour at the original site) throws off cells into either the bloodstream or, more commonly, the lymphatic system (a drainage system in the body, rather like the veins, that runs parallel to the circulatory system). Cells seeding off from the main cancerous tumour become deposited in areas of the body remote from the primary site. Once they have lodged in distant tissue they start to grow, forming a secondary tumour. Each type of cancer has a tendency to form secondary tumours in certain types of tissue. For example, cancer in the bowel tends to cause secondary growths in the liver; cancer of the breast often moves to the bones; cancer of the lung tends to form secondary tumours in the brain. However, these are not hard and fast rules, and a particular type of cancer can spread to a number of different sites.

Malignant tumours are fatal in a number of ways. Firstly, and most importantly, they seem to have an ability to suck the nutrients out of the system so that they grow at the body's expense – the cancer gets bigger as the patient gets thinner. Secondly, they can erode into important organs, preventing them working properly; and, finally, they can exert the same pressure and hormonal effects that benign tumours also exert, often made more complex because, being more primitive tissue, they can produce hormones that are wildly different from those normally produced by the tissue they come from.

Malignant tumours also cause problems because they invade and destroy the tissues that they have formed in. Frequently they cause more pain in the secondary site than they do in the original site – bone pain from secondaries can be particularly severe.

What sorts of cancers give rise to headaches? The answer is actually quite complex. *Any* tumour inside the skull can cause pressure on the brain, both locally and by obstructing the outflow of cerebro-spinal fluid – and in raising the pressure within the skull, benign tumours can be just as bad as malignant ones. A rise in pressure causes dull persistent headaches, but by the time headaches happen, other symptoms have usually occurred – such as weakness in an arm or leg, or changes in vision or speech. In addition, with a malignant abnormality there may be loss of weight, together with a general feeling of exhaustion and malaise.

Tumours inside the skull can be primary; in other words, they arise from the tissues inside the skull, such as the brain or its surrounding coverings; but more often brain tumours are secondary. Cancers which commonly manifest themselves in the brain include cancers of the breast and the lungs.

Don't forget that there's more to the head than just the brain. Malignancies can also affect the bones of the skull – usually secondary cancers, though primary tumours can arise in the sinuses. Secondary cancers can affect the bones of the spine, and primary tumours, both benign and malignant, can also affect the pituitary gland, which is a gland underneath the main part of the brain. The pituitary's job is to secrete hormones which control growth, reproduction, and water balance, among other things. Headaches are common with pituitary tumours, both benign and malignant.

Diagnosis

First, your doctor will take down your history. The first sign of a brain tumour is *not* usually a headache but rather, neurological features such as paralysis, altered vision or speech, vomiting, or altered levels of consciousness. Often these problems are intermittent, rather than constant. Pituitary gland problems usually show up as changes in the menstrual cycle, abnormal growth, or sometimes diabetes.

Other things that point to tumours are the existence of a previous cancer which is known to spread to the brain or bones, and a history of wasting or loss of weight, especially if coupled with a continuing sense of weakness or malaise. These are all symptoms which can point towards a tumour of the head or neck. On the other hand, as you will immediately recognise, most of these symptoms can occur completely separately from a brain tumour, and it is unlikely that your doctor will be able to diagnose a brain tumour without doing a lot of complex tests.

The first thing your doctor will do is to arrange for a blood test to check the Erythrocyte Sedimentation Rate (ESR). This is a broad method of working out whether there is anything odd going on in the body, and simply measures the speed with which the red cells in the blood sink to the bottom of a tube of blood. Although a raised ESR means there's something abnormal going on, a normal ESR doesn't necessarily exclude a malignancy, unfortunately.

Next, your doctor is likely to get an X-ray, though this doesn't give anything like as much extra information as you might think. Secondary deposits of cancer in the skull bones usually show up clearly, as punched-out areas where bone has been replaced by non-bony, malignant tissue. In addition, the X-ray will also show the shape and size of the cavity of the hollow in the bones, under the brain, where the pituitary gland sits. Tumours of the pituitary often alter the shape of this cavity.

On the other hand, simple X-rays are often unhelpful in spotting tumours of the brain itself; sometimes areas of the tumour will show up as white flecks on the X-ray, but because the consistency of a tumour is very much like the consistency of the brain itself, simple X-rays can't show the difference between the two.

If the symptoms point towards a tumour of the pituitary, then your doctor will measure the levels of various hormones in the blood.

Much more sophisticated tests are now available for example, a CAT scan (Computer Assisted Tomography).

MRI scans are amazing in their ability to show up detail in soft tissues. X-rays can't do this easily – most soft tissues in the body look exactly alike to X-ray. MRI scans are being used more and more to find the cause of problems deep within the body, without needing to stick in tubes, or perform operations to look around.

Finally, the doctor can organise an Electro-encephalogram (EEG) to measure the electrical activity of the brain. This can sometimes help to localise the site of a problem.

Although brain tumours are not common, they are not that rare, either. They are, unfortunately, *extremely* difficult to detect in their early stages. Often, the first inkling of a brain tumour is through some odd neurological event. Perhaps you have a stroke-like attack that goes away after a couple of days, though this is more likely due to a Transient Ischaemic Attack (TIA). Perhaps there is an attack of epilepsy occurring in someone who has never had epilepsy before; a first migraine occurring after the age of fifty may also be the first inkling of a brain tumour. As a general rule, any migraine which starts after the age of fifty should be treated with suspicion, and fits starting in adult life ought to be thoroughly investigated.

But even by this time it may be too late to save the patient. By the time a malignant tumour has progressed to the point where it is causing fits, paralysis or migraines it has often become incurable.

But all is not gloom – some types of brain tumour can be successfully treated. Let's run through the list:

• *Benign tumours* are relatively easy to treat. Simply removing them relieves the pressure on the brain and, provided the abnormal tissues have been completely removed (which is usually not too difficult to achieve), they are unlikely to re-grow again.

• *Malignant tumours* affect two main groups of people – children, and the elderly. Because children don't usually get strokes or episodes of abnormal consciousness, it's often possible to spot a brain tumour earlier in a child than in an elderly person. And the earlier the diagnosis, the more chance there is of doing something about it. Even so, by the time a malignant brain tumour is producing symptoms it may already be too late.

CHLOE

Chloe is a little girl of nineteen months. One day she fell over, hit her head and then vomited a couple of times. Her mother brought her to the doctor, just to be on the safe side, but as Chloe hadn't been knocked out, and there was nothing unusual found when examining her, her doctor suggested that Chloe's mother just keep an eye on her, and bring her back if necessary.

All was well, but a few days later Chloe did it again, this time falling off her toy tricycle. She seemed a bit dazed afterwards, even though there was no obvious bump on the head, and her doctor began to get suspicious. Was it the bump on the head that was causing the droopiness, or was there something else that was causing Chloe to fall and bump herself? It's common for epilepsy to start at this age, so her doctor sent Chloe up to the hospital. But they could find nothing and sent her home again.

A few days later Chloe became lethargic, went off her food, was wobbly and unsteady on her feet, and vomited continuously for twenty-four hours. It was now obvious that there was something seriously amiss, and she was re-admitted to hospital, where a CAT scan showed she had a large tumour at the back of her brain.

In addition, the tumour was obstructing the outflow of cerebro-spinal fluid (CSF), the fluid which bathes the brain. In Chloe's case the tumour was blocking the drainage of CSF, so the pressure inside her brain was going up and up. No wonder Chloe was irritable, drowsy, and unsteady!

A few days later Chloe had brain surgery. The tumour was large, and like a cabbage; although there was a lot of tumour, it was attached to the rest of the brain only by a small stalk. The surgeons were able to remove the tumour easily and completely, and then scraped away as much as they dared of the place where the stalk was attached to normal brain tissue.

The tumour was sent to the laboratory to be examined under a microscope and to everyone's relief it turned out to have a very small likelihood of malignancy; as a result Chloe's doctors decided she didn't need any further treatment, such as radiotherapy or chemotherapy.

For a few days after the operation Chloe was on steroids to reduce post-operative swelling in the brain, but this was soon discontinued. In addition, the CSF could drain properly because the pressure of the tumour on the drainage channel had now gone; so the pressure on the brain from inside subsided. Consequently, drowsiness, irritability, unsteadiness and vomiting – went away.

Chloe is now back at home. She's suddenly starting to talk very volubly and learning lots of new words! Obviously she's going to need follow-up treatment for some time to come – but it all looks very hopeful indeed.

*Chloe's case illustrates how a benign tumour can have tremendous effects on the way the brain functions, and how, when it's removed, all those effects go away. It also shows yet again how headaches are **not** early symptoms of a brain tumour. Vomiting, irritability, drowsiness, paralysis or being off balance are much more likely to occur first.*

It's harder to spot tumours in adults, simply because for every tumour there are hundreds of conditions which initially produce similar symptoms,. Upon diagnosis, however, treatment can sometimes be very successful, as we'll see later.

ALBERT

Although he'd been well all his life, at the age of seventy-one, Albert discovered that he couldn't remember the names of objects – or more specifically, he couldn't manage to **say** the names, even if he knew what he wanted to say. Because of the suddenness of onset his doctor thought that he had probably had a small stroke, and started him on a tiny dose of aspirin to thin the blood very slightly.

A few days later, he had what appeared to be another minor stroke; he was suddenly taken unwell, and again had an episode when he couldn't speak, though he was able to understand what people were saying to him. There was no lack of power in his limbs, and the doctor again felt that he had probably had a further small stroke, perhaps more like the Transient Ischaemic Attacks (TIAs) that occur when tiny clumps of platelets temporarily block an artery in the brain. Exactly as so often happens with TIAs, Albert had several more attacks, recovering between each of them. All his blood tests were normal, too.

Shortly after this his condition started to deteriorate: he became weak in the right hand and arm, and didn't respond to movements on the right side of his visual fields. Then he started to get severe headaches. Only now did it begin to look as though he was suffering not from a series of strokes, but instead from a tumour; this was confirmed on a CAT scan, which showed a large malignant growth on the left side of the brain, with swelling and water retention of the brain around it.

Unfortunately, the cancer was inoperable, but this didn't mean that Albert was beyond the reach of treatment. Far from it. The associated water retention and swelling around the tumour was causing excessive pressure on the brain. His doctor started him on the drug dexamethazone, and it was almost like waving a magic wand. Instead of being confused and unable to express himself, as he had previously been, he became clear-minded and his speech returned almost to normal. He no longer had headaches, although he was unable to read. He was well enough to enjoy life, and he felt comfortable.

This lasted for some weeks, but then he started to deteriorate more quickly, and the headaches started again. His doctor fitted him with a device to deliver a slow continuous supply of morphine, and a sedative underneath the skin. This provided Albert with continuous pain relief, and made him feel relaxed and restful until he died peacefully a few days later.

Albert's case clearly demonstrates the difficulties of diagnosing a brain tumour early enough to do anything about it. By the time he had even the very first symptoms his brain tumour was already inoperable. In addition, his severe headaches didn't come on until very late in the illness, occurring **after** the development of those signs that indicated his tumour.

*In a nutshell, Albert's case shows that brain tumours –
especially in the elderly – are nearly always inoperable by the
time they give rise to enough symptoms to be diagnosable, and
that headaches are not an early symptom of a brain tumour.*

Types of tumour

Tumours inside the skull can arise from the meninges (the coverings around the brain), the blood vessels, the pituitary gland, or the brain substance itself. By far the most common malignant tumour is a secondary tumour; these are most common as complications of lung cancer, but they may come from any organ in the body. After secondary cancer, the most common primary cancer group are called the *gliomas,* which are tumours of the nerve cells themselves. After this, tumours arising from the meninges are the next most common.

The exact symptoms produced by a tumour depend entirely upon where it is, what it's pressing on, and what structures it may be invading and destroying. Tumours at the front of the brain can produce a progressive change in personality, or alterations in the emotions, giving either euphoria or irritability. Further back, tumours can produce epilepsy and/or weakness of the limbs on the opposite side of the body.

Tumours in the side part of the brain called the temporal lobe can produce progressive inability to speak, and sometimes hallucinations; and tumours low down at the base of the brain cause a rise in pressure within the brain. This can lead to a condition called hydrocephalus (water on the brain), which causes severe headaches and vomiting, and which, in small children, can cause progressive enlargement of the head. Coordination is often a problem for people who have tumours in this position.

Benign tumours are relatively easy to treat and some malignant tumours respond to treatment, but others are relatively resistant. Surgery is usually the best treatment for benign tumours; malignant primary tumours can be successfully cut out, but the surgeon won't want to remove too much of the brain tissue, and it may be difficult to remove a malignant tumour completely. Often surgery is used to begin with, then chemotherapy or radiotherapy afterwards. Surgery is seldom used in *secondary* tumours; these are often multiple, and impossible to remove completely.

The response to treatment depends very much on the exact type of tumour; tumours arising from the same type of tissue in two different patients may have quite different sensitivities to treatment. The response to treatment is very much an individual matter and doctors in the cancer clinics will often try a particular course of treatment, and then adjust the treatment according to the individual response.

What else could it be?

It isn't always easy to know when a headache *isn't* caused by a brain tumour, because the symptoms overlap with so many of the other possible causes of tumours. For example, brain tumours can cause paralysis or weakness of arms and legs, and alterations to the speech, and so can *migraines, strokes,* and *Transient Ischaemic Attacks* (TIAs). Brain tumours can cause vomiting; so can migraines and *meningitis.* The headache of a brain tumour is indistinguishable from many other types of headache – *tension headache,* in particular – and the continual throbbing of the headache of *high blood pressure* is much the same.

However, as noted earlier, brain tumours are rare. Unless you have a history of cancer somewhere else, or gross alteration to your movements, sensations and level of consciousness, a brain tumour is unlikely. Obviously you will want to talk to your doctor about it, but the vast probability is that the cause will be something much less frightening.

ALICE

Alice is a solicitor aged twenty-six. She'd had a boney lump removed from her pelvis which, to everyone's surprise turned out to be a malignant tumour and she was being followed up, just to make sure everything was all right.

She'd recently been on holiday in the Mediterranean, where she'd been taken ill. A golf fanatic, she played a full round in the heat of a Mediterranean summer. That evening, while in a restaurant, she had progressively felt more and more unwell. She developed a bursting headache and eventually blacked out. Fortunately, there was an English ambulanceman nearby who observed what happened to her; he reported that Alice hadn't had a fit or wet herself; she appeared just to have fainted.

The headache passed off, but two days later she woke in the middle of the night with another extremely painful, bursting headache. As soon as she got back from the holiday she went to her doctor, anxious to know whether the dehydration she suffered was responsible. But this wouldn't explain why she woke up in the middle of the night with a headache.

Her doctor examined her, but could find nothing wrong; her blood pressure was normal, she had no abnormalities of movement, and the back of the eyes (which often show changes if there are problems within the skull) were completely normal. Nevertheless her doctor had a feeling all was not right. The symptoms didn't fit together. There had been no flickering lights in the visual field, so Alice's headache was unlikely to be migraine. Her blood pressure was normal, so it wasn't that. And the pain wasn't coming from her neck, either.

Episodic violent headaches – especially ones that make you pass out – are moderately suspicious, especially if there is no hint of migraines, blood pressure, or a sub-arachnoid haemorrhage. With a sinking heart, his doctor referred her urgently back to the doctor who had done the original operation, in order to get some special tests carried out.

> *To everyone's surprise, all the tests came back negative. To everyone's delight, Alice does **not** have a brain tumour – even though there were so many indications that she might have. Compare her case with the case of Albert (see pages 154-5) in whom at first there was no inkling of a tumour, and who yet died of one.*

Orthodox treatment

Orthodox treatment depends very much on the type of tumour, and its site. In an operation, a benign tumour is often easy to winkle out of its surrounding capsule. Once the tumour has been removed, the pressure on the brain tissue is reduced, and the brain can get back to working in its normal way again.

A benign tumour in the pituitary can also be removed, in an operation going through the top of the inside of the nose and approaching it from underneath.

Often it's not possible to tell whether a tumour is benign or malignant until, at operation, bits of it can be snipped out and looked at under the microscope (a biopsy). Even if the tumour is malignant, all is not lost. Removing the area containing the tumour may be enough to get out all the cells, particularly if it is the primary site. Giving radiotherapy or chemotherapy afterwards may also help to kill off any remaining malignant cells.

Where the cancers are secondary treatment is quite different. Once a tumour has moved to the brain, it is likely to have spread elsewhere; and there won't be just one growth within the brain. There will probably be a number, scattered throughout the brain tissue, all growing independently of the others. Clearly it's not possible to remove all these secondary deposits in an operation. Therefore, we usually try to kill off secondary growths with radiotherapy or chemotherapy.

Radiotherapy involves shining various types of high-powered electro-magnetic rays (or in some cases, nuclear particles) at the tumour. Chemotherapy involves giving anti-cancer drugs, which are often very potent and also very toxic to normal body cells. Both these therapies work because cancer cells grow much more rapidly than do nerves (in fact nerves hardly grow at all). So, by specifically attacking those cells that are rapidly dividing, we target the effects of the chemicals and the X-rays on to malignant cells rather than those which are normal.

Chemotherapy and radiotherapy do, however, have the disadvantage of interfering with rapidly dividing *normal* body cells, such as the gut, hair follicles and bone marrow. This is why chemotherapy can make you temporarily bald. Both types of therapy can make you feel nauseous and generally unwell.

The big advantage of chemotherapy is that it attacks the cells that are rapidly dividing *wherever they are*. It doesn't matter if one or two little groups of cells have seeded off and stuck in a part of the brain, well away from the other growths. The chemotherapy will get to those cells and will kill them off just as effectively as if they were part of the main group of malignant cells.

It's a common mistake to think that surgery is better than radiotherapy or chemotherapy 'because you can be sure everything's been taken away'. In fact, this isn't true. Although surgery may appear to remove everything that is malignant, this is not always possible. When there is doubt, chemotherapy and radiotherapy can often mop up cancer cells which the surgeon has not managed to remove.

Hormone therapy can also play a part, especially in secondary cancers derived from breast cancer. Many breast cancers need oestrogen to survive and by giving the anti-oestrogen drug tamoxifen, oestrogen receptors on the malignant cells can be blocked.

What about treatment of the headache from a brain tumour? The method of treatment is entirely dependent upon whether the tumour is benign or malignant. The pain of a benign tumour is almost always due to a general pressure rise within the skull, whereas local pressure gives localised side-effects – such as inability to speak. (This is why headaches are usually a later symptom, while localised effects on the brain occur earlier in the illness.) Remove the tumour, and the pressure goes away.

With a malignant tumour, pain is also usually related to pressure; but, in this case, it may be much harder, if not impossible, to remove the tumour. If the tumour is so far advanced, or else in such a position that surgery is impossible, then there are several courses of action that your doctor might take. Anything that shrinks the tumour is likely to remove or reduce the amount of headache, so radiotherapy, chemotherapy, or hormone therapy may help. In addition, steroid treatment may reduce the pressure; in particular, the drug dexamethasone can be amazingly effective in reducing the pressure within the brain, thus reducing headaches and vomiting, and allowing the brain generally to work much better.

But what about those many cases where the primary tumour has spread too far, or else the tumours are secondary and have got out of control?

Surprisingly, aspirin is enormously important for pain relief. While 'strong' drugs such as morphine are sometimes unable to provide adequate pain relief, simple analgesics such as aspirin can do the trick. The pain of secondary cancer of the bone is often markedly improved with aspirin, which can make all the difference.

Self-help
The best way to avoid problems caused by cancer of the brain, skull or neck is not to *worry* about them. There are more people who suffer from worry that they have cancer of these organs than there are people who have the cancer itself!

Self-help comes down to being realistic. By all means tell your doctor of your fears, especially if you have symptoms that could be the result of a brain tumour.. And you should certainly see your doctor if you have persistent symptoms and have previously had cancer elsewhere in the body.

But as far as your headache is concerned, be prepared to be reassured by your doctor, and don't worry about it.

Complementary treatment
There are many side-effects to orthodox medical treatment that can be relieved by complementary therapies. Radiotherapy often causes itching skin, soreness around the area being treated, and a general feeling of tiredness. Cystitis, diarrhoea and fear, are also common symptoms. Chemotherapy can

cause nausea, loss of appetite, hair loss and soreness of the digestive system (ulcers and lesions). The trauma involved with all of this, as well as the general debilitating effects on the system, can cause headaches as well.

While complementary therapies do not (or at least should not) claim to cure cancer, certain therapies can help the body fight the disease, and recover from orthodox treatment. It is important to talk to your doctor and your complementary therapist about all the treatments you are undergoing. In disease as serious as cancer, mismatched treatments can be fatal.

Aromatherapy is an excellent way to relax and recover, but should never be undertaken immediately after chemotherapy. Bathing and massage can often irritate sore skin. The best means of using the oils is inhalation – a vapouriser or a gentle bath blend – perhaps rose and geranium, which may help fight fear and depression, and fennel to help with nausea. Niaouli and tea tree have been used in Europe to reduce surface burning during radiation treatment, and lavender has been used to treat radiation burns. Rosemary is said to stimulate re-growth of hair. Lavender applied to the nostrils or in the bath with camomile, can reduce the headaches linked with brain cancers.

Acupuncture is valuable when dealing with the side-effects of cancers, as listed above, and will help to relieve pain and depression. There are, controversially, reports from China that indicate that acupuncture stimulates our body's anti-cancer substances. Chinese acupuncturists also claim that it boosts the body's immune system.

A homoeopath will prepare a package of remedies individually suited to your symptoms. These might include galium album, clematis and echinacea.

Medical herbalism can relieve some of the symptoms of cancer, and encourage the immune system to work against it. All treatment must be tailored to complement the orthodox treatments being received. There will be options for pain relief, depression (St John's wort) and nausea (ginger, peppermint or fennel), and calendula promotes healing of skin. Echinacea and garlic, taken internally, improve resistance to secondary infections. There are many many options to help your body deal with the cancer and the side-effects of treatment – both of which can cause headaches.

Nutrition is particularly important in cancer. A strong, healthy constitution is much more likely to have a fighting chance, and to respond better to treatment. Pain can be kept at bay by daily doses of phenylalanine, Supplementation of selenium may also help. under the guidance of a clinical nutritionalist. Some research suggests that it affects enzymatic processes that may inhibit the activation of some cancer cells. There is no doubt that it does have some anti-cancer properties. A good B-vitamin supplement will also help deal with the feeling of malaise, and Vitamin D is said to be useful. Sensible eating, perhaps a macrobiotic diet , is beneficial to some cancer patients.

Reflexology can help deal with the emotional repercussions of cancer, and speed up recovery after an operation.

Chapter Thirteen

TEMPORAL ARTERITIS

Connective tissue in the body consists of strands of tissue lying between and inside the organs. Like all other parts of the body, the connective tissue can go wrong, and there's a group of conditions called the *connective tissue disorders,* in which the body becomes allergic to elements of its own connective tissue. As connective tissue is found in organs throughout the whole body, the inflammation this causes can be widespread. Fortunately, they are quite rare and only one of the connective tissue disorders – temporal arteritis – is a significant cause of headaches. It's not a common disease, but it's important as, untreated, it can cause blindness, almost overnight.

The temple is the area of your head roughly between and above the eye socket and the ear. Across each temple runs the temporal artery. In temporal arteritis, the connective tissue inside this artery becomes very inflamed. As a result, the artery becomes much more prominent and very tender to the touch; at the same time there may be a severe headache. You may lose weight, and feel generally unwell in a non-specific way. There is often generalised scalp tenderness, and your muscles may ache over the whole of your body. And, finally, some patients get severe aching in the jaw muscles, on chewing. This ache quickly disappears when they stop chewing, and returns when they start again.

The importance of temporal arteritis lies not in the headache, but because it's not just the temporal artery that is affected. The single artery which supplies the eyeball, the *ophthalmic artery* can also become inflamed; when it does it swells up on the inside, and in doing so blocks itself off, reducing or cutting off the supply of blood to the eye. Unfortunately, the retina is very delicate. It can't survive for long without a blood supply, and if its blood supply fails, blindness can result, overnight. It's a worrying prospect; fortunately, the doctor can stop this happening, provided the diagnosis of temporal arteritis is made quickly and treatment with high dose steroids started immediately.

Temporal arteritis typically affects those over sixty. It's not always an easy diagnosis to make; the symptoms are often vague, and could point to a number of potential causes. Clinically the most significant pointer is that the temporal arteries are prominent, and *tender,* though it's not always easy to determine whether tenderness over the temples is due to tender arteries or underlying tender *muscles,* in spasm, as in a tension headache.

To clinch the diagnosis the doctor will take a blood sample and measure its ESR (Erythrocyte Sedimentation Rate). High ESRs occur in only a few types of illness – connective tissue disorders, cancers, rheumatoid arthritis and severe long-standing infections. For the doctor, pain in the side of the head, tender temporal arteries, and a high ESR confirm the diagnosis.

In the past, one of the ways of making the diagnosis was to take a small piece out of the temporal artery itself and look at it under the microscope. (Technically this is called taking a biopsy.) Interestingly, after this procedure some cases seemed to improve simply because the biopsy had been taken!

Over the years, temporal arteritis is sometimes a self-limiting disease; about a third of patients can eventually manage without their steroids, but it may take as long as seven years before steroids can safely be withdrawn. In two thirds of cases, it isn't possible to withdraw steroids at all. However, just because the disease may eventually go away doesn't reduce the need for steroid treatment while you've got it. If you don't take the steroids you may become permanently blind, without warning, perhaps overnight.

Although steroids reduce the risk of blindness, giving them doesn't seem to shorten the life cycle of the disease itself. Naturally the doctor will want to use as low a dose as possible, to reduce side effects. However, the dose mustn't be brought too low or relapses can occur.

Again, untreated temporal arteritis can progress to blindness. Unfortunately, once you've gone blind from temporal arteritis, nothing can be done to bring back your sight. Once the supply of blood has been shut off to the retina, the retinal cells die. They can never grow again, or be replaced, even if the blood supply to the eye is restored.

Type of headache
The pain can be throbbing over the eye, or in the temple region – but the headache can just as easily be in the back of the head or neck. Locally, however, the temples are often tender; so is the scalp.

What else could it be?
The pain from temporal arteritis is relatively non-specific and many other causes of headache can imitate it. *Tension headache* (which is often perceived in the forehead and side of the head) gives the same type of pain, often with tenderness of the *muscles* in the temple. In temporal arteritis, however, the artery itself is tender. Also, temporal arteritis is almost unknown under the age of fifty five, whereas tension headache is often seen in much younger patients.

Cancer is also a possible alternative diagnosis, because weight loss, a general feeling of being ill, loss of appetite, and a high ESR are often features of cancer. However, cancer doesn't cause tenderness of the temporal artery, nor does it cause the stiff generalised muscle ache of temporal arteritis.

Orthodox treatment
As with all the auto-immune illnesses, high doses of steroid usually sort out the problem very quickly indeed; the pain goes, the ESR drops, the headaches disappear and the risk of blindness vanishes. The good news is that the response is speedy: the bad news is that you may need to take steroids for a long time – months and years, possibly even for life, but the choice is stark – take the steroids or risk losing your sight.

One way to monitor the progress of the disease is by repeatedly measuring the ESR. The initial dose of steroids will be high, maybe as much as sixty mg in twenty four hours. As soon as steroids are given the high ESR quickly reduces, and the doctor will adjust the dose of steroid according to whether the ESR has gone back to normal or not. The dose needed varies from patient to patient.

Once the dose has been adjusted your doctor will want to monitor the progress of the disease regularly. Good control of temporal arteritis is achieved through a combination of monitoring the ESR and making sure that your symptoms don't return. At the same time your doctor will want to make sure that you are on the minimum dose of steroids that is compatible with achieving both these objectives.

Treatment is often long term, possibly even for life, though sometimes it is possible to tail off the steroids entirely after some years. Please note: after long term use of steroids, stopping or reducing the dose should *always* be done *very slowly*, and only *ever* done with the express permission of your doctor.

Self-help
If you think you've got temporal arteritis see your doctor *immediately*.

<u>Complementary treatment</u>
Like any of the other emergency conditions, temporal arteritis is too dangerous to waste time trying complementary therapies. Any delay in giving steroids to someone suffering from temporal arteritis may result in permanent blindness. If you suspect that you are suffering from this condition, consult your doctor, or the emergency services immediately.

Following the illness, you may benefit from some complementary therapies, to reduce the fear of recurrence, and the stress involved in any frightening illness, and to stimulate your body's ability to heal itself, and react well to the medical treatment you are receiving.

Acupuncture, acupressure and reflexology, will reduce the headaches that accompany stress, anxiety and fear. All offer relaxation therapies.

Bach flower remedies can be taken internally, or rubbed on pulse points immediately following an attack, and any time that fear or shock threatens to set in. Certainly many of the flower remedies can treat the subsequent psychological effects of temporal arteritis, particularly if there is any partial blindness, or simply fear of the disease recurring.

Rejuvenating aromatherapy treatments would include massage, baths or vapourisation with: sandalwood, frankincense, jasmine, rose, lavender and neroli. There are also oils which will deal specifically with your symptoms, whether they are persistent headaches, depression, lack of energy or general pain. Consult a registered practitioner for a customised programme.

A good vitamin and mineral supplement will help restore a weakened system, and royal jelly is a good all round nutrient source.

See the section on strokes, for more ideas about dealing with post illness symptoms.

FRED

Fred is a cheery old age pensioner, now in his seventy fifth year. Five years ago he came to his GP complaining of tenderness over both temples, together with pain over the eyes. The pain was intense, and his temporal arteries were very prominent and tender to the touch.

Clinically it looked as if Fred had temporal arteritis. The ESR was 75, so the doctor gave Fred a prescription for prednisolone (a cortico steroid), of forty mg a day.

Three days after starting the steroids his pain had almost gone. He felt very much better in himself, though there was still an ache behind the eyes first thing in the morning; by now the temporal arteries were much less prominent.

Over the next two months his doctor gradually reduced his dose of steroids to fifteen mg a day without incident; five months later he was down to ten mg a day. Two years later, Fred had had no further problems and no return of his symptoms, so the consultant suggested that it would be worth trying to withdraw the steroids completely.

Fred's GP had to do this slowly, warning Fred to contact him immediately if his symptoms returned, and monitoring his progress with regular measurements of the ESR. In addition, if the steroids were reduced too quickly, there was a possibility that Fred might collapse.

So Fred carefully reduced his daily dose of steroids by one mg every fortnight. Unfortunately, every time he went below seven mg a day Fred's eyes started to become sore again; and, after a discussion, everyone (including Fred) decided that it would be far better to give up any idea of reducing the dose any further. Fred is happy to take this relatively low dose of steroids for the rest of his life. He knows the consequences if things go wrong, and he would rather be on a low dose of steroids like this than risk losing his sight.

Fred's GP is happy too. He knows Fred is now on the lowest possible safe dose of steroids; and just needs to see him from time to time for a blood test.

Chapter Fourteen

EYE PROBLEMS

The eyeball is a sphere about the size of a ping-pong ball. Light comes in through the transparent *cornea,* which begins the process of focusing. Behind the cornea, the coloured *iris* controls the amount of light allowed in through the black hole of the *pupil.* Behind the pupil, the *lens* focuses light on to the light-sensitive *retina,* which lies on the inside of the eyeball, at the back.

Between the lens and the retina the eye is filled with a clear jelly-like fluid called *vitreous humour,* while in front of the lens is a much thinner liquid, the *aqueous humour* .

The pupil changes size in bright or dim light in order to control the amount of light falling on to the retina. In dim light the iris relaxes, pulling back to leave a large central pupil, which lets in more light. In bright light the iris contracts, narrowing the pupil to little more than a pinhole, and cutting off most of the light.

GLAUCOMA

High pressure inside the eyeball is called *glaucoma.* It tends to attack those who are over the age of forty, and there is a genetic element involved, so if any of your relatives have glaucoma, you have a higher chance of suffering from it yourself.

Aqueous humour (the liquid filling the front part of the eyeball) is constantly being created by the iris, and it constantly drains out of the eye through channels at the base of the iris. If this drainage channel gets obstructed, this fluid has no way out. Fluid is difficult to compress, and because aqueous humour is still being created, when its outflow is obstructed the pressure inside the eyeball rises dramatically.

Normally, the onset of glaucoma is quite subtle – the raised pressure in the eye gives no symptoms, except that the eyeball feels slightly more firm to the touch. However, this excess pressure has an unfortunate effect on the delicate light-receptive cells of the retina; these cells are very susceptible to pressure and are damaged, and even killed off, if the pressure rises for any length of time. The visual field (the amount you can see with your eyes stationary) become smaller and smaller, and 'holes' develop as the cells in the retina are gradually and progressively destroyed. Usually this destruction starts at the outer edge of the visual field so its effects are hardly noticed at first by the sufferer. But it's easy for an optician to test the visual field, and the changes will be very obvious. If left unchecked, a glaucoma sufferer will eventually lose his sight.

Although glaucoma is usually a slow, silent disease, in cases where the pressure rises swiftly, it *can* strike suddenly. The word *acute* means 'of sudden onset', and *chronic* means *long-term and continuing*. There are two types of glaucoma: chronic glaucoma (i.e., continuing and long-term), and acute glaucoma (i.e., sudden).

In *acute glaucoma*, the eyeball suddenly becomes excrucuatingly painful and tender. Sometimes the pain radiates into the head or chest, but most of the time it appears to come from the eyeball itself, which is very tender to the touch. The pupil is irregular and often oval instead of round, and can have a crinkly edge. The iris may be dull grey, cloudy, or grey-green, and streaked with blood vessels. All these changes happen to the structures situated underneath the cornea – the clear part of the eye. Redness of the *white* of the eye is not related to glaucoma; this is conjunctivitis, which is quite different.

Sudden onset of glaucoma like this is very rare, but exceedingly painful. The patient will get sudden *severe* pain in the eye; he may also see coloured haloes around bright lights, either before or during the attack, and then the vision in the affected eye will get slowly worse until in a really bad attack he can barely make out the difference between light and dark.

If glaucoma isn't treated properly, it may result in blindness. Chronic glaucoma can be just as devastating to the vision as the more painful acute variety. *Chronic* glaucoma is a long-term rise in eye pressure; while *acute* glaucoma is an episode in which there is a sudden increase in pressure – often on top of chronic glaucoma that existed already.

For various reasons, some people permanently have a higher-than-normal pressure inside the eye. On its own, a chronic glaucoma like this can be painless, but in the long term the extra pressure will still damage the retina.

In acute glaucoma, the drainage of aqueous humour is *suddenly* interrupted, and so the pressure inside the eye rises quickly, causing pain and altered vision.

Why should the pressure rise inside the eyeball? In chronic glaucoma it may be because there is a general furring up of the holes from which the aqueous humour drains – but we're not completely sure. Acute glaucoma is different, and patients who have these sudden attacks often have a slightly smaller angle between the base of the iris and the eyeball. When the iris opens to let in more light, its muscles retract, folding up on themselves rather in the manner of an Austrian blind. In people with a narrow angle at the base of the iris, the folded iris more easily obstructs the exit channel for the aqueous humour.

Acute glaucoma occurs almost entirely in people with this narrow drainage angle, which is more easily obstructed by the retracting iris. Those who are long-sighted are more at risk because they tend to have a smaller-sized eyeball, with a shallower front part to it.

The first attack of glaucoma often starts when the light fades, which causes the pupil to dilate and the iris to open out. An alternative reason for glaucoma starting can be emotion, such as fear, which also causes the pupil to open and the iris to retract. As the pressure begins to rise at the beginning of an attack, the patient starts to see haloes round bright objects – and then the pain sets in.

Type of pain
In acute glaucoma the pain is appalling, and often all that the patient can do is lie down in agony. He will probably be nauseous and vomit. The pain starts in and around the eye, though it can be felt in other places such as forehead, neck or even chest. Vision may suddenly go, to the point where you can only just perceive light, and light may hurt your eyes.

What else could it be?
Light can hurt the eyes in a number of conditions – such as *meningitis* – but this is quite different from the severe pain of glaucoma, where the eyeball itself is tender to the touch, and where the vision is blurred or fading.

The pain of glaucoma centres on one eye (sometimes both). This is exactly the same as the pain of *migraine, or cluster headache* which also seems to be centred on one eye. Similarly, referred pain from a severe *tension headache* or *neck problem* may also seem to be coming from the eyeball itself. *Sinusitis* can produce pain that is near to the eye socket.

A history of seeing haloes round lights, pain in the eye, and dimness of vision, plus a family history of glaucoma, all point in the direction of an acute glaucoma attack. The most obvious signs to the doctor are the changes that are happening within the eye itself – the dimness of vision, the cloudiness of the pupil, the irregular edge of the iris, and the increase in pressure. Glaucoma can also be spotted with the *ophthalmoscope* – the torch-like piece of equipment that the doctor uses to examine the eyes – as glaucoma produces characteristic changes in the retina.

Orthodox treatment
Fortunately, treatment for glaucoma is effective, but it's important to start it as soon as possible, in order to minimise damage to the sensitive retina. Because a retracted iris blocks the drainage holes and increases the pressure, we want to keep the iris contracted and the pupil small, so that the muscle of the iris keeps out of the way of the drainage holes. Therefore, your doctor will give eye drops that cause the iris to close up to a pinpoint. Frequently a drug called pilocarpine, or another called timolol, are used to do this. Either or both are given regularly, as drops may be all that is necessary to ensure that the pupil remains small.

If the drops don't work, a drug called acetazolamide can be given in tablet form, to reduce the pressure by reducing the formation of aqueous humour. Sometimes even this is not enough, and then an operation (a sclerectomy) to make a small, artificial drainage hole may be necessary. After this operation, even if the iris does dilate in dim light, it will not block the drainage holes.

Self-help

As with anything, prevention is better than cure. If you have a family history of glaucoma, then make sure you get your eyes checked regularly.

It's important to have your glaucoma diagnosed, because you can do many things to reduce the number of attacks. Anything which causes the iris to relax and the pupil to open decreases the drainage of the aqueous humour and may cause an attack. Low levels of light cause the pupil to open up, but there's no need to go around constantly seeking bright surroundings, because the eyedrops will constrict the pupil very adequately.

More importantly, many drugs have the side-effect of relaxing the iris. Atropine is one. Some medicines have atropine-like side-effects, including many anti-depressants. Your doctor will be able to tell you about any possible side-effects that the drugs you are taking might have.

If you have glaucoma, it's worth reminding your doctor about it *every time he prescribes for you.* It's easy for your doctor to forget you've got glaucoma when he's treating you for, say, abdominal pains.

What about treatment of the acute attack? Fortunately, acute attacks are rare, now that we detect and control chronic glaucoma. Obviously, in an acute attack you need the doctor urgently. In a sudden attack of glaucoma, heat is sometimes effective. You can apply heat safely to the eye in the following way. Get a bowl of near boiling water, and a wooden spoon. Wrap some cotton-wool around the end of the spoon, dip it in the water and *gradually* bring it near to the *closed* eye, keeping the eye as hot as you can bear. When the cotton wool pad starts to feel cool, dip it back in the water and repeat the process. Also, a pad over the affected eye will stop light getting in, helping in those cases where light itself is painful.

Both these methods should only be employed to relieve the pain while the eye-drops are taking effect. They should not be used instead of proper medical treatment.

Complementary treatment

Acute glaucoma is a medical emergency. If you are suffering from any of the symptoms, contact your doctor immediately. While awaiting attention, belladonna can be taken in homoeopathic *doses every fifteen minutes. Pain and fear can be controlled by Bach flower remedies, especially Rescue Remedy, which can be rubbed into the temples while waiting for help.*

Because eye drops and, in severe cases, a minor operation, deal so effectively with glaucoma, there hasn't been a great need for the alternative options found in complementary medicine.

However, acupuncture can deal with any pain following attacks, as can shiatsu. Both claim to open channels within the body, hopefully preventing further blockages.

Elderflower gel can relieve any pain or discomfort caused by glaucoma. Lavender, camomile, melissa, basil and clary sage in the bath or in a vapouriser will help to relieve the headaches caused by glaucoma. Wormwood on cotton wool reduces eye inflammation.

See the post-illness suggestions in chapter Nine, for general tips to recovering from sudden attacks on the system, and maintaining health and well-being.

EYE STRAIN

Focusing

Normally our eyes work well, bringing an image of what we're looking at into crisp focus on the retina at the back of the eye. Objects at different distances have to be brought into focus differently, and the way the eye changes its focus is by altering the shape of the lens inside it. Contrary to what most people imagine, most focusing is done by the cornea: the lens merely adds the finishing touches!

The lens is a squashy bag, stretched outwards by being attached round the whole of its circumference to a circular muscle, which is itself attached on its outer margin to the inside of the eyeball. When the muscle contracts it reduces the size of the central hole. This means that the lens isn't pulled outwards as firmly. As a result, the tension on the lens slackens off, allowing it to change from being thin into being fat and bulky with a more highly curved surface. Because a fat and bulky lens bends the light more, when the lens is fat it can bring nearer objects into sharp focus on the retina. When the muscle relaxes the central hole opens, and there is a greater pull on the outside of the lens, causing it to become less globular and more disc-like.

However, sometimes we don't focus quite as well as we would like. In older age, the pliability of the lens may be reduced so it can't focus properly and you may need glasses to see for both distances and close-up. Secondly, because of the way the physics of focusing works, those with slightly smaller eyes tend to be long-sighted, and those with bigger than average eyes, short-sighted.

In addition, the lens or cornea may not be perfectly symmetrical, in which case *astigmatism* occurs. This means that the eye can't focus on both vertical and horizontal lines at the same time. Further, because of the physics of light and lenses, focusing is more critical if the aperture of the lens is large. This makes it harder to focus in dim conditions, when the pupil of the eye opens and more of the lens is used to collect light. A slightly short-sighted person may find that he can focus on distant objects in bright light, but cannot in dim light. By experience we soon find out that we can see slightly better by half-shutting our eyes and peering. This, of course, tenses up all the muscles round the eye and can cause headaches.

Constantly refocusing the lens also causes discomfort. If the muscles of the lens are constantly altering focus, they will become fatigued, especially in the case of astigmatism. Just as tiring are the effects of trying to focus on an object that is just outside the normal focusing ability of the eye. The extra muscular effort that we use on these occasions can cause considerable discomfort and pain in the eyes – the so-called 'eye strain'. This is usually much worse after long periods of reading or other close work, and goes away after a period of rest, when the eyes are used for less concentrated activities. The ache can be in the eyes, in the forehead, or in the temple.

A quick way to check whether this is happening to you is to look at a book at your normal reading distance and then bring it towards you until it's about half as near. If you feel pain in your eyes when you try to look at the printing at the nearer distance, then you may well be suffering headaches due to eye strain.

People who are short-sighted usually have no difficulty in close work and reading, and it is interesting that the pain of eye strain usually affects only those who are long-sighted, or who have astigmatism. Pain usually occurs only where there are *minor* eye problems, because only this type of problem can be removed by muscular activity.

Finally, eye strain also occurs if your glasses are no longer right for you; perhaps they are over-strong, or else you've had them a long time and they're too weak. You may also find your eyes aching the first time you use new glasses, but as you get used to them this should go away – by the end of about a week. If the discomfort persists, check with your optician that your glasses have been made to the correct prescription.

Don't forget, too, that eye-sight can change quite rapidly. Regular visits to the optician are the only way to be sure that your glasses are still appropriate.

The treatment for these eye defects is quite simple; make sure that you go to an optician regularly and, if necessary, obtain spectacles.

Complementary treatment
There are a number of tried and tested home remedies for eye-strain. Try lying down with a cucumber slice on each eye which is cooling and refreshing. A camomile tea compress or rinse eases painful eyes and eye muscles. Witch hazel can be used as a compress for strained eyes. Rosehip teabags over the eyes for fifteen minutes relieves strain.

You can also take eyebright internally to strengthen eyes. Ruta, a homoeopathic remedy, may help relieve eye-strain after reading, etc. Arnica, nat mur or phosphorus may also be suggested.

Relaxation will help ease eye-strain.

Rubbing your temples with jasmine, camomile or lavender essential oils will relieve headaches caused by eye-strain. Shiatsu can ease tired and swollen eyes.

SQUINT
Each of our eyes has six muscles which move the eyeball to point in the direction we want to look. Normally these muscles work in concert, so that both eyes move to fix on the same object, but when one or more muscles are paralysed, too short or too contracted, a squint results. Again, minor degrees of abnormality can be overcome by using the muscles of the eye more than usual; the extra muscle tension from doing this is likely to cause headaches.

There are two ways to treat a squint: firstly, to go on using the eyes, using procedures and exercises to strengthen the muscles; secondly, if necessary, to operate on the eye muscles to re-position them so that the eye no longer turns in (or out).

One word of warning: The way in which the brain processes information means that a child with a squint soon learns to ignore the information coming from the squinting eye, *which may therefore go blind*. It is therefore enormously important to spot a child who is developing a squint.

The critical time can be surprisingly early in a child's development. Before the age of seven it is often possible to correct a squint, so that the child no longer ignores information coming from the squinting eye.

Even though a child may have *vision* out of each eye, still she may well not develop proper depth vision, especially in those squints that always were constant.

Large squints are therefore a considerable hazard to the development of normal vision, but squints like this don't usually cause headaches. It is the minor degrees of squint that cause the excess muscle tension associated with headaches.

Type of headache
The headache of eye-strain is at the front of the face and forehead. It is often worse after reading, or other close work.

What else could it be?
Tension headache is often perceived over the forehead or round the eyes. *Temporal arteritis* is associated with tenderness of the arteries in the temples – and also, unfortunately, with sudden blindness.

Many people with headaches ask if it could be due to eye-strain: the only sure way to find out is to see an optician and get a full check on your eye-sight, including (in children) a test to check for squinting.

Self-help
If you have symptoms that sound like eye-strain – pain in the eyes, which is worse after reading or intensive close work, and which goes away after a period of rest – then the remedy may be simple. Have your eyes checked. And use the glasses that the optician suggests.

The biggest problem comes with those whose vision is good enough to do without glasses on most occasions, but not quite good enough to be able to see properly without screwing up the eyes slightly.

Dim light makes focusing that much more difficult and someone with more or less normal vision in bright light may be quite severely short-sighted under dim conditions. A person like this may only need to use her glasses in dim light – such as in theatres and cinemas, when driving at night, and also when watching television. However, if she doesn't use her glasses in dim conditions, she's likely to get tense muscles from straining the eyes.

This obviously brings up a convenient way to reduce eye-strain – don't work in dim light. The older we are, the more light we need in order to see properly and if we can't see properly we tend to peer and strain and tense up those muscles around the eye again. To read clear print, a sixty-year-old person will need up to fifteen times as much light as a child at school, and ten times as much light as a twenty to thirty-year-old.

Special problems with spectacles

Two specific problems that have a direct bearing on headaches can arise when using spectacles. Firstly, as more and more people are using computers it becomes important to be able to see the screen clearly. We look at the computer screen from considerably further than the distance at which we read a book, so glasses that are correct for reading may not be quite right for looking at the computer screen. If you seem to get eye-strain after a lot of computer work, it may be a good idea to get the optician to check your eyes at the distance at which you normally view the computer screen. In some circumstances, and particularly when you are doing a lot of work at the computer or VDU, it may be appropriate to get glasses specially made for that purpose.

ALAN

Alan is a fifty-year-old man who works in the civil service. He was suffering from headaches and eye-strain. His work involved using a computer, but he found it difficult to focus on the screen because the glasses he used didn't seem to be quite right. If he didn't use glasses then he couldn't see his papers properly, and if he used his reading glasses he couldn't see the computer screen or his clients. In fact, he'd got into the habit of pulling his reading glasses halfway down his nose and peering over the top of them in order to try to get all the various things he needed in focus at the right time. Then, because his glasses were so far down his nose, when he wanted to look at papers in his hands he had to throw his head back to view them through his reading glasses.

Even so, when he looked at his computer screen or the top of his glasses, most of the world was slightly fuzzy, so he screwed up his eyes in order to bring the tiny lettering on the screen into focus. Once he realised his headaches were a mixture of eye-strain, reflex spasm of the muscles around the eyes, and neck strain, his problems became much simpler. His doctor suggested that Alan tell his employer of the difficulties he was having, and make sure that he had an optician's appointment. This he did, and he returned with a set of glasses that were appropriate for reading at the distance of the computer screen. These he found much more comfortable and was able at long last to get the computer screen in proper focus.

As a result of getting the right glasses, he no longer had to screw up his eyes, or tilt his head; his headaches improved without the need for any medication.

A specific problem causing headaches can occur in some people who use bifocals. The line between the lower and the upper lenses creates an odd blurred effect, and it isn't easy to look at something through this area of the glasses. Unfortunately, the normal angle at which we hold the head means this line often falls just at the top of the page we're trying to look at. It is not uncommon to see people with bifocals putting their head back slightly in order to be able to read the top few lines of the piece of paper they're holding in their hand..

Unfortunately, bending the head backwards in this way strains the joint between two vertebrae in the neck which, after a period of four or five years, can give rise to headaches. It is much better if you keep your head where it ought to be and use your hands to move the book down slightly so that you can read the top line of the page without cocking back your head. Alternatively, get a multi-focal lens with a gradation in strength over the whole of the visual field, with no sharp cut-off. Because there is no cut-off line there is less need to cock the head back.

Glare
Too much light can cause just as many problems as too little light: too much light causes us to screw up our eyes tightly, causing muscle tension and headaches.

What else could it be?
Quite a number of conditions causing headache can also give eye symptoms. These have all been covered in other areas of this book.

• *Pain radiating from one eye can occur as a result of migraine or cluster headache.*

• Herpes zoster, (*shingles*), is a painful skin infection which can attack both the eye, and the skin of the forehead above the eye.

• *Cervical spondylosis* and *arthritis of the neck* can in certain circumstances cause severe spasm in the muscles of the neck, which creates pain that appears to radiate out of one eye.

• Pain behind the eyes or just above the eyes in the forehead is often associated with *muscle spasm* in the neck, particularly the upper part of the neck. *Tension headaches* caused in this way often cause eye pain.

• Although flashing lights in the eye tend to be associated with migraine, in pregnant women they can also be associated with *pre-eclampsia.*

• Blurred vision can be associated with focusing problems that require spectacles. It can also be a symptom of *high blood pressure, acute glaucoma*, and *uraemia.*

• A *tumour of the pituitary gland* can 'pinch' the visual field to produce 'tunnel vision', in which there is loss of peripheral vision. Sometimes a *brain tumour* stops the patient seeing one sector of his visual field.

• *Permanent* blindness can occur in *temporal arteritis* and glaucoma (see above); and *brain and pituitary tumours* can each cause progressive blindness as a result of pressure on the nerves. Usually the loss of vision is progressive, but sometimes can be halted or reversed by prompt treatment. *Temporary* loss of vision with a headache is usually caused by *migraine*.

Chapter Fifteen

DENTAL CAUSES

There are two main dental causes of headache – toothache and an abnormal bite.

TOOTHACHE

Occasionally toothache can mimic a headache. The teeth are notorious for causing pain which is felt in a completely different site; the technical term for this is *referred pain*. The teeth can cause referred pain in wildly different sites and this is the reason why dentists sometimes find it hard to isolate which tooth is the source of the pain, and may drill several fillings out before they find the culprit.

A small amount of dental decay (otherwise known as caries) at the bottom of an otherwise normal-looking and well-filled tooth can cause tremendous pain when it extends to infect the pulp space deep within the tooth (the pulp space is the only live bit of the tooth). In turn, infection of the pulp space can track down to the very bottom of the tooth and cause infection in the jaw. Infection here is called an *apical abscess*. The pain of an infected or decaying tooth can be referred into the head or the neck, and in some cases can mimic headaches, particularly tension headaches and sinusitis.

Toothache can be diagnosed where there is obvious infection or decay in a tooth; or where the tooth is tender on being knocked or touched. One of the first features of a pulp space infection is that the tooth feels as though it has lifted up slightly, and is more easily banged by the opposing set of teeth when clenching the teeth together. An apical abscess can also make the gum tender at the level of the top of the root of the tooth, about a quarter of an inch below the gum margin. In the very late stages of an apical abscess there may be an obvious boil or discharging abscess at this site. This is called a gum boil.

What else could it be?

Dental pain can be confused with *sinusitis*, especially as dental pain (particularly where there is pulp space infection or an apical abscess) is often made worse by putting the head between the knees; dental pain and the sinusitis pain behave identically in this situation. *Tension headache* can imitate dental pain, too, but here there are trigger points on the neck, face or scalp – touching these exacerbates the pain. However, because of the way in which pain is referred from teeth, it can often cause reflex spasm in muscles at some distance from the actual site of the pain, so local tenderness in the muscles of the head or neck does not necessarily rule out a dental cause.

Treatment
Obviously dental work is required; to scrape out the inside of the infected tooth, maybe root-fill it, or perhaps perform an *apicectomy*, if there is an apical abscess. .

Self-help
Simple, minor tooth decay doesn't cause pain. The problems occur when nothing has been done and the decay has been allowed to advance. So, simply have regular dental check-ups and brush your teeth regularly with a fluoride toothpaste.

Brushing your teeth *properly* is important. It's not just the teeth that you need to clean, but also the gums. It's worth remembering that as many teeth are lost by gum disease as they are to tooth decay. Unfortunately, it is all too easy for scraps of food to collect between the tooth and the gums, where they begin to fester and set up an infection called gingivitis. Gingivitis can be almost as painful as toothache: typically it's much worse with hot and cold foods, and can be eased substantially by careful attention to brushing the teeth.

Complementary treatment
Obviously severe toothache caused by decay should be treated by your dentist, but there are a number of treatments for pain and inflammation that will provide some relief during attacks. Cloves have an analgesic oil contained in them and they can either be bitten whole, next to the offending tooth, or their oil can be applied neat to the painful area.

An infusion of marshmallow and sage can be used as a mouth rinse, and then swallowed. Mint also has antiseptic and analgesic properties and can be chewed or sucked at the site of the pain. Gum disease can be treated by chewing tarragon, sage and thyme, or by rubbing oil of thyme into the gums. Vitamin C is essential to gum health, so ensure you are getting enough.

Rinse your mouth daily with hypericum and calendula, mixed with cooled, boiled water, to prevent infection. A hot compress of camomile over the cheek, will ease the pain and draw the infection to the surface, if an abscess is present.

There are many different homoeopathic remedies available – and they will deal specifically with the kind of pain you are suffering, whether you have abscesses, or gingivitis, etc. Some suggestions are arnica, kali phos, silica and camomile. There are even homoeopathic remedies to deal with the fear of dental treatment, and discomfort following treatment.

Reflexology can sometimes ease toothache, Acupressure and acupuncture can deal with local pain, and also fear, tension and headaches.

ABNORMALITIES OF THE BITE

The second dental cause of headaches is a poor bite. For most of us our bite is something we take for granted. We just close our teeth together, and that's it. In fact, we only notice our bite if we've been for dental work where either a more prominent tooth has been removed – so the mouth closes slightly more than it normally did on that side – or else we've had a filling which has been left ever so slightly proud and suddenly our teeth seem to bang together, with the jaw rocking around on that slightly protruding filling.

Because we're not normally aware of our bite, abnormalities here can have very subtle effects. There are two areas that can cause difficulties. The first is when the jaw over-closes – perhaps too many teeth have been removed, or else you've always had a slightly asymmetric shape to your mouth or teeth. But for whatever reason, you may end up with a jaw that closes slightly more than it ought to. This puts stress on the joint between the jaw and the skull – the *temporo-mandibular* (TM) joint. You can feel this joint very easily, just in front of the ear canal. Try putting your finger into your ear, and open and close your mouth; you will feel the joint moving underneath.

The TM joint can become strained in a number of ways. If it closes more than it should, eventually it gets accustomed to working from an abnormal position and the stresses occurring within the joint can cause pain locally. As soon as the temporo-mandibular joint (TM) becomes painful, it will start causing spasm in the muscles surrounding it. This spasm may radiate pain into the head and cause headaches; in fact, some TM joint strains can even trigger off migraines.

Another cause of TM joint pain is when one side of the jaw closes properly and the other side doesn't, so there is a rocking effect. Finally, the TM joint, like any other joint in the body, is susceptible to arthritis. Inflammation within the joint, and wearing-away of joint cartilage, can be potent sources of discomfort. It can also dislocate, either with a blow, or on wide yawning.

Clicking noises within the joints can indicate problems of arthritis, but can also occur where there is excess muscular tension.

Orthodox treatment

Changing the angle and level of the bite can be very effective. Altering false teeth; or filing off proud bits of filling may all settle the bite down into a much easier, more balanced state that causes much less strain at the TM joint.

Alternatively, your dentist may want to put in a bite-raising appliance, which is about an eighth of an inch thick, made of clear acrylic, and fits over the back four teeth (usually of the upper jaw). Its function is simply to prevent the jaw over-closing. It isn't easy to eat with a bite-raising appliance such as this, and so it is often worn only during the night. (For some reason people tend to clench their jaws at night.) Even if a bite-raising appliance is used only at night, it can give marked relief during the day.

The object of using a bite-raising appliance is to re-position the jaw in the TM joint socket, altering both the range of movement of the joint and the pressure points within the joint. This relieves the stresses on the joint, and stops the pain.

TM joint problems are made much worse by stress: stress increases the level of muscle tension, which causes the joint faces to be rammed together more firmly, thereby causing more pain and damage. Therefore, stress management will help to relieve the pain of TM joint problems.

Type of pain

TM joint problems can give rise to several different types of pain – local, sharp, stabbing pain within the TM joint itself, often accompanied by dull, sore, muscle-contraction pain radiating over the sides of the face and head. In extreme cases, it can also trigger migraines.

Self-help

Make sure that you get regular check-ups, and don't assume that because you've got a complete set of false teeth you can't have a dental cause for your headache. If you've had your false teeth for a very long time – and, particularly if you have a lot of thinning of the gums as well, or if your false teeth don't fit as well as they used to and slip around your mouth rather more than you would like – then it's time to go to your dentist for a check. Do tell him if you are suffering from headaches, because although dental causes of headaches are not all that common, if there is a dental cause and you don't get it sorted out, you'll continue to suffer.

Complementary treatment

Obviously the only way to treat temporo-mandibular (TM) joint problems is by having specialised work done by your dentist. Until the work is done, however, headaches can be controlled by a number of different therapies.

Any of the analgesic aromatherapy oils will help to ease the pain – try bergamot, camomile, lavender, marjoram and rosemary in the bath, rubbed gently on the jaw area in a light carrier oil, or in a vapouriser.

Bach flower remedies can be taken before any dental treatment (to help alleviate fear). To soothe bruising following dental treatment, take arnica in homoeopathic doses. For shooting nerve pain, try hypericum, or belladonna.

Osteopathy or cranial osteopathy can be successfully used to treat skeletal pain. Acupuncture and shiatsu can also bring relief. Gently exercising the joint can help relieve some kinds of pain; and a medical herbalist might suggest an infusion of any of the following: balm, camomile, lavender, rosemary, skullcap, white willow and vervain.

Since the headaches are often caused by stress – jaw-clenching, etc – relaxation therapy and biofeedback are recommended.

Chapter Sixteen

EPILEPSY

Individual nerve cells within the nervous system are well insulated from their neighbours. Normally, impulses pass from one nerve cell to another only at special points called synapses, where the electrical impulse from one nerve is briefly converted into a chemical pulse, which then passes across the gap between the two cells and stimulates special receptors on the nerve on the far side. As a result of this chemical stimulus, the second cell sends an electrical signal along its own length, to be passed on to further nerve cells via more synapses.

In practice it is a great deal more complicated, in that each nerve cell has many synapses on it of many different types, and it will only send off a new impulse if enough of the synapses on it are stimulated at the same time. Because these nerve cells are well insulated from one another there is no direct transfer of electrical impulses from nerve cell to nerve cell – between the cells, impulses are only transferred chemically, at the synapses.

In epilepsy and the various forms of neuralgia this well-ordered system breaks down. Some of the cells in the brain may become irritable and start giving off large quantities of spurious electrical impulses. If this happens in a nerve that normally senses touch or pain, we will perceive this extra nerve traffic as pain in the area that the nerve normally supplies. This is termed neuralgia (which, broadly speaking, is severe spasmodic pain in the area supplied by one or more nerves).

Sometimes the irritability of nerves is so great that the 'insulation' material between them breaks down and the electrical nerve impulses bypass the synapses and jump directly to surrounding nerves, stimulating them. In turn, these nerves become over-excitable and cause the insulation around them to break down, causing the layer of cells next to them to become over-excitable ... and so on. In this way, a spreading wave of electrical activity, starting at a small focus within the brain, can spread to overwhelm the whole brain. This is epilepsy. There are many types of epilepsy, depending on where the original irritable cells are situated.

Epilepsy and neuralgia can cause headaches and head pain in three different circumstances.

• Firstly, neuralgia in nerves supplying the face, forehead or scalp can cause severe head pain.

• Secondly, epilepsy can cause headaches, for two quite different reasons, one common, and one very rare. To begin with, headache is common *immediately after a major fit* has occurred. Secondly, temporal lobe epilepsy can, on rare occasions, cause headaches. The temporal lobe is an area of the brain lying slightly behind the temples. It is a part of the brain which is responsible for quite complex functions. Epilepsy in this region has a completely different effect from epilepsy elsewhere and, very rarely, temporal lobe epilepsy can cause headaches.

EPILEPSY

Epilepsy can be divided into three main types:

• Petit mal is characterised by a sudden loss of consciousness lasting for a very short time – perhaps a quarter of a second to a few seconds. These are often called 'absence seizures' and during an attack the patient may suddenly stop talking in mid-sentence and then pick up from where he left off. Occasionally the muscles go limp and the patient drops down to the floor. Attacks like this are normally not followed by headaches.

• Grand mal epilepsy is what most people normally associate with the idea of 'somebody who has fits'. A grand mal attack may be preceded by an aura, an overwhelming feeling in which the patient becomes aware that an attack is pending; then he loses consciousness, falls to the ground, and goes into spasm for up to thirty seconds, during which time he stops breathing and goes blue. Then generalised jerking of the limbs begins.

A variant of grand mal epilepsy is Jacksonian epilepsy, in which the twitching starts in one small part of the body, gradually spreading towards the trunk and eventually involving the whole body: consciousness is eventually lost.

After a grand mal fit, the patient is very drowsy, is sometimes confused, often has a generalised headache, and usually wants to sleep off the attack, which he will probably do quite successfully without any need for interference.

• Temporal lobe epilepsy can be much harder to recognise, because the symptoms can be quite different. There may be visual hallucinations, which can consist of flashes of light or balls of fire, or even more complicated hallucinatory events. There may be disorders of smell and taste, automatic odd behaviour (such as suddenly undressing in public); occasionally there may be outbursts of aggression, or rage – or even attacks of laughter. Finally, temporal lobe epilepsy doesn't necessarily progress to a fit.

There is a crossover in symptoms between temporal lobe epilepsy and migraine; sufferers from temporal lobe epilepsy can get severe headaches, preceded by an aura with visual hallucinations – just like migraine. Usually muscular shaking and loss of consciousness gives the clue to the diagnosis, but sometimes a full-blown fit doesn't occur. Just to make things more complicated, very occasionally a migraine can end with a fit.

Usually the diagnosis of epilepsy is easy to make; either there has been a full-blown fit (grand mal) or else short episodes of loss of consciousness. If there is any doubt, an electro-encephalogram (EEG) may quickly show what is happening by monitoring the electric activity within the brain.

Most people with epilepsy had their first attack before the age of twenty. Why certain people are susceptible is unknown, though a brain injury does predispose to attacks. Sometimes attacks can start out of the blue in adult life, and then go away again within a few months. I suspect that some of these cases are the after-effects of viral infections in the brain.

Epilepsy usually starts in childhood, but the first fit has to be distinguished carefully from a fit due to meningitis; it's also important that fits from febrile convulsions (fever) aren't mistaken for epilepsy, and vice versa. Febrile convulsions are always associated with a rise in temperature and never last beyond the age of seven years. (They never lead on to epilepsy.) On the other hand, epileptic attacks occur out of the blue, unrelated to temperature.

It is unusual for epilepsy to start after the age of twenty. When it does, the doctor has to be careful to make sure that there is no underlying disease causing the epilepsy, such as a tumour. Epilepsy can also arise as a result of abnormal blood vessels stimulating the brain; and from scars in the brain caused by head injuries, operations, small strokes, and sometimes even strokes following migraine.

The doctor will want to fully investigate a first fit. A young child with a first attack of convulsions needs to be admitted to hospital for a lumbar puncture, to ensure that the fit isn't due to meningitis. In an older person it's much easier to be sure that a fit isn't meningitis, so there isn't quite the same rush to investigate. CAT scans and MRI scans will help to pinpoint any abnormality which is triggering off the attacks, and can be used when the EEG points to unusual brain-waves. CAT scans and MRI scans are also very useful in adults who have developed epilepsy, where the doctors are particularly concerned that there isn't an underlying tumour.

Emergency treatment of a fit

Never try to force anything into the mouth in order to stop the tongue being bitten or to hold the teeth apart. This advice used to be given in older first-aid books, but is now thought to be wrong. Instead, make sure that the person who is suffering a fit is moved out of any dangerous situation; for example, pull them away from live wires, off the railway track, out of the way of machinery, or out of water. Other than that, it is best to leave them alone and wait for the symptoms to die down. Once the attack has passed it may be appropriate to turn them on their side in the recovery position, placing them three-quarters prone.

The recovery position is ideal for someone who has lost consciousness or is drowsy. Any vomit will drain away, rather than lying in the back of the throat where it will choke them. The recovery position also allows the tongue to drop forward, maintaining a clear airway through the throat.

Where someone is already known to have fits and can be taken home there is usually no need to call an ambulance or get medical assistance unless something else has happened which complicates the situation; for instance, where the patient has injured themself, or where they are continuing to fit without stopping, or if there is anything else that makes you feel that the situation is not as it should be.

Cause
Epilepsy can have a number of causes. Severe head injury, meningitis, encephalitis, brain tumours, surgery to the brain and strokes can all produce scars on the brain which can in some circumstances act as triggers for epileptic attacks. However, by far the most common type of epilepsy seems to be caused by unknown factors. Some people just seem to have a nervous system where certain nerve cells fire off inappropriately.

Type of headache
If a headache follows a fit it is likely to be generalised and not particularly severe.

What else could it be?
Usually there is no difficulty in establishing that the headache has followed a fit. On the other hand, there are some similarities between migraine and epilepsy – principally that both of them may have an aura (especially visual) beforehand, an inexplicable sensation in which the patient knows that he is just about to have another attack; and in some cases of temporal lobe epilepsy there isn't a full-blown fit. An EEG will often sort out the difference between the two.

Orthodox treatment
Some epileptic attacks can be traced to a brain tumour, an abnormal set of blood vessels, or a scar on the brain and occasionally these can be removed surgically, with good results.

Where there is no identifiable physical abnormality triggering the fits, the treatment of epilepsy is by using one of the many anti-epileptic drugs available, such as phenytoin, carbamazepine, phenobarbitone, sodium valproate, vigabatrin, primidone, clonazepam or ethosuximide. These are often used in combination.

Self-help
Epileptic attacks are usually random, but in some people can be triggered by external events. Flashing lights are one; going without food is another; becoming stressed a third. It's interesting again how closely the triggers for epilepsy mirror the triggers for migraine. Once you know your triggers, then try to avoid them. However, this isn't always possible, and sometimes conditions at work – especially lighting – can increase the possibility of epileptic attacks occurring.

Flicker can be a potent trigger for fits, and one potential cause is the television/computer VDU. Have you ever been in a darkened room where the only source of light has been a television? If the room is lit only by the television, this means that the whole room is flickering. Watching television like this may precipitate an attack in those who are susceptible. Therefore, always have a light on in the room where you are watching television, as this prevents the flicker between bright and dark.

Working with a VDU, especially one in which there is high contrast, can also cause fits, particularly at those times when the screen is changing quickly. One note, though: flicker is reduced when contrast is reduced. Simply turning down the contrast and turning up the brightness may make all the difference between a screen that triggers off epileptic attacks and one that doesn't.

The final self-help technique is to accept with good grace that you have epileptic attacks and that you may have problems for some considerable time. Don't try and give up your epileptic medication without consulting your doctor. In fact, try to take your medication as regularly as possible, because the more constant the supply of anti-epileptic drugs in your bloodstream, the less likely it is that you will have any attacks.

<u>*Complementary treatment*</u>
Complementary treatment, as the name suggests, should complement orthodox medicine, particularly in the case of epilepsy, which should never be treated without the supervision of an orthodox doctor.

Currently under investigation is the role of Vitamin E in controlling seizures. It has been reported that epileptic children have abnormally low levels of Vitamin E; until this research is confirmed, it certainly won't hurt to ensure that you have an adequate intake. Vitamin E occurs naturally in foods like wheatgerm, apples, spinach and eggs.

Supplemental taurine, an amino acid, seems to be beneficial in the treatment of epilepsy. Studies are being carried out to see whether this acid can in fact be more useful than standard anti-convulsants.

Bach flower remedies can be rubbed gently into the temples and other pulse points of someone suffering seizure : these flowers have a soothing effect, and prevent shock and anxiety from setting in. Constitutional use of the remedies may also prevent an attack, if emotions are a trigger.

Constitutional treatment by a homoeopath might be successful. Specific remedies may include ignatia, belladonna, or aconite.

Vitamin B6, magnesium, calcium and zinc supplementation have proved helpful in some cases but Vitamin B6 can be toxic in excess: consult a registered practitioner for advice first. Reflexology may prevent attacks in epilepsy-prone patients, with specific massage and affirmation. Dance/music therapies can control stress, which often precipitates an attack. Any relaxation techniques will be useful in dealing with stress.

Finally, although a registered aromatherapist can suggest a specific oil, or blend of oils, suitable for treating the precursors to, and the effects of, an epileptic attack, this treatment must always be supervised. There are a number of essential oils that can provoke a fit in epileptics, and these are: fennel, hyssop, wormwood, sage and rosemary. Lavender, however, is said to be anti-convulsive and can be safely taken, a few drops at a time, in the bath.

Herbalists might suggest camomile tea, or roman camomile essence, to encourage relaxation; see the suggestions for tension headaches, on page 601, for further ideas about how to encourage relaxation, and prevent tension developing, which may be a trigger for attacks.

Cranial osteopathy claims to help epileptics by reducing the tension in the muscles of the skull, and encouraging the patient to relax.

Chapter Seventeen

PSYCHOLOGICAL CAUSES OF HEADACHES

It's sometimes very difficult to know just where to draw the line between what is normal and what is abnormal, especially where mental processes occur. For example, tension and stress occur in all of our lives at some point – but although mentally we are wearied by them, the fact that we are tense or stressed doesn't necessarily mean that our mental processes are abnormal. In fact, some stress is necessary constitutionally to our bodies. Nevertheless, excess tension and stress can make us ill, and if we don't recognise and deal with it, we can become exhausted mentally or physically.

Anxiety is similar – undue anxiety can be an altered way of thinking, in which we get anxious and stressed without any external triggers. At this point anxiety becomes a psychological problem.

In practice, it isn't easy to define the point at which these processes become part of illness behaviour. Tension headaches can occur in those who, psychologically speaking, are completely normal; in others, they can be part of an anxiety state. Therefore tension, stress, tension headaches, stress management, and relaxation techniques apply both to healthy and to psychologically unwell people. Don't assume that because you're stressed you necessarily have a psychological illness – you probably don't. Nor should you think that because you get tension headaches you're psychologically unwell; again you may well not be. However, if you are aware that your mental processes aren't quite what you would like them to be, and that your anxieties or your inner turmoil are such that *they,* rather than tension itself, are the underlying problem, then read on.

There is a definite group of people who have headaches due primarily to psychological illnesses. It is a gross misconception to say that these headaches are 'all in the mind'. It's all real pain; it's just produced differently.

Some people have headaches that are *entirely* caused by muscle spasm from mental tension, but there is often a mixed cause; any underlying neck injury will magnify, and be magnified by, the excess muscle tension caused through stress.

There is a second psychological cause for headaches, which is much more difficult to understand. This occurs when there is no apparent external source for the pain, and no muscle tension, either. It would be easy to think that pain like this really was all in the mind, but to the sufferer the pain is extremely real, as real as any other type of headache. We'll come to this subject in more detail later.

ANXIETY AND DEPRESSION

There are two main psychological causes of mental tension – anxiety and depression. You might think that they were opposites, like chalk and cheese; however, this is not the case. Paradoxically, those who are depressed are often anxious as well; and often those who think that they are anxious are actually, underneath it all, depressed.

Symptoms of anxiety/depression

Anxiety and depression are actually part and parcel of a single disease, not surprisingly termed anxiety/depression. Some sufferers exhibit more anxiety than depression, others do the reverse. Most have a bit of each.

Let's get rid of one misconception: depression isn't the same as sadness. Those who've experienced both say that sadness is an *enriching* experience – albeit an unhappy one – whereas depression is empty and numbing. Telling a depressed person to 'cheer up, you've nothing to be depressed about' is like hitting him in the face with a bucket of cold water, and about as helpful.

Symptoms of depression vary from person to person: the predominant symptom is early waking (perhaps at three or four a.m.) when you wake up tired, yet unable to get back to sleep again. You may find it difficult to get to sleep, or have an overwhelming sensation of tiredness, with lack of concentration, irritability, lack of sexual drive and exhaustion. You may experience a feeling of despair, often made worse because you know you've nothing in particular to be depressed about. You may have a sense of hopelessness, and of the uselessness of everything, or have a fear of death; you may have developed phobias, obsessional behaviour, or have a permanent sense of tension and anxiety. Often people with depression want to cry, but somehow can't manage to do it.

There is often a daily variation in the intensity of whichever symptoms you have; they are either much worse in the morning, and much better in the evening, or vice versa. In addition to these mainly mental feelings, there may also be body malfunctions – headaches, alterations in weight, gross tiredness which isn't relieved by sleep, palpitations, sweating, diarrhoea, constipation, a permanent sense of a lump in the throat, or a choking feeling. In the more severe cases you may feel paranoid – feeling your friends are avoiding you, or talking about you behind your back; you may even start to hallucinate and hear voices when there is nobody there, though in depression this is relatively *un*common.

There is often a slowness of thinking and lack of creativity, which means someone with a creative job, such as an artist or writer, is often more quickly affected by depression than someone with a manual job. This *doesn't* mean manual workers get less depressed, but their ability to work is less immediately affected.

Finally, and paradoxically, a person with depression can also be *agitated:* this is of great importance, because often agitation and tension are treated with antianxiety drugs which can sometimes exacerbate the underlying depression. Frequently, people like this are better treated with anti-depressive medication. This sorts out the underlying depression, and then the super-imposed anxiety goes.

One symptom that particularly concerns us here is the extra muscle tension that occurs in anxiety and depression; this often manifests itself as backache, neckache, or headache. While it *is* possible to get pure anxiety on its own, a good proportion of cases of long-standing tension headache have their roots in an *underlying* depression.

Headaches aren't actually more frequent in depression than they are at any other time – it's just that the sufferer perceives them more clearly, and reacts to them more often. There are two possible reasons for this. The first is that in depression there is a reduction in a brain chemical called '5-HT', and we think that perception of pain is greater as a result. The second reason (probably saying the same thing, but from a psychological viewpoint) is that in depression, a greater awareness of your body's functions occurs. This can easily become a vicious circle. You worry that the headache may mean something awful, like a brain tumour; which causes further anxiety, which in turn perpetuates the anxiety/depression syndrome. There are certain times when depression is more likely to strike – in adolescence, at the so-called 'mid-life' crisis, after times of intense stress, or lifestyle changes such as bereavement. In women, there may be a relationship to the monthly cycle, often being worse pre-menstrually, and at the menopause.

Why does depression occur?

In the brain messages are passed electrically along the nerve cells, but on reaching a junction between two nerve cells this electrical impulse is converted into physical form. Chemicals called *transmitter substances* are released by the first cell and travel across the synapse, to land on special receptor sites on the second cell. Here they either excite the cell or inhibit it, depending on their function. Each nerve cell may have hundreds of synapses on it, and will only fire off its own impulse if it receives enough incoming signals at the same time. In other words, nerves in the brain act not just as passive carriers of information, they also filter the information before passing it on.

The transmitter chemicals are stored in tiny bags inside the ends of the nerve cells. However, sometimes these transmitter substances don't seem to work as well as they should. Perhaps the nerve cell isn't producing as much transmitter chemical as it should; or else the receiving nerve isn't as sensitive as it could be; or alternatively, the first nerve cell has been stimulated so much that it has partially run out of transmitter chemicals and can no longer pass on the messages.

In depression it seems that there isn't enough transmitter substance to go round, so messages can't pass freely round the brain as they once did; as a result, thinking becomes an effort, and the emotions are dulled. This neatly explains how and why we may get depressed.

Some types of depression (particularly manic depression in which episodes of depression alternate with periods of excessive activity) undoubtedly occur for genetic (hereditary) reasons, and there has been some interesting work among the

Amish community in America to show how this genetic predisposition to depression is passed on. But there is a second group of people who get depressed; and at first sight this appears to have nothing to do with transmitter chemicals.

People in this category become depressed for psychological reasons: they worry about things, perhaps becoming obsessed with a problem that they can't solve, and have ideas, thoughts and anxieties racing round their head. You might think that depression which was entirely related to an outside event – such as bereavement – would have little or no effect on the transmitter chemicals. Not so! This is a good example of how transmitter chemicals can be used up by excess brain activity. In fact, the brain isn't inactive – it's simply having all its energy short-circuited in an attempt to deal with an insoluble problem. It's exactly the situation that happens in your house when someone switches on the washing machine: for a moment all the lights may dim, because most of the energy in the electricity supply is being diverted to making that huge motor start up, so there's much less left for the lights.

Exactly the same thing happens within the brain: so much mental energy is being used up trying to solve this unsolvable problem that there isn't much left for anything else. All this excess internal activity in the nerves is merely going round and round in circles, depleting the transmitter chemicals and making them unavailable for use in other situations.

There are therefore two main ways we can help people with depression. The first is to put back some of these transmitter chemicals (or else make the existing transmitter chemicals work more effectively); the second is, where appropriate, by counselling or psychotherapy to try to solve some of the problems that are rocketing around the subconscious. If successful, it will leave the brain cells free once again to pass messages on in the normal way.

Many anti-depressive drugs improve the brain's supply of 5-HT (one of the transmitter chemicals). This fits in neatly with the idea that the increased sensitivity to headaches in depression is due to a lack of 5-HT, making you both more depressed, and more sensitive to pain. Medicines to help restore some of the transmitter chemicals improve depression of both origins – biochemical, and related to external events. There are many non-brain causes of anxiety/depression, too. General physical problems such as lack of thyroid hormone (causing depression) or excess (causing agitation); kidney or liver disease; alcoholism; drug dependency; pre-menstrual syndrome (PMS); food allergies; lack of natural light during the winter in certain susceptible people, also called SAD – Seasonal Affective Disorder; and peculiar reactions to medicines, chemicals and food additives can all cause anxiety/depression. The treatment here is to remove or treat the cause wherever possible.

In many ways, depression is not a disease of the logic as much as disease of the emotions; it is often the inability to express those intense emotions that cause problems in the first place. Paradoxically, it is not the inability to experience joy that's the problem, but *anger*; and a fear of sadness.

Whatever the exact trigger, there is often a fear of the intensity of the emotions it engenders. For example, maybe you've just been bereaved – but you don't cry, perhaps through fear of making a scene, or because you are scared of the intensity of your emotions. When you do this, you put a clamp on your emotions, so your emotions are unable to change or move; the result is that although you're protected against the intensity of the sadness or anger that you feel, this emotional clamp also prevents you from becoming happy. Letting out these emotions, taking the clamp off so that you can first go *down* emotionally – by crying or expressing rage – means that ultimately you'll be able to come up again.

There are two ways to face your problems. Firstly, if you know what they are and can verbalise them, then concentrate on them and think them through. But be warned, facing your problems in this way is frightening: don't try it on your own, unsupported, especially if your depression seems severe.

Often these fears and emotions are too deep-seated to verbalise, and all that you are aware of is the emotion you feel, emotion that can't be put into words or reduced to logic. This is where things like art therapy can come in: by using music, art and dance, skilled therapists can help you express those inner feelings and let out those hidden emotions that have troubled you for so long.

Orthodox treatment

Treatment of anxiety/depression falls into three main areas. First, your doctor needs to be sure that there is no general physical cause for the depression – such as pre-menstrual syndrome (PMS), thyroid malfunction, etc. There is no point in undergoing psycho-analysis for anxiety if your anxiety is being caused by an over-active thyroid!

Assuming that general physical problems have been ruled out, if you have an obvious worry or precipitating factor then counselling or psychotherapy may help, so that you can talk through your problems, and be led to a deeper understanding of what you're afraid of. Then you can decide what to do about it. Thirdly, treatment with anti-depressive medication can put back the transmitter chemicals that are missing.

You might think that a patient with a psychological cause for her depression (such as an inability to cope with the break-up of her marriage) would be helped best by counselling and that medicines would be unnecessary. In fact, the opposite is true. What probably happens is this: the initial worries cause intense brain activity, which starts to deplete the transmitter chemicals. Then, because the brain chemicals are depleted, the patient is no longer able to think straight about her problems. Often the best way to help a patient like this is to prescribe anti-depressants for two or three weeks to replace the transmitter chemicals: then, once the brain can pass messages around itself properly, the patient has more energy to devote to solving those questions that caused her problem in the first place.

Those who have a natural dislike of medicines tend to throw up their hands in horror at an approach like this: but in my professional life, having tried both ways – counselling first, then medication; or alternatively medication first, then counselling – I've always had the best results from giving a high dose of antidepressant medication first, waiting for a week or two for it to take effect, and only then encouraging the patient to start approaching his problems.

BETH

Beth is a divorcee aged thirty-five, with two small children. For a long time she had been struggling along on her own, but eventually things began to overwhelm her. She started sleeping badly, felt tired all the time, and started to get headaches. She also felt very tense because her ex-husband was being very difficult over the way she was bringing up the children.

Finally she went to her doctor. The obvious clue was the continuing early waking and the perpetual sense of tiredness – Beth was depressed, and no wonder, with the problems she had on her plate at the time.

The first thing her doctor did was to reassure her that she was currently going through a bout of depression, but almost certainly it would get better with medication. He prescribed a sedative anti-depressant, and suggested that the daily dose should be taken an hour before Beth went to bed. In this way, the sedative effects would immediately help her problems with insomnia, both helping her to get off to sleep, and stopping her waking up quite so early in the morning. He warned her that the anti-depressant would take some time to act on the depression itself, and that she should expect to wait ten to twenty days before it started to lift.

Three weeks later Beth returned, a different woman. The headaches had gone, her sleep pattern had improved, she had got most of her energy back, and was now able to start dealing with some of the problems that beset her – particularly the ones involving her ex-husband.

Because she felt so much better she asked whether she could stop the anti-depressants. Her doctor told her that it wouldn't be a good idea: all that would happen would be that she would go back to her previous state. Instead, he congratulated her on her improvement – and said that he would probably want to continue the medication for a further three to four months. Beth was a little taken aback by this, but felt that her doctor knew best and agreed with his plan of action.

She came to see the doctor twice more in the intervening period, and her progress continued to be good. At the end of four months the doctor suggested that she should discontinue the anti-depressants, reducing them gradually over the course of ten days.

All was well. Beth discontinued the medication and found that she maintained her good progress; the headaches no longer troubled her, and, by now, she had managed to sort out some of the problems that were facing her.

Don't, however, expect anti-depressant medication to work immediately. It can take time to replace the chemicals that are missing or reduced – perhaps about three weeks. What *does* improve quickly is sleep. Some anti-depressants have sedative properties as well. Giving a sedative anti-depressant in a single dose at night helps the patient to sleep more deeply, which means that more refreshed the next morning, and better able to face the problems of the day.

Don't worry about the possibility of getting addicted to anti-depressant drugs – you can't. Although it's possible to become addicted to *tranquillisers*, addiction to *anti-depressants* is almost unknown. This is a good thing, because the best way to use anti-depressants is in high doses for several months at a time.

Several types of medicine are used in depression – older drugs such as amitriptyline and dothiepine have been used for many years with success; and now there is a new group of drugs called the *5-HT re-uptake inhibitors*, which look as though they could become the drugs of the future. As we've already seen, 5-HT is one of the transmitter substances in the brain. A re-uptake inhibitor simply stops the transmitter chemical re-entering the first cell, so that more of the transmitter substance lies around in the synapse, stimulating the second cell. Interestingly, drugs like this seem also to have a beneficial effect in some cases of eating disorders, and 5-HT is also thought to be one of the principle transmitters involved in migraine.

Because a large proportion of those with anxiety are actually suffering from depression, many people with anxiety can be managed on anti-depressants alone. However, some people may need tranquillisers as well, especially to help them sleep. There is a place for tranquillisers, but they have to be used in an entirely different way to anti-depressants; some tranquillisers can be addictive and are best used over very short intervals indeed.

Muscle relaxants can often help the patient with headaches due to anxiety and muscle tension, where simple painkillers cannot. These can be used at the same time as anti-depressants, and in a patient with severe tension headache a tranquilliser muscle-relaxant may be appropriate.

Finally, electro-convulsive therapy (ECT) is sometimes used in treating depression. In this the patient is anaesthetised and an electric shock is given to the brain, usually the side of the brain opposite to the speech centre.

Of late, ECT has had a very bad time in the media and some people have even called for its abolition. However, there are people – especially the elderly – in whom anti-depressant drugs don't seem to work particularly well, and in people like this ECT can often make the difference between a normal existence and continuous depression.

Counselling and psychotherapy

The counsellor or psychotherapist's job is to lead the client to see her problems more clearly, and make up her own mind on what to do about them.

There are many different types of counselling and psychotherapy: Freudian and Jungian psycho-analysis, psychotherapy, transactional analysis (TA), behavioural therapy, cognitive therapy, etc. They all have slightly different ways of tackling mental and emotional problems. Some of them – the analysis type – concentrate on the workings of the unconscious mind; psychotherapies are more concerned with conscious events; and behavioural therapy works through teaching the client to re-learn those responses which have been incorrectly learned in the past (for example, an irrational fear of spiders, when she knows that those spiders can't injure her).

Counselling is a complex affair, though the underlying concept remains the same – to identify those mal-adapted ideas, memories or attitudes which are contributing to the current problem. These mal-adapted responses are often based on fears and worries which have been buried in the subconscious, often because they're too painful or too terrifying to be brought out into the conscious. The psychotherapist's job is to allow the client to recognise these fears, bring them out into the open and examine them. When painful memories have been understood and re-interpreted they are usually much less threatening, and so the client doesn't fear his guilt so much, and can learn to deal with similar problems in a totally different way.

A highly recommended therapy is transactional analysis (TA), which is the nearest thing to do-it-yourself psychiatry there is. It's simple, and practical, and it helps you get to grips with your own problems. An excellent guide to transactional analysis is the book *Born to Win* by Muriel James and Dorothy Jongeward.

Whatever counselling system you choose, you will almost certainly need at least some professional advice; it is *impossible* to be objective about yourself (and even more impossible if you're anxious or depressed). You need the steadying, reasoned, objective assessment of a *competent* outsider. Otherwise you may go around trying to change the wrong things – or the right things, but in the wrong way.

Finally, beware of the amateur shrink! Counselling is complex and difficult – *and a counsellor can do damage*. Although humans can't remember physical pain (we can remember that we had it, but we can't recall the pain itself) we *can* remember mental pain. We can also re-create mental pain by re-living experiences that were mentally searing. A poor counsellor can do untold harm; by trying to force you into inappropriate responses, he can hinder your recovery, and it can give you further mental pain.

Self-help

Self-help in anxiety/depression has three main parts. First of all, be prepared to admit that you're depressed; secondly, don't wallow in it, but get professional help; and, finally, start helping yourself to get out of it. This is not the same as 'pulling yourself together', which doesn't work, mainly because it's directed at the wrong things.

Recognising that you have a psychological cause for your headache is the first step towards healing it. If you are constantly striving to prove that there is a physical cause as a way of evading your responsibility to tackle your psychological problems, then you will make no headway. For some reason society tends to make out that people with psychological problems are evil or guilty, while those with physical problems are not. It really isn't like that at all. True, you may have made decisions which, with hindsight, you realise have contributed to your own current unhappiness. But for many sufferers from psychological illnesses, sufferings have been imposed from outside – the woman who was abused as a child; the adolescent who doesn't love himself because his parents never really loved him; the man who is never allowed to show his anger because anger was always taboo in the family. Psychologically speaking, depression is often in-turned aggression – anger that you have not been able to express and so you turn it in upon yourself. So just because there is a psychological cause doesn't mean that you are necessarily guilty; certainly, no more than if you had broken a leg skiing.

The second part of self-help is to recognise that although you are depressed you *mustn't* wallow in it. Those who are depressed can get terribly self-absorbed with their depression and after a time some of them, as the saying goes, *enjoy* ill-health. Once you start wallowing in it you self-perpetuate the illness, and if you continue with the self-pity you're likely to find that you quickly start running out of friends.

The third self-help method is honestly and courageously to face up to the things that are bothering you. Often it is an unspoken subconscious fear that you are too frightened to approach; perhaps it's the fear of death; or that you can't adjust to your sexuality; or you feel worthless as a result of being unemployed; or maybe you just feel unloved and unlovable. Courageously going headfirst into whatever problem is bugging you is often the quickest way to get out of those types of depression which are purely psychological in origin. Trying to evade the problem merely prolongs the issue and will lead you into more misery.

This is not easy to do. Facing up to those fearsome problems that are so hard to handle that you try to forget about them and bury them in your subconscious, is a very frightening activity, and you will need a lot of emotional support to do it. Tackling deep-rooted, fearsome problems like this is often where professional guidance and counselling come in.

Finally, make sure you get enough exercise. The apathy of depression is quite enough to stop you doing things, but exercise really can make you feel a lot better. Physically speaking, exercise releases the body's own morphine-like chemicals (the endorphins) inside the brain, and these contribute to an increased sense of well-being. In addition, exercise uses up the extra adrenalin that will be swilling round your system if you're anxious.

Depression often has its roots in in-turned aggression – an inability to vent anger. Very often the condition can be improved by learning how to appropriately dissipate it. Assertiveness training is part of this technique – learning how *not* to be trampled on can be very important. It is all about making sure that you are able to put your point of view forward and be listened to. Some people were never taught to be assertive; they find themselves doing what others want simply because they've never learned to stand up for themselves.

Physical contact is often a necessity in cases of depression. We humans need the constant physical encouragement of human contact, and families and spouses can often help by making a point of touching. The hand on the arm, the arm round the shoulder, the kiss, the cuddle; these all say 'You're important to me, you're valuable *in yourself*' – sentiments that the depressed person longs to hear.

It will help considerably to express your feelings more often. In depression the emotions often get buttoned up, and expressing them can help (particularly as these emotions can be very strong in depression). In our stiff-upper-lip society, it's not always easy to let your emotions out, and expressing what you feel in art, music or dance may help. Art, dance and music therapy can be *extremely* helpful .

Although you might think that religion would be a consolation in depression – and sometimes it is – some depressed people perceive their religious beliefs as a burden rather than as a liberation. This is often tied in with a sense of guilt, worthlessness or failure. It is important to realise that these fears are a reflection of your *depression*, not an indictment of your *beliefs*.

Complementary treatment

Depression, especially when severe, is potentially life-threatening. Suicides can and do occur – in fact they're the largest cause of death in the teenage years. Don't use any of these complementary therapies until you've consulted your own doctor and asked his advice. The following approaches are complementary, not alternative; they should be adding to what your doctor is doing, not replacing it.

Almost every single alternative practitioner will vouchsafe his cures, so it is best to proceed with caution and consult a registered and preferably recommended practitioner at all times.

Complementary practitioners generally hold the view that tranquillisers and anti-depressants are counter-productive, for in the long run they don't cure the cause of anxiety, but simply mask its symptoms. Instead they may suggest herbs, for instance, that claim to treat the anxiety itself; these include balm, camomile, hops, motherwort, orange blossom, skullcap and vervain. The headaches of anxiety and depression are best treated by balm, camomile, Jamaican dogwood, lavender and white willow (aspirin in its natural form).

Clinical nutrition offers a Pandora's box of possibilities. Licorice is thought to have anti-depressant properties; magnesium is said to play a useful role in the treatment of depression, for it is known to be involved in the synthesis of some of the brain's neuro-transmitters. Vitamin B12 is the legendary doctor feelgood vitamin (used so excessively in the Sixties and Seventies). Vitamin B6 is also said to help in the treatment of depression/anxiety. In general, a consultation with a registered clinical nutritionist will ensure that no sub-clinical deficiencies are responsible for your anxiety or depression – which often can be biologically triggered.

Everyone's depression is different, and an aromatherapist would select oils suitable for your changing needs. Some suggestions might be camomile, clary sage, lavender, sandalwood and ylang-ylang – which have both sedative and anti-depressant qualities and so may be helpful if you are suffering from early waking or acute anxiety. Bergamot, geranium, melissa and rose are uplifting and anti-depressant; neroli and jasmine are beneficial when suffering from some of the more debilitating effects of anxiety/depression, such as extreme inexplicable fatigue, headaches, emotional instability, digestive troubles and broken sleep. Massage is important because of the physical contact and baths and vapourisation are equally effective. Baths are often a cleansing experience, and it can be a psychological boost to have one at the end of each day, to effectively wash away that day's troubles.

Osmotherapy, which is another form of scent therapy, based on slightly different principles to aromatherapy, has been used successfully in the treatment of anxiety/depression – even acknowledged and practised by some British hospitals. Certain scents may be as powerful as tranquillisers. In a hospital in Worcestershire in the UK, certain fragrances were used to reduce anxiety in patients, and a close correlation between the action of fragrance molecules and that of mood-altering drugs (like anti-depressants or tranquillisers) was discovered. A trained and recognised osmotherapist will be able to treat your individual symptoms. This is particularly helpful for those patients who have been addicted to tranquillisers at any time.

Bach flower remedies may be helpful in treating anxiety/depression, since they are claimed to affect the negative emotions, replacing them with a sense of calm. Try aspen for apprehension and foreboding, rock rose for extreme panic or terror, larch for despondency. Rescue remedy is a common standby for extreme anxiety or fear.

Acupuncture may also help with anxiety and depression.

Other complementary therapies include: acupressure, reflexology, counselling, the Alexander technique, T'ai chi, Transactional Analysis (TA), kinesiology and the relaxation therapies such as biofeedback,.

OTHER PSYCHOLOGICAL CAUSES

Almost all psychological causes of headache operate through the anxiety/depression muscle-tension path. There is, however, a tiny group of people whose headaches are completely psychological; there is no physical cause whatsoever, nor is there any evidence of anxiety, depression or muscle tension.

It's quite similar in many respects to phantom pain. A person who has had a leg amputated often finds to their great consternation that from time to time they get pain apparently coming from their non-existent foot – head pain of purely psychological origin is exactly the same. People who have headaches of purely psychological origin may be collecting their emotions and problems together and expressing them as a headache. These headaches are very real. They are also exceptionally difficult to deal with, and often need counselling and psychotherapy.

Associated problems

Stress is a constant problem in those with anxiety/depression: relaxation therapy will help. With increased tension comes the possibility of *high blood pressure* ; and increased muscle tension will exacerbate the muscle tension of *neck and spine injuries. Sleep problems* are frequently made worse by anxiety or depression.

Chapter Eighteen

HEADACHES IN WOMEN

Some types of headaches occur only in women. These are headache: caused by the contraceptive pill; from toxaemia in pregnancy; and related to the menstrual cycle.

A number of types of headache occur more frequently in women than in men – sub-arachnoid haemorrhage and migraine, for example. Other types attack men more often than women – such as cluster headache. And, of course, there are a large number of types of headaches which affect both sexes equally.

The female reproductive system is controlled by many different hormones. Each month during the fertile part of a woman's life, they cause a single egg to complete its development in one of the ovaries, and to be released into the Fallopian tubes which eventually lead to the womb. Two of the main female hormones, oestrogen and progesterone, are made in the ovary. Oestrogen is created by cells which surround the developing egg, while progesterone is released from the region formerly inhabited by the egg, after it has been released.

The whole cycle is under the control of hormones produced by the pituitary gland. One of its hormones, follicle-stimulating hormone (FSH), causes the egg and its surrounding cells to begin maturation. The female hormones are low in childhood, rising as puberty commences, and then (unless interrupted by pregnancy) continue to vary in a monthly cycle until the menopause. The time of the menopause is determined by the number of eggs left in the ovary ready to develop; when these run out, the ovary is unable to produce oestrogen and progesterone as it previously did, and the levels of these hormones begin to fall.

However, from time to time, hormone imbalances can occur. These can cause a variety of diseases, including abnormal monthly bleeds, pre-menstrual syndrome (PMS) and menopausal problems. Pre-menstrual syndrome and menopausal problems both include a wide variety of symptoms, including headaches.

HEADACHES RELATED TO THE MENSTRUAL CYCLE

Two types of headaches occur in relation to the menstrual cycle. These are *menstrual headaches,* occurring at the time of the monthly period and headaches occurring as part of the *pre-menstrual syndrome*, which typically occurs in the week or so *before* the period starts.

Pre-menstrual syndrome

Pre-menstrual syndrome (PMS) covers a wide variety of symptoms, the most common of which are irritability, breast swelling and tenderness, bloating, backaches, headaches, anxiety or depression, weight gain, food cravings, fatigue and abdominal bloating. Usually only a few of these symptoms occur in any one woman. Obviously, all of these symptoms can occur for other reasons, but in PMS the common factor is that the symptoms come and go in relation to the menstrual cycle, typically starting in the second half of the cycle and reducing or ceasing as or shortly after the period begins. In mild cases, the symptoms are only present for a couple of days before the period, but in severe cases the symptoms can occur through at least half and sometimes three quarters of the cycle.

Why does PMS occur? There are many theories, most of which revolve around imbalances of the female hormones. Note that word 'imbalance'; there isn't an absolute amount of each hormone that needs to be present, but a relative balance between them. The honest answer is that we don't yet know precisely why PMS occurs.

Orthodox treatment

One of the most potent ways to help sufferers of PMS is to make sure that both the patient and her family realise that they are dealing with a physical illness. The trouble with PMS is that sufferers feel that they're going mad. For women to *recognise* the fact that it's PMS, and to understand that her partner and her family also know that it's PMS, is a great relief.

Water retention is a common symptom of PMS. Certainly, giving a mild *diuretic* (a drug that encourages the kidney to excrete more fluid) often gets rid of PMS symptoms, especially bloating, weight gain and breast tenderness. *Vitamin B6* is also used in PMS, taken in doses of about 50mg–100mg per day. There is as yet no completely objective evidence that it works, though many doctors use it. Vitamin B6 is thought to exert its action on the brain, possibly by affecting the way in which the pituitary gland releases the hormones which control the female cycle. However, Vitamin B6 can cause inflammation of the nerves if given for long periods and especially if used in high doses. *Evening Primrose Oil* may help in some cases. Its active constituent, gamolenic acid, is now available on prescription.

As far as hormone treatment of PMS is concerned, one of the most helpful methods is to take extra progesterone in the week before the menstrual bleed starts. Progesterone is normally released from the ovary during the second half of a cycle, and the extra progesterone in tablet form boosts its effects. In severe cases it may help to add progesterone for two or even three weeks leading up to the period. *Extra oestrogens*, which *must* be used with extra progesterone (see below) can sometimes improve pre-menstrual symptoms. Oestrogen and progesterone together make up the combined contraception pill, so putting the patient on the contraceptive pill could help. Sometimes the preparations used in hormone replacement therapy (HRT) can also be used to boost the levels of oestrogen and progesterone in PMS.

Bromocriptine can reduce pre-menstrual breast pain, but it's not appropriate if you're planning a family.

Some types of *painkillers* such as *mefenamic acid* help reduce PMS symptoms, and relieve the pain of any headache directly. The drugs in this group are of a type often used to reduce inflammation in rheumatism and other musculo-skeletal problems. *Anti-depressants* may also be of use in some cases of PMS, especially where there are psychological symptoms such as anxiety or depression.

Self-help

Acknowledging that you are a PMS sufferer is a great step forward. It *doesn't* mean that you're hiding behind a convenient syndrome.

Diet can sometimes help. Follow the rules of low-fat, high-fibre, low-sugar diet, with lots of fruit and vegetables. Cut down on caffeine and alcohol, which will encourage mood swings. Keeping your sugar level as constant as possible may help; in some cases changing to a three-hourly starch diet, which includes lots of unrefined carbohydrates, will also make a difference. However, you'll have to make sure that your total daily intake doesn't rise and cause you to gain weight.

Complementary treatment

If you suffer from pre-menstrual craving for sweet things, a chromium supplement might help – this is because chromium is linked to our insulin levels, and this in turn controls the amount of sugar in our bloodstream.

Sometimes reducing fluid and/or salt intake before the period may lessen the sensation of bloating.

Relaxation and exercise, which both reduce tension, will help alleviate symptoms.

A supplement of Vitamin B6 can be helpful, starting two days before your symptoms normally begin and stopping just after your menstrual cycle has started. Evening Primrose Oil works for some women, taking it alongside Vitamin B6. Note that Evening Primrose Oil can cause fits in those suffering from temporal lobe epilepsy, so beware.

Acupuncture can help with many symptoms, including bloating (by helping the body eliminate excess fluid), cravings (by suppressing your appetite), mood swings (by calming your nervous system), painful breasts and headaches (through various methods of pain relief and reduction). Obviously, when the other symptoms of PMS are relieved, a great deal of pressure may be lifted from the sufferer. Simply controlling mood swings can provide relief from headaches by making the patient feel she is back in control of her own body – and that's a good starting point for banishing emotionally linked stress.

Aromatherapy has much to offer PMS sufferers. Geranium and rosemary are said to help prevent water retention. A head, neck and shoulder massage with lavender, sandalwood, camomile or geranium helps to relieve tension and relax the muscles, in the case of headache. Geranium, bergamot, rosemary and lavender (singly or in a blend) may act as stimulants to overcome lethargy and tiredness. Cold lavender compresses can relieve painful breasts. Where muscle tension is a feature, any of the manipulative therapies are likely to help.

Homoeopathy will work best if remedies are prescribed according to your specific symptoms – or group of symptoms. In general, however, lachesis and nat mur are used to relieve water retention; mood swings can be treated with kreasote, lycopodium and causticum; sore breasts may be relieved by pulsatilla.

The clinical nutritionalist might suggest some of the following. Vitamin B6 acts as a mild and natural diuretic, as does Fenugreek tea or dandelion root coffee. A low-fat, low-sugar, low-salt diet (as above) should be implemented, especially the week before, and the week of, your worst symptoms. Supplements of Brewer's yeast and adrenal glandulars can help with cravings and mood swings (included anxiety and depression). A calcium supplement, taken along with evening primrose, is said to reduce headaches by restoring the hormone balance between oestrogen and progesterone.

In terms of medical herbalism, you might try coughgrass and cleavers, drunk as a tea, which acts as a diuretic. Gentian can control blood-sugar levels; skullcap or oats can control mood swings; camoline, peppermint or feverfew can reduce headaches by improving circulation and relieving tension; and chaste tree or white deadnettle are said to improve the circulation, reducing congestion and pressure.

Royal jelly is also said to be helpful. Reflexology and biofeedback are also often recommended.

Headaches while menstruating

The period itself is a very stressful time in a woman's monthly cycle, especially on the first day. There may be abdominal pain, and a general feeling of being under the weather. This feeling tends to exacerbate any pre-existing headaches; sometimes the general lowering of the body's resistance means that ordinary headaches will occur more frequently at this time of the cycle. Migraines may occur more frequently in those who are susceptible

Because menstrual headaches occur as a result of a general debility of the whole system, rather than a specific hormone defect, with the exception of menstrual migraines, there is no specific treatment for them. Instead, the type of treatment used is related to the cause of the headache itself. It is very important to appreciate the difference – pre-menstrual headaches are treated by treating the pre-menstrual syndrome directly, while menstrual headaches are treated by treating the cause of the headache.

Menstrual migraine

Menstrual migraine is defined as migraine which occurs on the first day of the period (or on the day before or the day after). It is caused by the sudden drop in oestrogen levels that occurs at this time, and may respond to treatment with extra oestrogen – for example, in 'patch' form.

THE CONTRACEPTIVE PILL

There are two types of contraceptive Pill. The combined Pill contains oestrogen and progesterone, whereas the so-called 'mini-pill' contains progesterone alone. The mini-pill avoids the problems and side-effects associated with oestrogen, but at the expense of a slightly lower level of protection against pregnancy, and much poorer monthly cycle control.

There are many different versions of the combined Pill, varying in dose and type of oestrogen, proportion of oestrogen to progesterone, and so on. The combination that suits one woman may not suit another, so if you find one brand of Pill gives side-effects, often all that you need is to change to a different brand.

There are many potential side-effects of the combined Pill. These can include bloating and abnormalities of menstrual bleeding.

'Ordinary' headaches

Headaches can be a side effect of the combined pill, and if these are of a general, non-migrainous type, often all that is needed is to switch to a different brand of Pill containing slightly different amounts of oestrogen and progesterone. Often this makes all the difference and the headaches disappear. Occasionally switching from the combined pill to the mini-pill can do the trick.

Migraine and the pill

If you already suffer from migraine with certain types of aura, some doctors advise that you don't go on the Pill. There is no problem with those who get migraine without aura. However, a sizeable percentage of migraine sufferers find their existing migraines occur more frequently on the Pill. If you've had migraines in the past, then the treatment of the migraine itself is exactly the same as the treatment you've been accustomed to using.

On occasion, taking the combined pill can make your migraines less frequent or less severe. However there are two specific and potentially very dangerous types of headache associated with the 'Pill'. This is when a woman who has never had migraines before gets her first-ever migraine while taking the Pill. For reasons not yet clear, migraines which *start* on the Pill are potentially *very* dangerous and can lead to strokes. If you have a true migraine attack while on the Pill and you have *never* had a migraine before then you need to *stop the pill immediately.*

Having a first migraine attack while on the Pill means you should not take the combined contraceptive Pill again. The mini-pill only contains progesterone and is still acceptable, though it doesn't provide quite the same degree of protection against pregnancy. Exactly the same precautions need to be taken if your existing migraines suddenly change their nature (not their frequency) while you're on the combined Pill. The development of an aura where previously you didn't have one, numbness of fingers or lips, are reasons to stop the Pill straightaway.

Self-help
If you've had migraines in the past, before you went on the Pill, then you can continue to take the Pill as long as the nature of the migraines hasn't changed.

Complementary treatment
If you've had migraine in the past, then the same complementary treatments are likely to work if you're on the Pill. See the chapter on migraine for details of those therapies most likely to help.

TOXAEMIA OF PREGNANCY
During pregnancy, some women start to develop a syndrome call toxaemia of pregnancy. As yet, no one is completely sure why this occurs, but it is a very well-recognised problem. In its early form, there is puffiness of the ankles and the fingers, and weight gain, both of which are caused by water retention (oedema). Blood pressure rises slightly and there may be a little protein in the urine. Normally this settles with rest, but in its worst form (which is fortunately very rare) the patient gets a frontal headache, gross puffiness of her fingers and ankles, leaks protein into her urine, and her blood pressure continues rising. If this situation isn't checked, in extreme circumstances she may experience flashing lights in the eyes, together with a headache over the forehead and then have a fit. This condition is called eclampsia. After an eclamptic fit, the foetus has a high chance of dying – so too has the mother.

Thankfully, full-blown eclampsia is a very rare event, largely due to good ante-natal care. During routine anti-natal checks a woman's blood pressure is measured, she's weighed to make sure that she's not *suddenly* put on too much weight (which usually means that she's retaining water rather than that she's eating too much) and her urine is tested to make sure that there is no protein present.

A small percentage of pregnant women do get the symptoms of early toxaemia – a little swelling of the fingers, a slight rise in blood pressure, or perhaps a little protein in her water, but the early stages are relatively benign. *Pre-eclampic toxaemia* (PET) like this responds well to rest. In most cases, the blood pressure falls, the excess water is lost, and the leakage of protein stops. In more severe cases it make be necessary for the patient to be admitted to hospital for strict bed rest, sometimes under quite heavy sedation.

Although rest usually makes the symptoms of toxaemia go away, it's very often difficult to get a woman to rest in her own home. At least two hours lying in bed in the morning and two hours in the afternoon – may be all that is required to bring the blood pressure down. In early toxaemia, however, if the symptoms persist and the blood pressure continues to rise, then hospital admission is going to be necessary. In extreme cases it may be necessary to induce childbirth by medical means, to make sure that the baby is delivered as soon as possible; and in some cases an emergency Caesarian section is needed to save the baby's life or simply to prevent the blood pressure going even higher.

Full-blown toxaemia is a potential medical disaster, and must be treated as an emergency. On the other hand, although many pregnant women experience a few of the early symptoms of pre-eclampsia *very* few progress to the much more malign full-blown toxic stage. It is only in full-blown toxaemia that the frontal headaches occur, but if you're in the later stages of pregnancy and have developed any of the symptoms listed above, you should contact your doctor or midwife *immediately*

We still don't know why toxaemia occurs. It may be related to exercise and certainly it's helped by rest. Interestingly, its usually less common in subsequent pregnancies.

Finally, a small point needs to be made about blood pressure in pregnancy – the blood pressure rise caused by toxaemia is quite different from the blood pressure rise caused by 'ordinary' blood pressure. It is quite possible to have high blood pressure during pregnancy from 'ordinary' blood pressure without any problems: on the other hand a *rise* of blood pressure at this time may indicate toxaemia.

Type of headache
The headache is severe, and across the forehead, accompanied by flashing lights in the eyes.

What else could it be?
A *tension headache* produces a similar type of headache. *Migraines* can produce flashing lights in the eye, but the headache isn't at the front, but over one half of the head. The tests your doctor does of your urine, blood pressure and weight will indicate whether or not it's toxaemia.

Self-help
Make sure you get good ante-natal care, and try to rest as much as possible during the later stages of pregnancy, though this can be very difficult; and if your doctor is advising you to rest more because of a rise in blood pressure, then do please take his advice – it's important.

Some doctors feel it is caused by a lack of high-quality proteins (meat, fish, eggs, etc.) and will suggest a dietary change. Do try to eat a healthy, well-balanced diet. Light exercise can also help *prevent* PET, but once you're got PET, *rest* is essential.

Complementary treatment
Full-blown pre-eclamptic toxaemia, or full-blown eclampsia, must be treated by a doctor – and preferably in the hospital. However, there are some complementary measures that can be undertaken on a preventative basis.

Efforts to keep your blood pressure down should be made, and that includes watching your diet and taking measures to reduce stress. Avoid coffee, tea and alcohol, and in its place try soothing camomile teas, Dandelion root coffee is a mild diuretic, which may help control oedema.

Homoeopathy and acupuncture both offer therapies to deal with high blood pressure and pre-eclampsia, but the treatment will be tailored to your individual needs.

*Oedema can be relieved by massage of the legs with geranium and
rosemary essential oils. Lavender may relieve headaches, as can acupressure.*

MENOPAUSAL HEADACHES

Women are born with about two million eggs in their ovaries, in an arrested state
of development. During the reproductive years, one by one, about four hundred of
these eggs are stimulated to develop, mature, and finally be released into the
womb. The remainder degenerate and are absorbed. The cells around each egg are
important because they produce the oestrogen and progesterone of the female
cycle.

Quite simply, all that happens at the menopause is that the ovaries run out of
eggs. There are simply no more left to develop, and as a result, two things happen.
Firstly, there are no cells able to produce oestrogens, so the level of oestrogen
falls; secondly, the brain detects this and tries to stimulate the ovaries by making
the pituitary produce ever larger quantities of FSH.

This lack of oestrogen is the principal cause of menopausal symptoms. For
reasons that we don't yet understand, as the oestrogen level falls, the circulatory
system becomes unstable and as a result flushing and sweating occur. Other
symptoms of the menopause include: woolly-headedness, vaginal dryness, poor
memory, back pain, flooding (very heavy periods), depression, a general sense of
feeling unwell, and headaches. Sometimes migraine can start or worsen at this
time. However, simply providing supplemental oestrogen can bring the woman
back to her previously normal state.

Some women get many more menopausal symptoms than others. There are
those women who float through the menopause with grace and ease, while others
have a wretched time of it, with hot sweats that keep them awake half the night,
flushes that make them beetroot-coloured and mental befuddlement that makes
them think they're going mad. It's unclear why some people have such a difficult
time of it, and although in the past many doctors felt that there was a large
psychological involvement, it now appears in most cases that any psychological
effects of the menopause occur as a result of changes in the hormonal level.

Due to the effects of oestrogen, migraines are more common in women. It used
to be thought that the incidence of migraines declined at the menopause, with the
decline in oestrogen levels, but it now appears that this is not necessarily so. Some
women have fewer migraines after the menopause; but others have more, and a
small proportion of women find their migraines *start* at the menopause. In those
whose migraines have worsened, hormone replacement therapy (HRT) can bring
matters back to normal again.

If you're having headaches and you are also going through the menopause, then
your headaches may respond to hormone replacement therapy (HRT). Some
doctors believe that HRT should be given to every menopausal woman, to prevent
bone-related problems like osteoporosis (thinning of the bones that is increased by
oestrogen deficiency in menopause). Others feel that the menopause is a natural
phenomenon and shouldn't be tampered with unless a patient is having severe
symptoms. Most doctors probably fall somewhere between these two extremes.

Diagnosis of the menopause is not always easy. Menopausal symptoms may occur at a time when the periods are still relatively regular, and having normal or nearly normal periods doesn't mean you aren't entering the menopause. In addition, some women have already had their womb removed (hysterectomy), even though their ovaries may still be in place, so they don't have periods any longer. Apart from menstrual irregularities, most of the remaining menopausal symptoms can also be caused by non-hormonal circumstances. In other words, it's not always easy to be sure, from your symptoms alone, of the point at which you're entering the menopause. Sometimes it's necessary to do a blood test to be sure if the symptoms are likely to be related to the menopause or not.

There is a further problem in those who've had a hysterectomy. Even if your ovaries are left behind, those who have had a hysterectomy have a fifty percent chance of having their ovaries fail within the next five years – in other words, of entering the menopause. Without a womb you may not realise you're menopausal. A thirty-six year old woman who had a hysterectomy four years earlier might actually be going through the menopause.

It's easy for a doctor to work out whether or not you're menopausal. A simple blood test can measure the level of FSH (follicle stimulating hormone) produced by the pituitary. In menopausal women this level is always high because the pituitary is desperately trying to stimulate the production of oestrogen from the follicles in the ovaries.

If some or all of the symptoms mentioned in this chapter seem to fit you, it may be a good idea to go and see your doctor. Certainly, if you are having these symptoms and also getting headaches then hormonal replacement therapy (HRT) may well remove your headaches, as well as the rest of your menopausal symptoms.

Orthodox treatment

Treatment of menopausal symptoms is by replacing the oestrogen. Almost as soon as this is done, any true menopausal symptoms will disappear.

Oestrogens are powerful drugs and, used on their own, they can cause cancer of the womb to develop. But don't be alarmed, there's a simple way to get around this. Adding progesterone during the second half of your cycle removes this extra chance that you will get cancer of the womb. If you still have a womb in place, then you will need oestrogen *and* progesterone; if your womb has been taken away then you only need oestrogen.

CAROLE

At the age of forty-four Carole went to her doctor complaining that she had been feeling unwell for the past two or three months. She had been getting headaches and episodes when she became hot. She also had a lot of stress in her life.

Four years previously she had had a hysterectomy, but her ovaries had been left in place. The episodes of 'feeling hot' sounded very much like menopausal symptoms. Bearing in mind the fact that half the patients who've had a hysterectomy suffer ovarian failure within five years of the operation, her doctor suspected she was having an early menopause. He checked this by doing a blood test for FSH (follicle stimulating hormone) and the result came back as being abnormal. Carole's pituitary was desperately trying to stimulate the ovaries into action by producing a lot of FSH, but the ovaries were not responding. In other words, Carole's symptoms were caused by the menopause.

She was prescribed oestrogen in the form of patches, which she wore on her skin, replacing them every few days. Because she no longer had a womb, there was no need for her to have progesterone as well. Shortly after she started using the patches, her headaches and flushes started to go away and since then have not returned.

Although Carole is still under stress at home and at work, her case shows quite clearly how menopausal symptoms can cause headaches independently of stressful situations.

What are the benefits and problems associated with hormone replacement? Firstly, the menopausal symptoms go – all the physical and mental symptoms improve and there is often a feeling of well-being where previously there was a vague sense of malaise. Secondly, as the normal drop in oestrogen at the time of the menopause causes the bones to lose calcium, artificially prolonging the time the bones are exposed to oestrogen keeps them stronger for longer, and in later life reduces the chances of developing osteoporosis or of getting a fracture.

Hormone replacement therapy also massively reduces the chance that you will get ovarian cancer and it may also reduce the chance of heart attack.

The drawbacks of HRT are that the periods return again and there is a possibility of an increased chance of breast cancer. Overall, the statistics are in favour of the HRT user. The chances of dying following a fractured hip, from ovarian cancer, or from heart disease are all reduced by a greater factor than the chance of getting breast cancer from having HRT. About five times as many lives will be saved through using HRT by comparison with those lost by HRT.

However, HRT has not been in use long enough for us to be certain that there are no long-term side effects. Although HRT is probably safe for the first five years, and may well be safe for much longer, the statistics are not yet entirely conclusive.

If you would prefer not to be on HRT, but would like treatment for some of the symptoms, the drug clonidine may help with hot flushes; and oestrogen cream applied locally to the vagina may assist with vaginal dryness.

Self-help

Exercise and a sensible diet particularly one that is rich in calcium will help stave off the effects of osteoporosis. Iron and B-complex vitamins can help offset the anaemia caused by flooding. Deep breathing techniques can help restore control, when you are suffering from mood swings, or other emotional symptoms of the menopause

Because of the slightly increased chance of getting breast cancer, the mammogram (a sort of breast X-ray) should be arranged on a regular basis.

Don't hesitate to talk to a counsellor about the psychological symptoms of the menopause (anxiety, phobias, confusion, depression, poor memory, etc.). What you experience might be natural, but it is certainly not easy or pleasant. Storing up emotions, fears and depression will most certainly cause tension headaches.

Complementary treatment

Complementary therapies can help deal with some of the secondary effects of the menopause.

Acupuncture can stimulate the body to deal more effectively with anxiety, depression, stress and irritability. It is supposed also to improve the balance of hormones, which will reduce the symptoms of the menopause. Headaches and migraine can be relieved by treatment to produce the body's natural painkillers (the endorphins).

Aromatherapy can have a soothing effect – particularly techniques involving bath and massage. Analgesic oils such as lavender and camomile can be used to massage the head, shoulders and neck in order to remove tension and improve circulation. Headaches and migraine can be treated in this way. Clary sage is said to help balance hormones.

An osteopath or chiropractor can reduce the headaches and migraines triggered by stress or neck problems, reducing nervous pressure and tension.

A clinical nutritionist would probably suggest supplementary pituitary glandulars. Avoid spices, alcohol, caffeine and smoking, and reduce your fat intake – all of which help prevent headaches, by reducing the number of potential trigger factors.

A naturopath will suggest a healthy diet, exercise and regular sleep. Various dietary supplements might be recommended; in particular, the B vitamins, and Vitamins C and E.

An in-depth consultation would be required for a homoeopath to effectively relieve the symptoms of menopause. Cimicifuga might be suggested for psychological symptoms (which can just as easily cause headaches), sanguinara for headaches and hot flushes, cauophylum for tension and anxiety, and lachesis for headaches.

Sage has an effect on the oestrogen levels and can be used for problems associated with hormone imbalance. Angus castus, false unicorn, oats and St John's wort can all be drunk, or taken in tinctures. Skullcap may ease anxiety or depression. Geranium oil is said to affect hormone balance, and the essential oil of rose is supposed to have a toning effect on the reproductive system in general.

Vitamin E is said to keep your reproductive organs healthy.

Chapter Nineteen

HEADACHES DURING SEX

No, it's not a music-hall joke – headaches and intercourse do have a direct connection, rather than the proverbial inverse relationship! Of course, having a headache may prevent you from enjoying intercourse, and its a good excuse for avoiding it, but headaches can occasionally relate to the act of intercourse itself. In complete contradiction to the joke, headaches with intercourse are more common in men!

There are three types of headache that can occur at intercourse. The first is an *exacerbation of tension headache*, and in patients who get tension headaches, intercourse may bring on a dull ache over the whole head. It may be more severe than tension headaches previously experienced, and it is probably due (amongst other reasons) to over-dilation of arteries in the head.

The second type of headache is caused by a ruptured artery adjacent to the brain: a *sub-arachnoid haemorrhage*. Blood pressure rises during intercourse and this may be the final straw which causes an already weakened artery to rupture. (About one in forty cases of sub-arachnoid haemorrhage occur during intercourse.

The third type of headache, *benign orgasmic cephalgia* (which is a bit of a mouthful, so I'll call it 'true coital headache'), is actually quite rare. It's a sudden, explosive, one-sided headache coming on at intercourse, and lasting for a few minutes up to a few hours. Not only is it rare, it doesn't affect the patient every time he makes love. Some patients experience a period of several months during which they get this type of headache during love-making, but then the tendency dies away and they are no longer troubled. In other patients, the headache occurs only occasionally, but on a seemingly random basis.

What goes wrong?
Where the pain is a *tension headache* made worse by intercourse, the underlying causes are the same as for ordinary tension headaches. They are at least partially due to relaxation of the muscle in the walls of the arteries, which allows a higher blood pressure to be transmitted through to tissues which normally aren't accustomed to such high pressures.

With a headache from a *sub-arachnoid haemorrhage*, caused by a ruptured berry aneurysm (a balloon-like weakness or bulge in the blood vessel), the escape of blood into the area surrounding the brain, and the pressure it develops locally, are the root causes for the pain.

In the third type, *true coital headache*, no one is really sure what happens. There is a definite association of true coital headache with migraine, so it's quite possible that there is a common factor; blood vessels in the brain which are abnormally responsive in migraine may also be reacting too quickly to changes in body chemistry that occur during intercourse. ('True coital headache' and 'exercise headache' may both be just variants of migraine.)

Type of headache

Tension headaches made worse by intercourse come on as a dull ache over the whole head, developing before orgasm. It may pulsate in time with the heart beat. The pain of a sub-arachnoid haemorrhage brought on by intercourse is typical of all other sub-arachnoid haemorrhages – a feeling of being hit on the back of the head or neck, followed by an explosive headache of immense severity.

The pain of a true coital headache is a sharp, one-sided, sudden onset, explosive pain which lasts anything from a few minutes to a few hours.

What else could it be?

There is no one disease called 'headache during intercourse'; headaches with intercourse could be any one of the conditions that have been outlined above.

Because a severe, sudden onset of head or neck pain *occurring for the first time* at intercourse could be due to a sub-arachnoid haemorrhage you must get medical help *immediately*. On the other hand, if you've already had headaches with intercourse, and this is just another of the series, then it is unlikely to be a sub-arachnoid haemorrhage.

Headache with intercourse is often due to (or made worse by) *tension headache*, and, depending upon the sexual techniques used and the position of the neck, it might also be related to previous *neck or back injury*, or *neck muscle spasm*, especially if the head is held in an abnormal position for some time. In particular, bending the head back for any length of time can induce severe neck pain of the muscle spasm variety. The distinguishing features of tension headache, neck injury and neck muscle spasm are that there is often a previous history of injury to the neck, local tenderness of the neck or its muscles, stiffness on bending the neck to the side, and the neck muscles can often be felt in spasm.

Orthodox treatment

If the headache is due to *sub-arachnoid haemorrhage* then medical treatment needs to be sought urgently; the patient will need an urgent operation to close the bleeding artery inside the skull.

Where the headache is an exacerbation of *tension headache*, all the treatments for tension headache will be helpful. And if the headache is related to neck or spinal injury, treating the underlying injury itself will reduce trouble in the future.

MOIRA

Moira is a cheerful, thirty-eight-year-old homemaker who began to get very upset because every time she and her husband made love she suffered from headaches. She was also becoming very worried – was it something serious?

The problem seemed to be worse as her excitement grew; as soon as she began pelvic thrusts or rocking movements she would get a dull pain at the back of her head which really put the damper on things.

Her blood pressure was normal; she didn't have migraines; and the pain wasn't severe enough for a sub-arachnoid haemorrhage. But in the past she'd had a bit of back trouble, and it was her osteopath that eventually found the cause of the problem – an area of inflammation in the middle of the back had caused the lining of the delicate spinal cord to stick to the inside of the bones of the spinal column. As a result, when she started rocking her pelvis, she pulled on this area of the back, which in turn pulled on structures higher up in the neck and brain, causing the pain.

Moira now knew what was causing the problem, so at least she could relax. Treatment was directed at mobilising the stiff middle part of the spine so that it could withstand much more bending and movement; attention was also given to the associated muscle spasms, which both limited the movement of the back and increased any spinal pain. Just knowing that the pain wasn't anything lethal helped Moira to relax even more; and knowing also what movements brought it on meant that she could adjust her methods of love-making so as to minimise the strain on her back.

True coital headache (i.e. neither a tension headache nor a sub-arachnoid haemorrhage) will go away of its own accord. On the other hand, knowing that you're going to get a belter of a headache is not conducive to marital intimacy, and is likely to turn you off sex altogether! So something needs to be done. In fact, the drug propranolol, a beta-blocker, is very effective in preventing these headaches occurring. It's not available over the counter, so your doctor will need to prescribe it. Taking a small dose regularly is all that is needed, and from then on intercourse should be pain free. This type of drug interferes with the contraction of the muscles inside the blood vessels, which suggests that the cause of true coital headache originates from the blood vessels in the brain.

Self-help
Well, you could always become a monk ... except that this is hardly an acceptable self-help technique!

Quite seriously, this brings up a most important problem; even if a serious cause for your headache has been ruled out, it is easy for a vicious circle to develop in which the pain associated with intercourse so puts you off sex that the next time you're so anxious about it that you get a tension headache. And, because you had a tension headache that time, you get one the next time, through worrying about it – and the time after that and the time after that.

To prevent this vicious circle from developing you need to do two things: firstly, recognise that your headache isn't life-threatening or serious, just painful. This will take at least some of the worry out of the situation. Secondly, start to treat the problem with whatever medical, alternative and self-help techniques are appropriate.

In true coital headache, it's important to reassure yourself that the tendency to have headaches at intercourse lasts only for a short time, seldom occurs at each act of intercourse, and – most important – can be prevented with drugs. Just knowing that it is harmless, that it will eventually go, and that there are good medical treatments that can stop the headache starting, may all be enough to help you relax and minimise your headache.

True coital headache is not the same as tension headache and so relaxation techniques are unlikely to be so important, although they may help a bit, especially if you're getting wound up about the problem. On the other hand, because there is a relationship between true coital headaches and migraine, maintaining good control of your migraines may reduce the frequency of true coital headaches.

EWAN

Ewan is a slightly shy, married, thirty-year-old who came somewhat sheepishly to ask about his headaches. He was very embarrassed about it, the more so when it transpired that they were worst when he made love to his wife.

He'd been having headaches like this for some time and now he was convinced that he had something really wrong with him. In addition, the pain was beginning to put him off intercourse, because every time he and his wife began to make love he knew the pain would just get worse and worse.

He described the pain as being in the back of the head, coming on slowly, and with a rhythmic pulsing quality in time with his heart beat. It was also noticeably worse if they slept in and then made love in the morning.

Ewan was obviously a tense man, but his blood pressure was normal, he didn't suffer from migraines, and the pain was really an enlarged version of the tension headaches he had from time to time. A brief neurological examination was completely normal, as well.

Ewan had tension headaches which were being exacerbated by intercourse. On being told there was no physical abnormality he relaxed visibly. Now that he knew he wasn't likely to die in the middle of it, he could approach love-making without fear.

Ewan was shown how to feel for the painful trigger points in his neck muscles. His doctor suggested that it would help to reduce the tension in these muscles – and hence the headaches – if he got his wife to massage his back and neck, and especially these trigger points, before they made love. This is an occasion where massage with an aromatic oil such as ylang-ylang can be very appropriate. In fact, they found that massaging each other in this way was a very gentle and appropriate beginning to foreplay, and led naturally on to further intimacy. In particular, it helped Ewan to begin love-making in a much more relaxed state, which immediately reduced the level of his tension headaches.

Finally, Ewan was given some simple advice about ways to avoid tension, and this, together with a little analgesia an hour before he was likely to make love, was enough to put the break on his headaches; in turn, the improvement convinced him that he wasn't suffering from some incurable or dangerous disease.

Complementary treatment

If the headache is due to a sub-arachnoid bleed you need medical attention urgently; complementary therapies are not useful until after help has been sought and attention given.

If the headache is an exacerbation of a tension headache, all the complementary therapies listed in the chapter on tension headaches will help.

In the meantime, however, there are numerous things that can be undertaken – many of which can enhance sexual intercourse. Try massaging (or having your partner massage) around the back of the neck, temples and eyes with a blend of basil, camomile, coriander, lavender, melissa or clary sage, in a grapeseed or avocado carrier oil. Eye compresses of camomile or rosemary can help, if you use them for twenty minutes or so when the headache sets in, or following intercourse.

Tea tree, geranium, niaouli or lavender on the lamp or radiator beside the bed will provide a stimulating aroma, as well as working to relax you. If you are worried about sexual performance, try a bath with ylang-ylang (a known aphrodisiac) or rose (for women, in particular).

Acupressure can be done between partners, as can reflexology – both of which are relaxing and preventative. Soft music will release tension, as will candlelight – romantic and therapeutic.

Regular courses of feverfew may help to prevent headaches during sex, in the same way it can control migraine. Acupressure and shiatsu are helpful for long-term conditions, and osteopaths and chiropractors can also pin-point a musculo-skeletal cause that orthodox medicine might just have missed. Psychotherapy can help you deal with feelings of fear or apathy surrounding sexual intercourse. Often deep-rooted feelings can be the cause of physical pain.

Associated problems
High blood pressure is a predisposing factor for a sub-arachnoid haemorrhage. *Neck and spine problems* can trigger off pain during lovemaking.

Chapter Twenty

HEADACHES IN CHILDREN

Headaches in children are somewhat different to headaches in adults. To begin with, children often have an ache in the abdomen, rather than the head, during fevers – so a child going down with a mild flu-like illness will complain of a tummy-ache. In an adult this would be a headache. This phenomenon is quite marked, and the younger the child the more likely they are to complain of abdominal rather than head pain in generalised infections.

This is particularly true in the case of non-specific illnesses such as viral infections, urinary tract infections, and so on. It makes diagnosis more difficult, of course, because many abdominal illnesses can also cause abdominal pain, and these have to be excluded from the diagnosis.

A useful point is that a tummy-ache that is really a 'headache in disguise' is always felt around the middle of the abdomen. When asked where it hurts, the child will always point to his navel. Some abdominal illnesses can also cause central abdominal pain, so it doesn't exclude other things; however, what you can confirm is that if abdominal pain is somewhere *other* than the navel, then it's unlikely to be caused by a temperature/infection alone. To make matters even more complex, not all children perceive general pain in the tummy – some have headaches, just as adults do. A useful rule of thumb is that the younger the child, the more a headache is likely to mean something other than just a mild infection.

A specific variety of this perception of abdominal pain is abdominal migraine. This behaves almost exactly like migraine, except that the pain is centred in the abdomen rather than the head. It has the same time span as an ordinary migraine, and seems to be a childhood equivalent.

The second reason why children get different types of headaches from adults is because children suffer from a different range of illnesses to adults. This means: more fevers, more tumours, fewer neck injuries, hardly any strokes and no menstrual or pre-menstrual problems before puberty. Eye problems and, behavioural problems also cause specific difficulties in childhood. The pattern of children's headaches reflects these differences.

Let's look at each of these causes in turn.

INFECTIONS

Headache from fever occurs much more frequently in children, for two reasons. Firstly, an infection in a child usually causes a much higher fever than the same infection would in an adult: a mild viral infection producing a temperature of only 99.5° F (37.4° C) in an adult might produce a fever of 103° F (39.4° C) in a child.

Secondly, the higher the temperature, the more powerful the headache, and children get many more high fevers than adults. As we've just seen, part of this is because some illnesses produce high temperatures in children, and not in adults. But there is a second and more important factor at work: children are simply much more vulnerable than adults to being infected by the germs that are present in the community at the time. The reason is quite simple. A person is vulnerable to any illness he hasn't met before, but once he's had the infection, he develops immunity to it, so he can't get it again. This is why (with very few exceptions) it's only possible to have an illness like mumps once. After the initial infection the body recognises the mumps virus, and on every subsequent occasion that this virus tries to gain entry, the immune system locates and neutralises it.

Lastly, and very importantly, don't forget meningitis is a cause of fever and headache. Meningitis is more common in children, so get into the habit of checking for a stiff neck *every time* your child gets a temperature. That way, if it *is* meningitis, you'll be giving your child the best possible chance of getting over it. Meningitis in the very young doesn't always give a stiff neck: a bulging fontanelle (the soft bit at the top of a baby's head), vomiting, irritability and/or drowsiness, are among the things to look for. And remember that in meningitis *immediate* medical treatment may save your child's life.

But meningitis is rare. Don't get over-anxious about the possibility of your child having it. Just check that neck, routinely, *each time* he or she gets a temperature.

TUMOURS

Sadly, brain tumours are more common in younger children, certainly during the first five or so years of life. There are good physiological reasons for this – tumours are essentially disorders of cell division, where the cell doesn't know how to stop dividing. During the development of the baby in the womb, and then in the first few years of life, a great deal of cell division occurs. If cell division goes wrong it may manifest itself as a tumour. In addition, the immune system (which has a large part to play in detecting and removing malignant cells) is immature and perhaps doesn't recognise altered, cancerous cells for what they are.

After the early part of childhood, tumours generally reduce in frequency and the incidence of cancer only rises again in later life. This too is understandable because in later life the immune mechanisms of the body start to break down and cancer cells may no longer be as easily recognised and dealt with.

HYDROCEPHALUS

Hydrocephalus is another condition which is largely a disease of the very young. Cerebro-spinal fluid (CSF) is created in chambers called the ventricles, deep within the brain, and flows out to the outside of the brain through a small set of channels.

Here it bathes the brain, and then passes down the spinal canal, where it is re-absorbed. If there is an obstruction to the exit of CSF from within the brain, the pressure inside the head rises and as a result progressively blows the brain up from the inside, like a balloon. This is hydrocephalus, sometimes known as 'water on the brain'. Obstructions to the outflow of CSF include: a congenital narrowing of the drainage canal; a tumour which is pressing on the outflow tract; or, after meningitis, which has scarred the outflow tract so that it becomes blocked and can no longer drain the fluid properly.

The effects of hydrocephalus vary according to the age of the child. In the very young child the skull bones are separate, fusing together as the child gets older. In a very young child who hasn't yet fused her skull bones, this extra pressure distends the brain and also makes the skull swell. Because the skull can swell, the pressure on the brain doesn't rise that much, so this doesn't give as much pain as you might imagine. However, in the older child where the skull bones have fused, a rise of pressure within the ventricles squashes the brain against the unyielding inside of the skull, causing severe headaches, vomiting and other symptoms.

The treatment is to release the pressure, usually by putting in an artificial drainage tube called a shunt, to drain the excess CSF away. Often these shunts work for a number of years, and then become gummed up, but by then the skull and brain may have grown sufficiently for the normal drainage channels to reopen.

Hydrocephalus can also occur in adults, principally because of tumours which block the drainage of CSF. The reason hydrocephalus is more common in children is that it is associated with certain types of malformation that exist at birth, especially those related to certain types of spina bifida (a disorder of the spine and spinal cord). The increased incidence of brain tumours in childhood also means that there is more chance of a tumour obstructing the drainage channel. Meningitis, which can 'gum up' the drainage channel, is also more common in earlier life.

ABDOMINAL MIGRAINE

Although children often have 'headaches' in the abdomen, we are not yet sure whether abdominal migraine is a normal migraine that is just perceived in the stomach (as with other general pain in children), or whether it is an entirely separate variety of migraine. At first you might think it strange for a migraine to cause abdominal symptoms. However, even in the adult, migraine is not *just* associated with headache. The absorption of food and medicines from the stomach is considerably delayed, there is very often vomiting, and it may well be that the headache of migraine is merely the most prominent part of a condition which actually affects a great deal more of the body that just the head. It isn't surprising that the abdomen would hurt if there were problems of absorption within it and there are also food-allergy components to the cause of migraine.

Abdominal migraine follows much the same pattern as 'head' migraine. The time scale is much the same; there is often sickness and nausea; but, the aura and visual disturbance don't occur. Abdominal migraine responds to many drugs that help in adult migraine – particularly painkillers, metoclopramide (an anti-nauseant), and at times, non-steroidal anti-inflammatory drugs (NSAIDs) such as ibuprofen.

Only a proportion of childhood migraineurs get the abdominal form of migraine; the remainder get 'normal' head migraines. Nor do people with abdominal migraine continue with abdominal migraine all their lives. Often the migraine is converted to the 'normal head form, or stops altogether.

EYE PROBLEMS

At least some headaches in children occur because of unsuspected eye problems. Squinting or focussing difficulties cause headaches when they are *minor,* because the child can compensate for the problem by tensing up the eye muscles or peering. This leads on to tension in the muscles of the eye and face, and to tension headaches. Major degrees of abnormality in the eyes *don't* cause headaches, simply because the child can't compensate by tensing up his muscles, so he doesn't try.

Every year many children are unexpectedly diagnosed as being short-sighted when they and their parents didn't think that anything was wrong. Often it's only spotted because the child doesn't seem to be doing well at school. Then someone thinks to check whether she can read the blackboard – and she can't. The trouble is, if the child's vision has always been that way she doesn't know any better; she thinks vision is like that for everyone, so she doesn't complain.

Minor degrees of squinting can also remain undiagnosed for a considerable time, especially where the child can normally compensate for the squint by extra muscular action. Note also that astigmatism (an inability to focus on horizontal and vertical lines at the same time) is a particularly potent cause of headaches.

BEHAVIOURAL PROBLEMS

Tension headaches can occur in children just as in adults and this is the second most common cause of headaches, after the headaches of infections. The underlying causes can include fear of school, especially where there is bullying, or the child doesn't get on well with his teachers; it can be a reflection of family disharmony – parental break-up, relationship problems with brothers or sisters, difficulties with adjusting to a new baby in the family, the illness or death of a parent, or sexual abuse. Don't forget the effects of TV and videos – often younger children are exposed to material that is very frightening.

Tension headaches in children are a sign of unhappiness and stress. Gently talking through the child's worries may quickly point to what is wrong, but professional help may also be needed. It's important to remember that the tiniest changes in routine can all cause stress on a child. And stress, as we know, is the precursor to tension headaches.

EPILEPSY

Epilepsy isn't just a childhood disease, but most cases do start at this time. Epilepsy can cause headaches in the period immediately after a fit.

The most important thing you can do when your child is suffering from any illness is: *don't panic.* Even if they do occur more commonly in childhood, they are still rare. Deal with your child calmly and methodically. Assess his or her symptoms and if you are worried or in doubt call your doctor.

Chapter Twenty-one

MISCELLANEOUS CAUSES

THE BODY CLOCK

The body has its own natural rhythms and when these get out of synchronisation we can feel particularly unwell. When there is conflict between the body's internal clock and the external time by the sun, you can feel quite ill. This is the basis of jet-lag: your internal bodily rhythms say that it is ten-thirty in the evening, and time to go to sleep, while your eyes tell you that it is four in the afternoon, and you should be awake.

Body rhythms are very deep-seated and take quite some time to shift to the new local time. All sorts of biochemical events vary with the time of the day – levels of steroids in the blood; response to anaesthetics, and the ability to metabolise alcohol, for example. General mental processes are effected, too – so much so that some companies won't let their senior executives make any decisions at all within three days of flying across the Atlantic. Jet-lag is worse when you have to bring your body clock *forward*. So flying the Atlantic from West to East tends to be much more traumatic than the East-West journey. The symptoms of jet-lag include poor sleep and fatigue, difficulty in concentrating, headaches, loss of appetite and indigestion.

The greater the number of time zones you cross, the more you will be affected by jet-lag. Older people also suffer more than younger travellers. For short business trips you are best to try to keep to your old time, arranging meetings according to (home) times when you would normally be awake. But to minimise jet-lag when you want to adopt the new time, make a point of rigorously adhering to the new local time for all activities and make a point of re-setting your internal clock using the stimulus of light (see below).

We all experience a mild form of jet-lag whenever the clocks are put forward or back. Putting the clocks forward (in the Spring) is much more traumatic than when they are put back in the Autumn. It can take about a week to adjust to putting the clock forward.

Quite what regulates the body clock isn't completely understood, but it's related to the production of a hormone called *melatonin* by the pineal gland, which is in the middle of the brain. Left to itself, the body clock's normal 'day' is about twenty-four and a half hours; this internal clock is nudged into line with the solar day by the effects of sunlight and external social factors such as noise and eating. In fact, you can re-set your body clock by exposing yourself to sunlight at certain key times of the day. For example, one of the quickest ways to bring your body clock forward is to expose yourself to sunlight as soon as you get up in the morning.

When the body clock is out of line with the solar day we feel generally unwell. This is particularly noticeable in those who regularly have to go on to a night shift – nurses, police officers, some factory workers, for example – and it commonly takes them some time to change to the new rota. In the meantime, they get an irritable bowel, a general sensation of heaviness in the limbs, and headaches. All this occurs simply because they have suddenly swapped day for night and night for day.

There are two ways to help if you have to go on night duty. As far as possible try to minimise the number of clock changes you have to undergo. If you're on permanent night duty, five nights on and two nights off, don't try to change yourself round to an 'ordinary' day on your days off. Instead, go to bed at the same time throughout the week, whether you're working or not, so that there is some consistency about your life. In this way your body clock won't be pushed around too often.

Secondly, if you do have to re-orientate your body rhythms, remember that sunlight is one of the best ways to do it. Exposure to sunlight early in the day tends to make you want to go to bed earlier; exposure to sunlight late in the day tends to make you wake up later. It's very logical if you think about it.

Complementary treatment

Aromatherapists recommend that you inhale lavender upon your arrival, if you want to stay awake, and rose geranium, if you want to sleep.

There is a new theory that taking the natural hormone melatonin will help you get back to your own normal rhythms faster.

Tryptophan, an amino acid, has been used to treat jet-lag with some success providing deeper and longer sleep while travelling and on arrival.

EXERTION HEADACHE

Exertion headache is a throbbing pain which can be brought on by exercise – such as running, swimming, sexual intercourse or sometimes even by sneezing and coughing. It particularly effects men over the age of forty. The headache is usually throbbing, extends over the whole of the skull, and lasts for a few hours. It is often associated with nausea – and sometimes even vomiting – and the need to avoid bright lights (photophobia), which are painful.

Exertion headaches may actually be a rare form of migraine. Very rarely they can be associated with tumours or abnormal blood vessel formations inside the brain, and because of this it is wise for a full set of investigations to be carried out.

Treatment of exertion headaches can be surprisingly simple. For some reason indomethacin, one of the non-steroidal anti-inflammatory drugs (NSAIDs) seems to be very effective in removing the pain; aspirin can also be used. Beta-blockers, such as propranolol, may also help. In those cases caused by blood vessel abnormalities or tumours, surgery may be necessary.

Complementary treatment
Lavender oil, applied neat to the nostrils can have a powerful effect on exertion headaches, or try a tiny valerian tablet.

Exertion headache shares a lot of similarities with migraine and may be a rare form of it; it is also identical to true coital headache.

HYDROCEPHALUS

Cerebro-spinal fluid (CSF) is formed inside the ventricles, which are spaces deep inside the brain. From here it moves slowly outwards and downwards, passing out through a narrow canal to enter the space around the outside of the brain and spinal cord. It is then gradually absorbed into the veins which line the inside of the skull.

The weak link in the chain is the canal connecting the ventricles with the outside of the brain. If this is obstructed, CSF cannot get out from the inside of the brain. Unfortunately, this fluid continues to be formed, gradually increasing the pressure within the brain, blowing it up like a balloon. This condition is called hydrocephalus, commonly known as 'water on the brain'.

Conditions that obstruct the outflow of CSF include a congenital narrowing of the drainage channel; a tumour pressing on the channel; or, after meningitis, which scars the canal so that it become blocked and can no longer drain CSF properly.

Hydrocephalus is a disease which affects those at the extremes of life. It is common in young children because they are more prone to those conditions which obstruct the outflow canal. These are congenital malformations, meningitis and brain tumours. Hydrocephalus also occurs in adults, but is significantly different from that in children. Most childhood tumours are tumours of brain tissue itself, whereas in adults many tumours are secondary growths spreading from other parts of the body. Hydrocephalus in adults gives severe headaches, with vomiting and confusion. Again, the skull is unyielding, and the brain tissue is severely compressed by the rise of pressure. Treatment is difficult. If by any lucky chance it is due to a benign tumour obstructing the outflow canal then it can be removed, but often hydrocephalus in adults occurs from inoperable malignant tumours.

Benign intra-cranial hypertension

Benign intra-cranial hypertension is a permanent rise of pressure within the CSF, but without any obstruction of the drainage (outflow) canal. It is more common in obese women; occasionally it occurs following pregnancy or miscarriage; it can also be related to brain infections and mild head injuries in certain people.

Intra-cranial hypertension causes generalised swelling in the brain, due to the presence of excess water, a condition called oedema. Its symptoms are very similar to the effects of hydrocephalus in an adult – there is headache, vomiting and impairment of consciousness.

Benign intra-cranial hypertension responds well to steroids and they can often keep it completely under control.

Lumbar puncture headache
The brain floats inside the skull – moored in the cerebro-spinal fluid (CSF). If CSF is drawn off, then the brain tends to sink down inside the skull, pulling on its moorings – and this is exceptionally painful.

Normally, of course, this doesn't happen. However, when a lumbar puncture is performed some of the CSF fluid is drawn off. This causes the brain both to tug on its moorings and also to swell slightly to make up for the fluid that has been drawn off. This hurts. It is quite common for a headache to develop for twenty-four hours, following a lumbar puncture, while the body is replenishing the level of CSF. During this time the patient is encouraged to lie still and flat (he usually wants to) and the headache is usually lessened if the patient stays in this position, lying in bed.

PAGET'S DISEASE
Paget's disease is a relatively rare condition which typically affects old people – men more than women. It causes thickening and bowing of the bones, particularly the long bones of the legs. It also causes thickening of the skull bones, which can cause headaches that are felt deep down inside the skull, often towards the back. Basically, new bone is produced faster than old bone is destroyed. Deafness is common, and in a small number of cases Paget's disease leads on to a bone tumour.

The characteristic features of Paget's disease are that the thickened skull bones increase the size of the head; this thickening can be seen clearly on X-ray. There are also special blood tests which can diagnose Paget's disease.

Paget's disease is rare and can be helped by giving injections of the hormone calcitonin, which encourages the bones to absorb more calcium. Analgesics may be prescribed to deal with the pain.

Complementary treatment
Constitutional homoeopathy might help, and extra Vitamin D, which has a similar action to calcitonin, is often recommended.

URAEMIA
The kidneys are responsible for filtering the blood, removing excess water and waste products. Badly diseased kidneys can't do this properly: they can't concentrate the urine, and they can't excrete waste products properly and the condition called *uraemia* results.

Uraemia comes on slowly and is accompanied by a large number of other symptoms – protein in the urine, weakness, high blood pressure, anaemia, loss of appetite, nausea and vomiting, diarrhoea, itching, hiccups, and sometimes confusion. Headaches are common – both from the uraemia (and all the other changes) and also because of the rise of blood pressure.

Severe kidney failure is not necessarily a disease of older people; it does occur in younger people. Sadly, in uraemia there is little that can be done to improve the kidney's function. Sometimes low protein diets reduce the amount of urea that is formed; in the later stages careful control of the amount of fluid that you drink can also help; but, if you're getting a headache from uraemia then there are only three things that are likely to cure you: dialysis using an artificial kidney or a technique called peritoneal dialysis (whereby fluid is pumped in and out of artificial holes in the abdominal wall) or else a kidney transplant.

Long-term untreated urinary infections can damage the kidneys and cause them to fail, so it is important to make sure that infections in children and young people particularly are fully treated, and that the infection is completely gone from the urinary system. Otherwise, if the infection is left to grumble on for month after month, and year after year, it may damage the kidneys progressively.

However, don't get too alarmed about this. Intermittent attacks of cystitis or other urinary tract infections will not produce this sort of damage to the kidneys. It is not the frequent infections that do the damage, it is the *continuous,* unremitting infections, present for months and years that damage the kidney in this way.

Therefore, as far as prevention is concerned, if you are prone to infections in the bladder make sure that you go to your doctor to get appropriate antibiotic treatment. This will remove the infection and stop any possibility of damaging the kidneys.

Complementary treatment
Constitutional homoeopathy can be helpful for both preventative measures and treatment of existing uraemia.

RESPIRATORY FAILURE
Far and away the biggest causes of respiratory failure are bronchitis and emphysema. In both cases the tubes leading to the inside of the lung get blocked with excess mucus; the delicate lining of the bronchii which transports mucus away is damaged and so the mucus remains where it is. Finally, when the air gets down deep into the lungs it can't enter the blood easily.

The main cause of bronchitis and emphysema is smoking. *All* smokers eventually get a certain amount of bronchitis, although only a small proportion get full-blown respiratory failure.

The chief symptom of respiratory failure is progressive breathlessness. Usually this comes on slowly. At first the shortness of breath is only slight, associated with exertion, but gradually preventing the patient from undertaking normal day-to-day activities. The shortness of breath increases until eventually the person is breathless, even at rest.

There are two varieties of respiratory failure, depending upon how the control mechanism for breathing copes with the problem. The type which concerns us here is when the level of carbon dioxide in the body rises greatly. When this happens the patient becomes blue around the mouth, lips and tongue, and has a headache; there may also be restlessness, anxiety, delirium and drowsiness.

Obviously illness like this must be treated by a doctor, possibly even in hospital. Oxygen therapy may help, but for complex physiological reasons it isn't always possible to give large quantities of extra oxygen. Inhaled steroids and drugs to open up the airways may sometimes be helpful in bronchitis; physiotherapy to help clear mucus from the lungs is often useful.

Bronchitis and emphysema can place a great strain on the heart; added to this, the tobacco that causes the bronchitis also furs up the arteries of the heart, so patients with respiratory failure frequently have a degree of heart failure. Controlling the heart failure may help the respiratory failure.

In the long run there is little we can do to help those who have respiratory failure. It is so sad to see someone in this situation, knowing that it has almost always been caused by the patient himself ... through smoking.

Self help

Respiratory failure can be prevented, and that means no smoking. And the sooner you give up, the longer your lungs are likely to last. Tobacco smoke contains carbon monoxide which also poisons the red cells and stops them carrying oxygen. In the long-term, carbon monoxide also causes furring up of the arteries in the heart.

If you have respiratory failure you can also help yourself by keeping as relaxed as possible. The more anxious you are the more tense your muscles will become, and the more you tense your muscles the more oxygen you use up and the more carbon dioxide you create.

Complementary treatment

If an attack of bronchitis or emphysema comes on, get plenty of bed rest, with a hot water bottle on your chest. Steam inhalations are also helpful to loosen the phlegm. Avoid damp, cold and dust. There are a number of homoeopathic treatments for bronchitis and emphysema – including aconite, belladonna, kali bichrom or pulsatilla. You will need a full consultation to receive the most useful treatment.

Under the care of a registered practitioner, Vitamins E, A, C and D can be supplemented, and zinc can help. Extra iron is often recommended.

Oils of eucalyptus and hyssup are expectorant. Cloves and eucalyptus can be steeped and drunk as a tea, with lemon. Teatree and oregano oils are a good choice for the vaporiser.

Chapter Twenty-two

WORK-RELATED HEADACHES

Headaches can occur at work for a wide variety of reasons, and for our purposes it's simpler to classify headaches by what triggers them off. In all cases of work-related headaches, treatment follows the same principles – identify the trigger factor, and then deal with it. This sounds simple, but isn't always easy in practice.

Work-related headaches fall into four main categories, according to the type of trigger causing them. These are:

• Musculo-skeletal and ergonomic problems (the relationship between the worker and his or her environment)

• Light, noise and vibration

• Chemicals, including allergies

• Stress

If you're getting a lot of headaches at work then it's worth thinking carefully about whether any or all of these items apply to you. Sometimes the answer is easy: a headache coming on whenever you go into the factory's paint shop, or one that always occurs when you've been using the computer, is easy to sort out.

However, there are traps. Obviously, a headache which seems to come on at work is likely to be directly related to work conditions. But headaches may occur when stress is *removed*, so a headache which occurs at the weekend can be due to *relaxation* from tension from work. Don't forget, too, that in allergies the body can be supremely sensitive, and traces of work chemicals that are taken home on clothing or overalls may continue to cause symptoms at times away from work.

Allergies can create diagnostic traps, too; for a start, in allergies the cause-and-effect relationship can be altered by constant low doses of exposure to the offending substance. You might imagine that if you're very allergic to a substance then your reaction is likely to be brisk, and directly related to your exposure to it. This is absolutely correct, *but only if you have been away from the substance for some time*. In this case, exposure to the substance you're allergic to *will* produce a sudden and often intense reaction. However, if you are constantly exposed to a substance to which you are allergic there is a more random pattern of reaction, combined with a general malaise. Therefore, if you're allergic to the chemicals exuding from the new carpet in the office, you may feel generally under the weather while at work, with headaches coming on more or less at random, unrelated to the time of day, or the day of the week. Often it's only when you go on holiday, away from the offending chemicals, that your headaches and other symptoms go away, returning when you go back to work. But isn't it easy to blame the headaches on going back to the stress of the office? This is where physical and psychological causes for headaches overlap.

Discovering the root cause of headaches at work can sometimes be easy; on other occasions you may need a great deal of patience. You need to change things one by one: for example, altering only the position of your computer, or making a point of not going near the chemical store, or avoiding the new reception area.

Altering a lot of things at once may get rid of your headaches, but finding out which of the ten items you've altered is the culprit may be difficult. If you've altered the position of your computer at the same time as staying away from the reception and avoiding the paint shop – and your headaches clear as a result – then which of them is the actual cause?

ERGONOMIC AND MUSCULO-SKELETAL PROBLEMS
This particular cause of headaches constitutes a massive topic and has already been touched upon earlier in the book.

LIGHT
Too much, or too little light can cause headaches. Factors such a the contrast of computer screens and the glare of sunlight are covered elsewhere on this book.

Fluorescent Lighting.
Although fluorescent tubes appear to be giving off a steady shadowless light, in reality they flicker one hundred times per second. Because the retina smooths out these little bursts of light, normally we're not consciously aware of the flickering. However, this flickering still has a very special and very odd effect. When you switch your gaze from one point to another, the eyes move in a smooth line; however, if the fluorescent light is in its 'off' phase at the time you are about to look at another point in the room, your eyes can't see it, and will overshoot it slightly. When the light comes on a hundredth of a second later, your brain realises that it's overshot the mark and starts moving your gaze back again until it gets to the right position.

Therefore, under fluorescent lights your gaze is constantly overshooting and needs constantly to be corrected. Making these extra corrections is tiring on the eyes, and is one of the reasons why so many people find working under fluorescent lights irritating and tension-making.

There is a very quick way to stop this happening – double the frequency of the current in the lights. Then the fluorescent tubes flicker at two hundred cycles per second, which is too fast to allow the eye overshoot to occur. Working under fluorescent lights like this is much more restful, but lamps like this are more expensive than the ordinary sort.

NOISE

Noise is like glare – the more there is, the more tension it inspires. Part of this tension occurs reflexively. The eardrum is the receptor for sound inside the ear, vibrating as sound waves impinge upon it. The movements of the eardrum are picked up by a tiny bone called the *malleus,* which then transmits the vibration to two further bones in the sensory part of the ear. Attached to the malleus is a small slip of muscle called the tensor tympani. When this muscle contracts it pulls on the malleus, preventing both it and the eardrum from vibrating too much. This has the advantage of being able to damp down loud sounds so that the delicate sensory mechanism inside the ear doesn't get overwhelmed.

The *tensor tympani* is a muscle like any other muscle, and after a time it too can go into spasm and get tired in the presence of constant loud noises. In addition, reflex contraction of the muscles around the neck, head and face also occur where there is constant loud noise. This muscle tension serves to cause headaches.

Noise is also wearing just because it *is* noise – it stops us concentrating and makes it difficult to make out what other people are saying. This acts as a further source of stress, and where there is stress there is increased muscle tension. Yet more headaches result. (This is even more the case when the noise is an irritant, such as a baby's cry, where in addition to the noise there may be feelings of anxiety, stress or guilt at being unable to do anything about it.)

For most types of noise-induced stress the cure is simple: reduce excess noise wherever possible. If you're working in a noisy environment, then by law your employer will be required to supply you with ear defenders. *Wear them!* If you don't you may permanently damage your hearing.

Of late, excess noise has found a place in the office, with the arrival of the computer printer. The daisy-wheel printer, which gives high-quality characters, is like a manic version of a golf-ball electric typewriter; a dot-matrix printer gives off less of a clatter, more of a constant whine. Both these printers can be extremely annoying in the office environment. The cure is simple: buy a printer hood. This is an acoustic shield, which fits over the printer, yet allows you to see what is being printed. Alternatively, buy a bubble-jet or a laser printer, which are virtually silent.

VIBRATION

Vibration is really noise that we feel rather than hear. Vibration acts directly on the muscles and joints, irritating them, and if there is a pre-existing joint or muscle injury, vibration is likely to make it much worse. The frequency of the vibration is critical; certain frequencies are notorious for causing problems, such as low frequency – seven cycles (pulses) per second – which is quite literally gut-wrenching in high power. It's whether individual vibrations are just at the right (or wrong) frequency that determines whether they will cause trouble or not.

Vibration works its damage by setting the tissues in motion with ever-increasing force. It tends to come from machinery, but don't forget the vibration and jolting that can come from riding vehicles such as tractors and landrovers over rough ground. Normally these are provided with well-sprung seats, but if you are using vehicles off-road, do be aware of the amount of vibration and knocks that you can get. Being a passenger or a pilot in a helicopter, or in a low-flying light aircraft can also give you considerable vibration. Surprisingly, blows to the pelvis and seat can strain the neck considerably and headaches from neck joint injury and/or neck muscle tension can result.

Treatment is by avoiding vibration where possible. When this is impossible, reduce the amount of vibration transmitted through to your body. In particular make sure that your seat is well sprung. Cushions – especially air-filled rings – can damp down vibration and jolting very effectively. Thick gloves reduce the vibrations from hand held machinery. If you're doing a lot of running or walking on hard surfaces, cushion the effect on knees and spine by using footwear with resilient soles – for example, trainers.

CHEMICALS

Chemicals can cause physical problems in just the same way that foods can. There are two routes: the first is a *direct pharmacological effect* where the amount of the response relates directly to the dose of the substance. The second type of response is an *allergic* effect, in which only a small amount is needed to trigger a large, maximal reaction.

However, in practice it is not always easy to separate pharmacological and allergic effects, particularly when dealing with chemicals which are very toxic, but which still work in a pharmacological fashion, so that only tiny doses are needed to do a lot of damage.

Because pharmacological and allergic effects work on the body in different ways, it may help to know by which route a particular irritant is working. For example, antihistamines may help block an allergic effect, but are unlikely to help where a chemical is producing a direct pharmacological response.

These chemicals may produce 'ordinary' headaches, or act as triggers to produce migraines. Typical chemical agents that cause headaches include paint thinners; the petroleum-based products that exude out of paint after hardening; chemicals released from newly manufactured synthetic carpets; printing inks and chemicals used in photocopiers; the solvents used in dry cleaning; carbonless copying paper; duplicator ink, and, of course specific chemicals used in industrial processes.

Testing to find which chemical causes the damage must be done by careful elimination. Treatment is principally by recognising the cause and avoiding the trigger substances. Better ventilation may help considerably; extractor fans and air filters may be appropriate in some industrial processes. Wearing an over-garment that you *don't* take home will minimise your contact with splashed substances at work. Where the chemical is operating through an allergic route, anti-allergy measures will be appropriate.

BIOLOGICAL AGENTS

Fungi sometimes grow in air-conditioning systems, particularly where humidifiers are used, as the warm, wet conditions inside the humidifiers are ideal for promoting fungal growth. Contaminated air-conditioning and ducted warm-air heating can both pump large amounts of air polluted with millions of fungal spores around the building, and anyone who is allergic to these spores will react to them. Hay fever-like symptoms which start off at the time the air-conditioning or central heating is switched on may, in fact, be due to allergy to fungal spores sprayed into the air in this way.

Treatment is principally by recognising the cause of the problem and avoiding it where possible. Better ventilation may be all that is necessary. Proper anti-fungal treatment of air-conditioning systems; anti-allergic treatment such as antihistamines, etc. may be needed; in severe cases of allergy to fungal spores, desensitising injections can be given, but only through your local hospital. Homoeopathic desensitisation may also work.

STRESS

Work is one of the biggest causes of stress in our lives. We can be stressed by the work itself: we worry whether we are capable of doing it properly, or whether we can get it completed on time, and what the boss or our peers think of our performance. Then there's the responsibility of being in charge of people, and the particular stresses of middle management – caught in the nutcracker between the demands of top management on the one hand, and the shop-floor on the other,

In today's world there's the increased threat of redundancy, or the related feeling that the continuation of you job is in the hands of people outside your industry – such as the banks – who may put you out of business.

Stress is a potent cause of headaches. Coping with stress is a large subject, and beyond the scope of this book. However, there are many very good book on alleviating stress available in all bookshops. The result of stress, tension headaches, has been discussed in detail in Chapter Three.

THE 'SICK BUILDING' SYNDROME

Reaction to synthetic fabrics and petro-chemical fumes, lighting flicker, allergy to fungi, and sensitivity to positive ions in the air can individually produce headaches in susceptible people, but more commonly one, two or more of them act together. A recently labelled condition is the 'sick building syndrome', in which people in a particular office find that just attending work makes them ill, with headaches, a feeling of malaise, sniffles, and maybe even a slight temperature.

Sick building syndrome has a very loose definition, but quite a number of problems are relevant: poor ergonomic design of the computers and office furniture; fungal spores in the air-conditioning system; windows that won't open so there are lots of positive ions inside; offices lit exclusively by fluorescent lighting; newly painted walls and new carpets that are giving off chemical vapours; and duplicators and photostat machines that exude chemical solvents. And, of course, it's made worse if some of the employees smoke.

The cure for 'sick building syndrome' is to remove as many of the unwanted sources of stimuli as possible – cleaning up the air humidifying system using anti-fungal agents; fitting non-flicker fluorescent lights; and making sure that windows can open to let fresh air in from the outside, both to provide more negative ions, and also to blow away petro-chemical fumes, fungal spores and tobacco smoke.

Chapter Twenty-three

FOOD, CHEMICALS, DRUGS, ADDITIVES AND ALCOHOL

Many substances can cause headaches, and these include chemical solvents, gas appliances, alcohol, certain foods, additives and preservatives, car fumes and drugs, both prescribed and over-the-counter varieties. Sometimes the headaches are caused by the sudden withdrawal of a substance to which you're addicted – such as caffeine; a food to which you're allergic; or one of the addictive drugs. In each case, the treatment is obvious.– identify the problem, and then permanently eliminate the offending substance.

Some of the reactions we get to chemicals are caused by a direct effect of the chemical on the body. The effect may be related to the dose we receive – a *pharmacological response*. In other cases the reaction is allergic. This works by a completely different pathway, with the offending substance triggering off the body's immune system. In this case you get a maximum response for anything other that the tiniest dose.

Although pharmacological and allergic responses work through completely different routes, *treatment* is much the same. The only difference between the two is that it will be harder to completely remove something to which you are allergic, because even tiny amounts of the offending chemical may trigger symptoms.

Let's look at some of the more common sources of chemicals that can cause headaches.

GAS

In the old days, town gas used to contain high quantities of carbon monoxide. These days, in Britain, we use North Sea (natural) gas almost exclusively. This type of gas contains methane, but no carbon monoxide. Methane is not a direct poison, though in high enough concentrations it can be dangerous simply because it can displace the oxygen from the air – during a large gas leak, for example. Inhaling pure natural gas would be fatal simply because it doesn't contain any oxygen.

In order for gas to burn properly, a good supply of oxygen is needed. If there's not enough oxygen the gas burns incompletely. When methane burns in a good supply of air it forms waste products of water (as steam) and carbon dioxide. However, if burning takes place in a poor air supply carbon monoxide will be formed.

Carbon monoxide is *very* poisonous; it poisons the system by interfering with the way oxygen is transported from the lungs to the tissues. Therefore you must ensure that your gas fire has an adequate supply of air, and a good, clean vent. The importance of not blocking up the ventilation bricks in a room with a gas fire is obvious. In small quantities it merely reduces the oxygen-carrying capacity of the blood, but in larger amounts it can kill. Continual exposure even to low levels of carbon monoxide can quickly poison a very large percentage of the oxygen-carrying capacity of the blood.

Carbon monoxide poisoning is not a permanent thing, and in small quantities it debilitates rather than kills. However, it is a potentially vicious killer, and the more carbon monoxide to which you are exposed at any one time, the greater your likelihood of dying. The symptoms of carbon monoxide poisoning are principally headache, drowsiness and befuddlement.

Carbon monoxide is also present in cigarette smoke. The amounts are too small to kill, but it definitely impairs the ability of the body to supply the tissues with oxygen.

THE THOMPSONS

Fred and Evelyn Thompson are a retired professional couple living in their well-maintained retirement cottage. Over a period of six months they began to notice that they were getting headaches after spending time in their lounge, and that there often seemed to be a funny smell about the place. This continued for many months. Eventually they commented about the situation to some friends, who suggested that leakage of fumes from their gas fire might be the cause.

So they called in the gas board to survey it. The inspector took one look at their fire and immediately told them not to use it, as it was extremely dangerous. It had been badly fitted, and, as a result, fumes were leaking directly from the back of the fire into the lounge; in addition, the chimney flue was inadequate, and the net result was that they were receiving an appreciable dose of carbon monoxide.

Naturally, they did as he suggested; they called in the builders to fit a bigger flue, and a gas board fitter to re-install the fire. Once this was done the smell of the fumes disappeared completely, and so did their headaches.

Orthodox treatment

Carbon monoxide poisoning is potentially fatal. If there is any question about the health of the patient – and especially where a young child or an older person is involved – you should call a doctor immediately. The patient may need to go to the hospital. In hospital, treatment is simple – giving high concentrations of oxygen increases the amount of oxygen carried by the blood (although the red blood cells which normally carry oxygen have been poisoned by the carbon monoxide, some oxygen goes along dissolved in the blood serum) and after a while the carbon monoxide dissociates from the red blood cells, which can then go about their oxygen-carrying work normally again. After a minor degree of exposure, the patient is usually back to full health in a couple of days. However, lack of oxygen quickly and often *permanently* damages the brain, and death or severe brain damage can follow in severe cases of carbon monoxide poisoning, as well as damage to other tissues due to lack of oxygen.

Self help

Don't close off ventilation holes in rooms with gas fires. *Do* get your gas fires serviced regularly. *Do* check the chimney flue for birds' nests and anything else that can cause pressure, which would force waste gases back into the room.

Don't use old-style open-flue water heaters (the type that get their supply of air from within the room) in bathrooms and other enclosed spaces. A sudden, massive build-up of carbon monoxide like this can kill the occupant in the bath. Closed-system burners are much safer. These are the so-called 'balanced flue' systems, where incoming air is drawn exclusively from the outside, and the exhaust gases are vented exclusively to the outside.

CAR FUMES

Exactly the same principles apply to car exhaust fumes as apply to gas. Incompletely burning petrol gives off carbon monoxide as a waste product, and even the best maintained car engines emit a certain amount into the atmosphere. If operated in an enclosed space (such as a garage with the doors shut) there is a quick build-up of carbon monoxide in the air. This is the reason why you should *never* start a car engine without first opening the main garage door. Any leakage of exhaust gas into the passenger compartment can create headaches through carbon monoxide poisoning. The level of exhaust gases in the passenger compartment can often be relatively high and if you're aware that your car always smells of exhaust fumes after a journey, then you are probably exposing yourself to progressive amounts of carbon monoxide. If you end up with a headache and nausea after every car journey this is additional evidence that you've got exhaust-leakage problems.

As well as carbon monoxide poisoning, you can also become sensitive to other chemicals liberated in the exhaust.

Self-help

Be aware of the potential problem. Check your exhaust pipe regularly and make sure that any holes or leaks are mended as soon as they're found. In addition, make sure that the engine is properly tuned. This reduces carbon monoxide emission to the lowest possible levels.

One particularly awkward situation concerns people who live or work in areas with a high degree of traffic pollution – those who work in underground car parks, near big roundabouts where the vehicles are likely to be stuck in traffic jams for long periods of time, or in narrow and enclosed streets that are poorly ventilated by the wind. Again the cure is quite simple – identify the cause of the problem, and avoid exposure to the offending substance. On the other hand, it is unusual to have problems with car fumes unless you are working in an enclosed space. Making sure there is good ventilation and, if necessary, installing decent extractor fans, can make a lot of difference.

Don't forget that you can become sensitive to petrol itself (see *solvents*, below). If you're getting headaches and there's no obvious leakage of exhaust gases into the car, but there is a smell of petrol, it may be that you are sensitive to the petrol rather than being poisoned by carbon monoxide. If your petrol tank is slightly leaky, petrol fumes may well drift into the passenger compartment – especially in hatchbacks, and cars with back seats that let down to allow a continuous space from the passenger compartment into the boot. Because the petrol tank is often situated underneath the boot, any leakage of petrol vapour into the boot in cars like these can quickly circulate into the passenger compartment. If you frequently smell petrol, get the engine and petrol tank checked out.

SOLVENTS AND OTHER CHEMICALS
Solvents come in many forms. Most are based on petro-chemicals (chemicals with a petroleum base) and are used as cleaning agents, as paint thinners, or in glues, etc. While solvents are usually harmless in small quantities, those working with the same solvents day in and day out may become allergic to them, and where there is a massive amount liberated (for example, in a car-spraying plant) good ventilation is essential. Similar problems occur with 'carrier chemicals' used in the home – wax polish sprays, and pressurised aerosols – as well as dry cleaning fluid, glues, deodorants, perfumes, and chemicals used in hairdressing salons (i.e., permanent waves and bleaches). In addition, chemicals exude from paintwork, artificial fibres (especially fresh carpets), and plastics.

Usually it's easy to show a relationship between exposure to the solvent and the headache. A headache that only begins at work may well be related to some chemical to which you are being exposed in the workplace. However, exposure at home can be more difficult to sort out. *Constant* low-dose exposure, especially with an allergy, can be difficult, because you may not be away from home for long enough to clear the chemical to which you are sensitive out of your system. Consider allergies as a cause if your headache goes away when you're away from home for a few days, and returns when you return.

However, things are not always as simple as this, because the headaches may be related to family stress, which is absent when you're away on business; or to the poor quality of your bed. Nevertheless, patiently working through the possibilities, eliminating suspect items one by one and putting them back in again after a few days may tell you what is going on quite quickly. From then on it's a matter of eliminating those things that seem to cause you problems.

Perhaps the most difficult situation is that of the worker who gradually becomes sensitive to solvents and chemicals he uses. A typical example is the professional painter who's become sensitive to solvents in paint. Constant low-dose exposure, even in well-ventilated rooms, will be enough to give him headaches, often apparently at random. Other groups who experience chemical sensitivities at work include those working directly with chemicals – in the photographic industry or the pharmaceutical and petrochemical industries, for example.

There is no real treatment for solvent-related headaches other than excluding them from your environment. If you are getting pharmacological-type problems (dose-related), simply installing proper ventilation hoods and extractor fans may be all that's necessary; but, if you are developing a true allergy, you may even need to change jobs. Homoeopathic desensitisation might just work.

ANNETTE

Annette is a forty-year-old secretary who began suddenly to suffer from headaches. They seemed to come on when she was in the company of a particular group of friends, and she began to wonder what the problem was. Some of the people were fellow-workers in the office. Were her headaches related to the stress of being at work?

After a time she managed to work out the common factor – perfume. She only got the headaches when in the company of people who were wearing a particular type of perfume, and provided they were not using the perfume that day, she wouldn't get any headaches at all.

By observing when her headaches occurred and asking her friends what perfumes they were wearing, she was able to identify the culprit.

Since discovering which perfumes gave her headaches, it's become something of a topic of conversation with her – and she's been interested to find out how many of her friends also got headaches from particular brands of perfume. The brand may vary from person to person, but the same brand consistently gives headaches in the same person.

MEDICINES

Many medicines can cause headaches. Sometimes these are 'purely' side-effects – what in medical terms are called idiosyncratic reactions: a patient gets a headache while taking a particular drug, whereas other people generally don't. Idiosyncratic reactions tend to be specific to a particular drug in a particular patient, and usually the onset of the headache is quite clearly related to the time when he or she started taking the medicine.

Some groups of drugs used in the control of blood pressure can cause headaches. As part of their normal action they alter the muscle tone in the arteries, which are the high pressure side of the circulation. Control of blood pressure is by means of muscles lining the walls of the smaller arteries (the arterioles). If these muscles relax, the bore of the arteriole gets bigger; if they relax too much, blood at a higher pressure than usual can flow through to the organ the artery supplies. In some cases this distends the organ unpleasantly, causing pain. This is particularly important in the case of those arterioles which supply the brain. Certain drugs which make the muscles in these arterioles relax cause a pounding headache to develop. The most noticeable drug to do this is glyceryl trinitrate (GTN), which is commonly used under the tongue to abort attacks of angina (transient heart pain).

GTN works by dilating the arteries of the heart so that more blood can flow through to the heart muscle; however, the same action also happens in the arteries supplying the brain. As his heart pain diminishes, the patient also gets a bounding headache for a short period of time, as blood enters the brain under higher pressure than usual. Although with ordinary GTN this bounding headache always goes away quickly, other slow-release nitrates taken by mouth act on the heart for a longer period – and can also produce headaches in susceptible people.

Other drugs used to control blood pressure can cause headaches as a side-effect, especially if they act by reducing arteriolar muscle tone. Many drugs used to control blood pressure act in this way, but the sensitivity of individual patients varies considerably and what may cause terrible side-effects in one may not affect another at all.

Again, the cure is simple – avoid the offending drug. However, *don't* suddenly discontinue a prescribed drug without first talking to your doctor. This can be very dangerous especially if you're taking something like beta-blockers. It's usually of little value to try to treat headaches caused by specific drugs. It's much better to avoid the culprit drug, and change to an alternative preparation.

The contraceptive Pill can exacerbate existing migraines, or even (rather dangerously) cause them to start in a patient who previously didn't have migraines. Please see the chapters on Migraine and Headaches in women for further details.

DRUG ABUSE

Drug abuse (of the so-called 'street' drugs such as heroin, bupenorphine, etc.) can cause headaches in two different ways. Firstly, the excess use of the drug can cause headaches directly; secondly, and rather annoyingly, withdrawal from the drug can also cause headaches.

The chief problems with drug addiction are in the withdrawal phase, where cramps, shivering, sweating, headaches and a sense of general malaise are added to an intense craving for the drug that has been removed. The cause of a headache like this is pretty obvious – and the treatment is *not* to give yourself more of the drug to which you're addicted, because this will only prolong the agony. Eventually you will have to go through withdrawal and the longer you've taken the drug the worse your symptoms will be. Many of the addictive drugs can cause headaches during the withdrawal phase, but heroin and bupenorphine (Temgesic) are particularly notable examples. Most of the orthodox medical treatments and complementary therapies to treat addictions will be helpful.

Complementary treatment
Counselling relieves the stress associated with withdrawal symptoms, and this support can relieve headaches triggered by emotional problems and tension.

Herbal remedies which are helpful in withdrawal from drugs (particularly narcotics) are oats, rosemary, balm and skullcap (to calm and lift the depression). Constitutional homoeopathy can help with the withdrawal process, as well as dealing with the symptoms.

Detoxifying and anti-depressant aromatherapy oils, like those suggested for smoking and hangovers, see pages 235 and 236, can have some effect, and analgesic oils, like lavender, bergamot and camomile can be massaged into the temples, skull and neck. Hot baths with any of the suggested oils can be beneficial, and also reduce any associated stress.

Really, any therapy that works for you, that will get you through the difficult withdrawal period, can be undertaken. All of the following therapies offer some treatment, and may be suitable singly, or in combination: acupuncture, acupressure, biofeedback, reflexology, dance, music and art therapies, relaxation therapies, medical herbalism, clinical nutrition, naturopathy, Bach flower remedies, counselling, T'ai chi and kinesiology.

FOOD

Food can cause headaches in a number of ways. Food sensitivities are however a very complex topic and I will only summarise the role of food and additives here, in order to set them in the wider context of chemical sensitivities.

Like any other chemical substance, food can cause problems in two ways. Firstly, there is a pharmacological reaction – where a substance in the food has a direct effect on the body's cells. A pharmacological reaction like this is always dose dependent – the more you take in, the bigger the reaction (at least, up to a point). The other way foods can cause trouble is when the body has become allergic to a specific foodstuff; when the food is eaten, the body recognises it as a potential 'foreign' agent, and mobilises the immune system to try to deal with it. Allergic reactions like this tend to be much more like an on-off switch – they trigger off a maximal reaction at very low doses.

As an example of the two ways in which foods can react, tyramine is a constituent of chocolate and cheese, and in certain people can cause migraines via the direct pharmacological route. Reducing the level of tyramine in your diet will reduce the migraines. On the other hand, some people are *allergic* to various foodstuffs; they may also get migraines, but the migraines are triggered in a different fashion and usually require much smaller doses to start them off. Many different types of foods can cause migraine like this and the tendency to react to a particular food depends if you've been sensitised (become allergic) to this food. In turn, this relates more to the individual's exposure to that food in the past, rather than to any specific chemical constituents of the food itself.

Food additives can cause problems in exactly the same way as foods.

Some foods and additives are much more potent than others in causing headaches. There is even the 'Chinese restaurant syndrome' – pressure in the face, pain in the chest and a burning sensation in the head and chest. This seems to be related to eating certain types of Chinese food, Wonton soup, in particular, especially when taken on an empty stomach. Only a certain group of people seem to be sensitive in this way; the offending agent is thought to be monosodium glutamate, which is often used in Chinese cooking. However, it may not be monosodium glutamate on its own that causes the problem; there may well be an interaction with other constituents of Chinese food.

Another food additive which can cause problems is sodium nitrite, which is used in cured meat products such as Frankfurter sausages, and luncheon meats. In some people, sodium nitrite can produce a similar headache, together with flushing and redness of the face.

The pattern of meals can also affect headaches. Some patients with migraine find that low levels of sugar in the blood can trigger off an attack, and so going without a meal may be hazardous. Note, however, that a migraine caused by the absence of food can also be caused by a food allergy; there is a distant relationship between food addiction and food allergy, and patients who are allergic often get withdrawal symptoms when they initially omit a food to which they are allergic from their diet. Therefore, a migraineur who develops an attack every time he misses breakfast *may* be triggering the attack by low levels of sugar in the blood, but it might just be that he's allergic to milk (or tea, or coffee, or marmalade, or pork or eggs) and is having withdrawal migraines as a result of not eating any for some time.

ALCOHOL

Alcohol is an interesting substance, in that it does exactly the opposite of what most people feel it does. For a start, while most of us think that alcohol jollies us up, it doesn't. It's actually a central nervous system depressant, but since it first depresses those areas that inhibit our behaviour, it makes people jollier simply by sending inhibitory mechanisms to sleep!

Alcohol is also not a thirst-quencher. It is excreted in the urine, and pulls a lot of water along with it at the same time, acting as a mild diuretic. The only reason why alcoholic drinks *appear* to quench our thirst is because beer and other dilute beverages contain large quantities of water.

Alcohol can cause headaches in three ways – through sensitivity to alcohol itself, from a hangover, and in an alcoholic as he or she starts to withdraw from alcohol.

Some people are simply sensitive to alcohol; in these people, alcohol can cause a severe headache which is obviously related to drinking. Alcohol can also trigger off cluster headaches and migraine attacks.

Headaches caused directly by alcohol may not be straightforward. For a start, we shouldn't really be talking about alcohol, but about the *alcohols* – for there are a lot of them. Often headaches that come on after drinking a particular beverage are caused not by the alcohol itself, but by a sensitivity to some of the other alcohols and aromatic chemicals produced during the fermentation process. Red wine is notorious for this. Often individuals will say that certain drinks always seem to give them a headache, while other drinks seem quite all right. This is because they are particularly sensitive to the specific mixture of alcohols and other ingredients in that particular type of drink. Mixers can also be headache-related; in particular, tonic water.

The treatment, obviously, is to watch out for those drinks, or combinations of drinks, that seem to affect you, and simply avoid them.

The second way in which alcohol can cause a headache is during a hangover. Some of the headache is due to the direct effect of alcohol and its breakdown products, but a good part of the headache of the hangover is caused by dehydration. As noted earlier, when alcohol passes out in the urine, it drags with it a large quantity of water, and after a binge (particularly a binge on spirits, which contain little water) the body can get quite severely dehydrated.

Interestingly, the headache of a hangover is at its worst long after all the alcohol has been broken down by the body. The other aromatic chemical constituents of the drink may also have an important role – which is why mixing your drinks can have such a devastating effect. Some oriental races have an inherited inability to break down any further some of the by-products of alcohol, which may explain why people in these groups are much more sensitive to alcohol than other races.

The headache of a hangover is throbbing, made worse by moving the head, and is often accompanied by nausea or vomiting. The headache occurs some time after alcohol has been drunk, unlike the migraines produced by alcohol, which occur more or less as soon as the alcoholic drink has been taken.

The third way in which alcohol can cause headaches is during the withdrawal phase, the drying-out process, from alcohol addiction. In some cases this headache may be 'allergy withdrawal' in nature: here there is both addiction and allergy to some of the other chemicals (not just the alcohol) in the preferred drinks. It sounds surprising that someone could be addicted to a substance he's allergic to – but it's true, especially for food-related allergies.

Self help

Pretty obvious, this one. If you know that a particular type of alcohol gives you problems, then avoid it. As far as hangovers are concerned, while the old 'hair-of-the-dog' remedy may work for a time (in other words, giving yourself a little bit more alcohol), it actually serves to perpetuate the problem, even if there are good homoeopathic and allergic reasons why this approach might sometimes work. (Giving a small dose of a substance you're allergic to may stop withdrawal symptoms – though it continues to perpetuate the allergy in the long-term).

The best way to treat a hangover is to avoid further alcohol, to drink plenty of fluid (non-alcoholic) and to take a couple of aspirin, as long as you're not sensitive to them (see below). Fructose (fruit sugar) may help lessen the effects of alcohol through biochemical effects, and honey and tomato juice are good sources of this. Paracetamol *can* be used for pain relief, but many physicians are wary of recommending paracetamol with alcohol because both chemicals damage the liver; after an alcoholic binge, paracetamol may be relatively poisonous. Even by itself, paracetamol can be a very dangerous substance, if it's used indiscriminately, at more than the recommended dose. A small amount, plus alcohol, could kill you, particularly if you have had any liver-damaging condition like hepatitis. There have been instances of people who have made a token suicide attempt, taking only a handful of tablets – say, ten – together with alcohol, and have died as a result.

On the other hand, aspirin can also cause stomach bleeding, especially on an empty stomach. The effects are worse in those who are especially susceptible or allergic to aspirin. Because alcohol itself can pickle the lining of the stomach and cause bleeding, aspirin needs to be used with care after a binge, particularly as gastritis commonly occurs at this time.

As far as headaches from alcohol withdrawal are concerned, this is a stage you may have to go through, though painkillers will certainly lessen the symptoms. Not everyone gets headaches during 'drying-out', and it depends – among other things – upon how long you've been a drinker. The shorter the time, the more likely you are to get headaches; those who've been drinking for a long time are more likely to develop restlessness, delirium and depression. In headaches caused by alcohol withdrawal, simple analgesics may be enough to get rid of the pain.

Complementary treatment

A hot bath with pepper or juniper is invigorating, particularly when suffering the effects of a hangover. Fennel oil can be inhaled to relieve nausea. A blend of juniper and fennel oils, used in massage, or in a vapouriser – even the bath – may also help.

Rose oil is said to affect liver function, easing nausea and headaches. Kola is a herb which contains a large percentage of caffeine; it is often used to treat nervous headaches and hangover in the short term. Valerian and lady's slipper, drunk as teas, can relieve the headache of hangover.

Baths with a few drops of essential oil of lavender can help to ease headache. Lemon in hot water, and hot peppermint tea can be drunk to alleviate discomfort. (Remember that peppermint will nullify the effects of any homoeopathic remedies you are taking.) Yarrow and elderflower are said to encourage the body to expel toxins caused by alcohol and its by-products.

In extreme cases, with shaking, vomiting and severe headache, Rescue Remedy, a Bach flower remedy, may help. Dilute in a glass of warm water.

Homoeopathy offers several cures for hangover; for example, hangover in the morning, after drinking spirits, would respond to nux. Other remedies might include capsicum and kali bichrom.

Deficiencies in Vitamins A, B, C, D and K, folic acid, bioflavanoids, iron, zinc, and potassium are very common in heavy drinkers. Ensure that you are taking adequate quantities of the above if you are a heavy drinker, or following a drinking session. Evening primrose oil is said to be useful in treating the symptoms of hangover, and it is claimed that Vitamin B15 (pangamic acid) can help ward off hangovers through speedy recovery from fatigue, and a beneficial effect on the liver. Nutritionists suggest that you take one tablet before your first drink, and one before bed.

Some people suggest that you drink a pint of mineral water before going to bed. The water should flush out toxins and prevent dehydration symptoms. Fizzy mineral water can ease stomach discomfort.

TOBACCO

Tobacco can cause headaches in two ways. Firstly, carbon monoxide is produced when tobacco is burned. Usually this doesn't cause a problem by itself, however, long-term exposure to carbon monoxide furs up the arteries of the heart, a condition known as arteriosclerosis.

Some people are allergic to tobacco smoke, and can get severe headaches when in smoky atmospheres. This effect seems to be allergic rather than pharmacological, so even a small amount of tobacco smoke will be enough to trigger a headache. The only true remedy here is to avoid smoky conditions.

Detailed methods to help you give up smoking are beyond the scope of this book, but the essence of them all is will-power. All the aids to stopping smoking will be completely useless if you don't try – hard! (And it is hard, too.)

Complementary treatment
Tobacco smoke is toxic because of the tars (cancer-causing substances), nicotine (artificial stimulation) and carbon monoxide. Smoking also increases the risk of heart disease, stroke, bladder disease and cancers of the stomach and the neck of the womb.

Regular exposure to smoke depletes the body of Vitamins A, B, C and D, as well as bioflavanoids and zinc. Do ensure that you are getting adequate quantities in your diet; if you are a heavy smoker you may need supplementation.

Acupuncture can help to relieve the pain of tobacco-induced headaches, and, if you are a smoker, help you to give up. Oats, skullcap and valerian will help deal with the headaches caused by exposure to tobacco smoke. A combination of colt's foot and plantain can be given to clear out the respiratory system after stopping.

Bach flower remedies can help deal with negative emotions while trying to give up smoking; for example, there is impatiens for impatience and irritability; gentian for despondency, and cherry plum for uncontrolled, irrational thoughts. Controlling your emotions will prevent them building up to become another cause of headaches. For irritability, B-complex vitamins. Niacin can be used under a doctor's supervision to detoxify the body.

There are numerous homoeopathic remedies available to help with headaches caused by tobacco withdrawal, passive smoking, and over-smoking.

An aromatherapist might suggest massage with anti-depressant oils like bergamot, camomile, clary sage, jasmine and rose. Detoxifying oils, used in the bath or the vapouriser, include fennel and juniper. All are useful for headaches caused by smoking, even passive smoking.

Reflexology offers a programme to help you give up smoking.

CAFFEINE-INDUCED HEADACHES
So you think you're not a drug addict? In fact, every society has its own legal drugs that produce either stimulant or sedative effects on the brain. In our society, three legal drugs that do this are caffeine, nicotine and alcohol.

Caffeine is present in coffee and cola drinks, and there are surprisingly large quantities in tea. Two cups of tea equals roughly one cup of coffee in terms of caffeine content. As most of the population of England drink several cups of either tea or coffee each day, this amounts to a sizeable daily dose of caffeine. Some people are much more addicted to caffeine than this and drink ten or twenty cups a day, to say nothing of additional cola drinks.

In many people this causes no effects whatsoever, but those taking large quantities of caffeine may get a condition called *caffeinism* which comprises agitation, restlessness, difficulty with sleeping, tremors and a headache. Reducing the dose of caffeine helps considerably; but those who regularly and often take in a lot of caffeine will get a withdrawal headache if they suddenly stop their consumption.

If you've got a headache from suddenly stopping caffeine, have a caffeine-containing drink. Then plan to reduce your intake to a more sensible level, doing so slowly and progressively. Be aware that as well as being · *addicted* to the caffeine (pharmacologically) you can also be *allergic* to the coffee or tea that goes with it. If you are really having problems with caffeine then you may need to cut out coffee, tea and cola drinks altogether and to try fruit squashes and mild herbal teas instead.

Complementary treatment
Caffeine acts directly on the nervous system, bringing about an almost immediate sense of thinking more clearly, and relieving fatigue. Caffeine stimulates the release of stored sugar from the liver, which accounts for the sudden, uplifting experience. Through this reaction, however, enormous strain is placed on the system.

Like any other drug, caffeine can be toxic if taken in quantity. And for the record, decaffeinated coffee is not an ideal substitute. The process by which the caffeine is removed from the coffee involves a number of chemicals and soaps, and these additives are notorious for causing headaches.

Peppermint tea is stimulating, and a tonic (although it shouldn't be taken with homoeopathic remedies). Mu tea can increase vitality, and dandelion root coffee is a delicious alternative to regular coffee – and a mild diuretic as well. Guarana is a popular supplementary pick-me-up with the healthfood gurus.

Acupuncture can increase energy, and relieve the headache associated with caffeine.

Chapter Twenty-four

WEATHER, ATMOSPHERE AND HEADACHES

There are many ways in which the weather can cause headaches. There are direct weather effect; i.e., barometric pressure, thunderstorms and ionisation of the air. Furthermore, the amount of sunlight you get – whether too much or too little – can be surprisingly important. Finally, hot weather can dehydrate you, which can directly cause headaches.

DIRECT WEATHER EFFECTS

Ions are atoms or molecules which have become electrically charged – either by the removal of one or more electrons (one of the atomic particles) which gives a positive ion, or by the addition of an electron (which gives a negative ion). Transfer of electrons like this is the basis for static electricity.

Are you one of those people who feel very oppressed when a thunderstorm is due? And afterwards, do you feel invigorated as the rain splashes down? If so, you may be sensitive to electrical charges. Before a thunderstorm, the air is heavily charged with positive ions, one of the two forms of static electricity. As the thunderstorm passes, the air changes from being positively charged to being negatively charged.

Typically, before a thunderstorm the hot, humid, oppressive, positively charged atmosphere makes certain people feel tense and on edge, and this edginess often manifests itself as headaches, which are relieved as the storm eventually passes over. If you're particularly sensitive to positive ions, and there's thunder in the air, try taking a shower. This can help for the same reasons that being near a fountain or a mountain stream can – sprays of water create negative ions, which will relieve your symptoms somewhat.

Offices and ions

Much the same thing occurs in offices, but on a smaller scale. Positive charges tend to build up because the insides of offices are usually dry, with the humidity artificially controlled down to a low level; and the petroleum-based materials from which office carpets, furniture and equipment are made encourage the build-up of static electricity. How many times have you walked across an office and felt a slight electric shock as your hand touched the door handle? This is static electricity building up on your body, often caused by the action of your synthetic-soled shoes on synthetic carpets.

Sometimes the static in an office fills the air with positive ions. Under these conditions the office feels oppressive and stuffy, and you may suffer constant headaches. You could counteract this feeling by opening the windows to let in some fresh air, but in offices with central air-conditioning, the windows are often sealed.

Devices called ionisers can sometimes help control this situation. These push out negatively ionised air to counteract and annihilate the positive ions floating around in the office air. However, ionisers are moderately expensive to buy, and are not necessarily going to make you feel much better. Do give them a trial run *before* you buy, to see whether they help you or not. (Ionisers may also help remove pollen and dust from the air, too.)

Barometric pressure

We often hear of old soldiers complaining that they feel their war wounds more when there's bad weather coming. Some arthritis sufferers also find that their joints are more painful when the air pressure is low.

The reason barometric pressure varies is simple enough. Water vapour, molecule for molecule, is lighter than the gases that make up the remainder of the atmosphere. Since water vapour displaces other gases from the air, damp air weighs less than dry air. 'Barometric pressure' measures the weight of the atmosphere pressing on the surface of the earth; so, in damp conditions barometric pressure is less, because the extra water displaces the gases in the air and makes the atmosphere above the measuring point that much lighter.

Quite why this should make joints more painful and war wounds more sensitive, no one knows. Is it the barometric pressure itself? Unlikely; it's probably the humidity of the atmosphere. Some people get headaches related to barometric pressure, being worse in damp conditions and better in dry ones.

SUNLIGHT

Sunlight can affect headaches in two completely different ways. Too much sunlight produces *glare,* while in certain people too little produces a condition called *Seasonal Affective Disorder*.

Glare

Brilliant sunlight causes glare. We respond to glare by tightly screwing up our faces in order to minimise the amount of light coming into our eyes. Over a short period of time, glare does no damage (provided you're not looking directly into the sun), but over a longer period, screwing up the muscles around the eyes causes tension headaches. The longer the glare continues the more likely it is to cause headaches.

Glare is essentially too much unwanted light, but it doesn't have to be a very sunny day to cause glare; the direction of light counts, as well. It's *unwanted* light coming into your eyes that determines whether glare is present; it's quite possible to have a sunny day in a Mediterranean country, with the sun at its zenith, and have little glare. On the other hand, you can experience glare by driving straight into the sun at three o'clock on a December afternoon in Manchester!

So what is it about light that makes it glare? The answer is two fold. Obviously the more light there is the more likely it is that glare will occur. However, a lot of sunlight falling on a landscape that is primarily dark *won't* cause much glare. It's the bounce-round of light reflecting on light surfaces that causes the difficulty; i.e., light coming off snow, off sand, off water, off light-coloured surfaces such as concrete paths and buildings, reflecting off windows, off the white pages of a book or newspaper, and off white garden furniture and walls. And anything that reflects sunlight as brilliant flashes of light makes glare even worse.

However, direct, intense sunlight isn't always necessary. A lot of glare is created when the sun is behind a thin haze of high cloud. This makes the whole sky radiate light, instead of it coming just from the sun. If you've ever been to an air show under these conditions, you'll know how much more wearing it is to look at aircraft against a bright white background like this, than it is to watch the Red Arrows against the backdrop of a deep blue sky.

What can you do about glare? The answer is quite simple – minimise the amount of reflected light coming into your eyes. For instance, if eating outside minimise glare by using a dark-coloured tablecloth and using pottery cups and saucers, rather than glasses or china which reflect light so much more. Putting up a parasol helps as well! And, if you have a particularly bright area in the garden (perhaps a patio with a white, concrete floor), avoid it during the brighter times of the day.

Sunglasses are very effective. Simply donning a pair of tinted spectacles may make all the difference and it certainly allows you to read a book more comfortably. Polarised sunglasses are particularly useful; they have a material within them which only allows light to pass through if it is vibrating at a particular angle. Basically this means that they can selectively cut out glare and reflected light, instead of just light in general. Tinted glasses simply reduce the total amount of light, which is of some benefit, but not as effective as polarised lenses.

Seasonal Affective Disorder (SAD)

Seasonal Affective Disorder (or SAD, for short) is a recently discovered cause of depression which is primarily related to a lack of sunlight. Sufferers from SAD find that they become lethargic and depressed around October. This feeling lasts until about April, when suddenly they get a burst of activity, their depression lifts and they feel normal again ... until the following autumn. SAD is now a well-recognised cause of depression, which can cause muscle tension and headaches.

Only a small proportion of people seem to be susceptible to SAD, which seems to be related entirely to the amount of light coming into the eyes. So, if you work outdoors, you're less likely to be affected, while if you work inside you could be afflicted that much more quickly.

The treatment, as you'd expect, is exposure to light; but the intensity of light is very important. Normal levels of artificial light, even in brightly lit surroundings, are simply not enough. In other words, what we *feel* is powerful artificial light is, by comparison with sunlight, very weak indeed.

There are special lights available to treat sufferers of SAD; these are called 'light boxes' and are of particularly high intensity. It isn't necessary to look straight at the box, as long as you have it in your field of vision. You could read, or watch television at the same time, for example.

What do you do if you are suffering from SAD? To begin with, make the most of any natural light you can, especially towards autumn and winter. Ensure that you have an outdoor hobby – walking, golfing, gardening – and make a point of going out in the sunlight whenever you can. Perhaps you could have your mid-day meal on a bench in the park rather than merely sitting in the office. Secondly, think about a winter holiday somewhere much sunnier, where there are longer periods of daylight, or a lot of snow (snow will tend to multiply the effects of daylight by producing a lot of glare).

Lastly, in cases where SAD has been diagnosed, your doctor can arrange light therapy in which you are exposed to artificial light of a sufficiently high intensity to counteract the effects of lack of natural sunlight.

DEHYDRATION

Excessive exposure to the sun causes headaches in two ways. It gives us headaches by inducing glare and it heats us up, dehydrating us and causing headaches as a result.

The human body is very good at controlling its own internal conditions, keeping the concentration of body fluids more or less the same and maintaining a constant temperature. The way we control our temperature is simple. It takes a lot of heat to change water into water vapour, so at the times when we're hot we sweat, which takes a lot of heat away from the body.

This can occur in one of two situations – when we're working very hard, producing a lot of excess heat as a by-product of muscular movement and also, and most importantly, when we can't become cool because we can't properly evaporate our sweat. This happens when it's very humid. Sweat can't evaporate easily into air that already carries a large amount of water, so it lies unevaporated on the skin, and we become all to quickly aware that we feel hot and sweaty.

Too little fluid in the body – dehydration – can cause headaches in its own right. In addition, sweat contains salt, and a large amount of sweating depletes our salt reserves. This in turn leads to an imbalance of body and blood chemistry, which can make us feel unwell.

Under hot, dry conditions you can lose a lot of fluid, and salt, without knowing. In conditions where the air is dry you won't be able to see that you are sweating.

Although natural weather conditions may not seem dry enough to allow dehydration to occur through insensible sweating (sweating we are not aware of), people in artificially dry environments can lose a lot of water without realising it. Any industrial environment where the air is artificially dried can do this; and because of the laws of physics, simply heating up the air in the room has the effect of relatively drying it out. Warm air can absorb more water than cool air. Therefore hot and/or dry environments may cause dehydration-type headaches; for example operating theatres, hospital wards, foundries, and certain industrial processes taking place in rooms with controlled low humidity.

How do you know if you're dehydrated? Simple. How much urine are you producing? And is it light or dark? If you are dehydrated your body will try to conserve fluid, so the kidneys will excrete very little urine. As a result, the waste products in your urine will be more concentrated, making it a darker yellow colour. On the other hand, (assuming you haven't got diabetes or kidney failure) you're unlikely to be dehydrated if you are going to the toilet several times a day and producing normal amounts of light-coloured urine.

The cure for dehydration is obviously to drink more fluid (preferably non-alcoholic), but do be careful. Drinking copious quantities of water at one sitting isn't good for you and can even be dangerous. Nor is it necessarily just water that you need; sometimes a little extra salt will be necessary to replace some of that lost in the sweat. Wear light clothes, but not synthetics, for sweat can't get out through this material. You're better off wearing, say, cotton or other natural fibres which can breathe. A wide-brimmed sun-hat helps, by keeping the direct heat of the sun off your head and shoulders.

You might think that if you're dehydrated you'd be very thirsty – and you might be – but only up to a point. Its quite possible to feel unwell from salt depletion and dehydration without necessarily being very thirsty.

To prevent dehydration, avoid caffeine and alcohol, which are diuretics. Should you become dehydrated, sachets of rehydrating salts are available from the chemist. Take them with a measured amount of water. In an emergency, you can make a version of this dilute liquid mixture yourself, with one pint of drinking water, one-quarter teaspoon of salt and one tablespoon of sugar. Sip slowly and frequently.

So, too much sun can give you headaches, working through a combination of mechanisms. Excessive sunlight can produce glare, which causes you to screw up your eyes, giving you a tension headache. Excess heat from the sun can dehydrate you and deplete you of salt, both of which can also give you headaches. Often headaches from too much sun are not caused by just one or other of these problems, but by both together. In addition, too much sun is tiring.

If you've had too much sun, go into a cool, less bright environment; perhaps take a cool shower. Drink adequate fluids, use sunglasses, and, if necessary, take a couple of tablets of paracetamol or (where appropriate) aspirin. You may find a short nap helps also. This is probably all that is needed to tide you over what is usually a temporary hiccup in the system.

Chapter Twenty-five

PULLING IT ALL TOGETHER

A current trend is to discuss *holistic* medicine as if it were something new, invented by alternative practitioners of the Seventies and later. Some people even seem to think that holistic medicine is a new approach, in comparison with orthodox medicine, which is deemed dry, mechanical and unrelated to real life.

In fact, nothing could be further from the truth. Orthodox medical doctors have known for a long time that your genetic make-up, your working environment, your marriage, your hobbies, the chemicals with which you're in contact, your thoughts and your concerns, in fact, your whole lifestyle, are all intimately bound up with whether you feel well or ill. Holistic, in terms of medicine, means caring for the whole person – mind, body and spirit. It is not the form of medicine that is holistic, but the attitudes and views of the practitioner – orthodox, alternative or otherwise.

This point is very important, especially for headache sufferers. *Good orthodox medicine is holistic, too.* It's all about treating the whole person, not just little bits of him. You don't have a headache in isolation. You are a person with a headache, and in order to understand and treat that headache we need to look at the whole of you, not just the bit from the neck up. Orthodox and complementary treatments all have their place in assessing and treating that headache.

There is a second reason why it is so important to consider all aspects of you and your condition – many people don't have headaches from just one single cause. Usually there are a lot of different reasons, and their effects all multiply together. Perhaps, you've identified the cause of your own headache as cervical spondylosis. But, if you look more closely, you'll find you get other headaches as well – those caused by tension, for example (a common fellow traveller with cervical spondylosis). Maybe you get the odd migraine, too, and of course there's the pain from that whiplash accident you had ten years ago, to say nothing of the fumes that you get from the old jalopy you drive, and the mid-life crisis you're currently going through ...

It's vital to emphasise the degree to which all the various causes of headache are interlinked and inter-related. Some are so tightly bound together that its almost impossible to disentangle them; for example, arthritis in the neck is almost inevitably accompanied by reflex muscle spasm, which gives tension headaches.

This is where *true* holistic medicine comes in, and by this I mean medicine which looks at every single aspect of the individual. In dealing with headaches it's important to recognise that both orthodox and complementary medicines may have a part to play; that environmental, working and living conditions are important; that psychological, social and spiritual factors are involved.

With a bit of luck, you've now worked out what is the main cause for your own headaches. Or, to put it more accurately, you have probably found a number of things that interact, and you're not yet certain which of them is the real culprit.

The answer, of course, is that you needn't try to find one culprit; *all* the various triggers may have an effect on you. You don't need to worry about whether you've mainly got a tension headache or whether there's a bit of migraine there as well. Instead, accept all these as possible diagnoses and go to work on each of them, one at a time.

Headaches have a nasty habit of not just adding together, but multiplying each other. It's surprising how often a small problem – such as a worn-out joint in the neck – can have such amazing knock-on effects. Maybe the amount of stress that you're under wouldn't normally give you a headache, except that having a worn-out joint multiplies the effects of the tension on your neck muscles, so that even a small amount of stress manifests itself as pain, which in turn will give more spasm, which gives more pain ... It's important to look at each and every one of the possible causes of your headache and try to deal with each of them, however minor each may appear to be.

In some cases, there will be one major cause for your headaches, plus a few minor ones, in which case removing the major cause may clear up the problem entirely. On the other hand, where there is no clear-cut single cause, the best treatment consists of trying to remove or minimise as many of the contributing factors as possible. You will probably find there comes a point where you have reduced the level of insult to your head and neck below the threshold for causing pain, and suddenly your headaches go away – or at least become manageable, which is half the battle.

DAVID

David was an intellectual type, accustomed to long hours poring over books and studying in libraries. A solicitor by profession, he had the typical stooping posture so common in those who do book work all day – head and neck bent over his chest.

David had continued with this bad posture for such a long time that his neck had become quite accustomed to it, but over the years its effects had taken their toll on his neck joints. By the time he went to his doctor he had a really troublesome neck. Any abnormal movement could throw it into spasm; five minutes of putting up curtains (which necessitated throwing his head back to look at the curtain rail) irritated his neck sufficiently to put the muscles into spasm for the next two days, and a tension headache was the result.

Any number of events could cause problems like this. He had difficulties every time he painted the ceiling; swimming breaststroke (with his head held up out of the water) arched his neck to much that he would get pain within a few hours, even after swimming in a warm swimming pool. And if he ever swam in the sea, where the cold water made muscle spasm occur more quickly, his neck would become painful within minutes.

Two events in his life showed just how irritable his neck had become. Anything round the lower part of his neck, such as a camera strap, or even prolonged walking while carrying a light bag in one hand, could throw his neck into spasm. Just walking around an historical exhibition with his camera round his neck had started off neck spasm that lasted two weeks. And on separate occasions he found out that his favourite hobby – narrow-boating on canals – also caused problems. Normally when piloting his narrow-boat he would sit sideways on the raised, box-like area beside his tiller, facing the middle of the boat, twisting to look out towards the prow. In doing this, he would twist his head slightly to his left. Holding this position for a number of hours gradually sent his neck into spasm, and within two days of the beginning of a holiday he was in pain again.

He also had a certain amount of osteo-arthritis, which meant that these changes in function of his neck were superimposed on top of some minor physical abnormalities. Consciously changing the way he stood and walked helped, but this could be of only limited assistance because of the underlying anatomical changes.

It seemed useful to attack the problems on several different fronts. First, his doctor encouraged him to become aware of his posture, and recommended that he see a teacher of the Alexander technique to help him re-learn how to stand and sit correctly. It would take David a long time to re-learn the movements and postures that he had so assiduously hampered with bad habits for the past twenty-five years.

Next there were more specific tasks to be learned. It's useful to be able to exercise by swimming, but not when it puts your neck into spasm, so David was told that if he swam he should either do breaststroke properly – putting his head in the water – or, alternatively, swim backstroke. In backstroke the swimmer bends his head forwards slightly, an excellent antidote for a neck which mostly gets into trouble on being bent back too far.

Next he was warned to be very careful of all those activities that required him to look up or bend his neck backwards in any way. If he had to do this for more than a moment or two, he should make a point of bending it forward again immediately afterwards and, if necessary, leaning his hands on top of his head, gently pulling his head down and *forward to stretch the muscles in the back of the neck. Side-bending the neck, moving his ear towards his shoulder, also helped, and he was encouraged to exercise the neck in three different planes of movement, which he found very helpful. In fact, after a time he learned to manipulate his own neck when he got into problems. Often when he had a sore neck, just by letting his head hang loosely to one side he was able to open up the offending joint, which usually gave a loud click, and immediately the pain in his neck decreased.*

Finally, David's doctor encouraged him to adopt a more symmetrical, balanced posture whenever he found himself in an awkward, one-sided position, such as when he was piloting his narrow-boat. Simply shifting to the other side of the boat from time to time helped, so that he spent equal amounts of time looking to the left and right. But it was important to start this before he started getting pain in his neck. Once the pain occurred the muscles were already in spasm and it would be much more difficult to get the neck to respond.

But there were other things to consider, as well. For example his slight short-sightedness made him screw up his eyes when watching television, causing headaches from muscle tension. This was cured by a visit to the optician. In addition, David gets the occasional migraine, especially with red wine, so this was something to avoid. And there was tension at home and at work that also increased his neck muscle spasm – attending to these, learning to take control of difficult situations, and also learning to relax, all helped enormously.

This is true holistic medicine – looking at *every* facet of your life and working out whether things are in order or not. Try it. Go through all the various trigger factors and see how many of them you can reduce or eliminate, without unduly affecting the quality of your lifestyle. You may be surprised how little you need to do to get rid of the headaches that have been plaguing you. Try changing the mattress in the bed, perhaps, or taking a little more exercise; keeping your weight down; getting a check-up or some tablets for your blood pressure, or some treatment for that pre-menstrual problem. Maybe it will involve re-assessing and working on the quality of your home life, the relationship with your husband, your job, your approach to middle age, your spiritual beliefs.

Once you've done all these things you will probably find that your headaches are very much better, and along the way you'll almost certainly become fitter, happier, more relaxed and have a greater sense of well-being.

FURTHER READING

COMPLEMENTARY MEDICINE

The Readers' Digest Family Guide to Alternative Medicine, edited by Dr Patrick Pietroni
The Alternative Health Guide, by Brian Inglis and Ruth West (1991)

SLEEPING PROBLEMS

Don't Just Lie There: Michael van Straten's Guide to Good Sleep, by Michael van Straten
(Kyle Cathie Ltd, 1990)
Healing Dreams, by Russ Parker (SPCK)

BACKS AND NECKS

Beating Back Pain, by Dr John Tanner MB, BS, BSc., The British Holistic Medical Association
(Dorling Kindersley, 1987)
The Back Shop Book: A–Z of Family Backcare, by Bonny Mounayer and Suzy Wynn-Williams
(Optima, 1989)
Banish Back Pain, by Roger Newman Turner (Thorsens, 1989)
Back in Action, by Sarah Keays (Century, 1991)

STRESS

Coping with Stress, by Helen Dore (Hamlyn, 1990)
The Successful Self, by Dorothy Rowe (Fontana/Collins, 1988)
Families and How to Survive Them, by Robin Skynner and John Cleese (Methuen, 1983)

ALLERGIES

Not All in the Mind, by Dr Richard MacKarness (Pan, 1976)
The Complete Guide to Food Allergy and Intolerance, by Dr Jonathan Brostoff and Linda Gamlin
(Bloomsbury, 1989)

DIET

The No-Diet Book, A Guide to Permanent Weight-loss Without Dieting, by Dr Michael Spira
(Fontana, 1982)
The Complete Hip and Thigh Diet, by Rosemary Conley (Arrow, updated 1993)
Healthy Eating: Fact and Fiction, Which? Books
(Consumers' Association and Hodder and Stoughton, 1989)

DEPRESSION AND ANXIETY

A Practical Workbook for the Depressed Christian, Dr John Lockley (Word UK, 1991)
Born to Win, by Muriel James and Dorothy Jongeward (Addison-Wesley, 1971)
SAD – Seasonal Affective Disorder, by Angela Smith (Unwin, 1990)
The Latest Help For Your Nerves, by Dr Claire Weekes (Angus and Robertson, 1972)

HEALTH AND EXERCISE

BBC Health Check, by Dr Barry Lynch (BBC Books, 1989)

PREMENSTRUAL SYNDROME

Premenstrual Syndrome – How to Beat It, by Dr Ian Simpson and Wendy Holton
(Peter Andrew Publishing Company, 1992)

EXERCISE

Physical Fitness – 5BX 11-Minute-a-Day Plan, exercises developed by the Royal Canadian Air Force
(Penguin)

USEFUL ADDRESSES

ALCOHOL

Al-Anon
61 Great Dover Street, London SE1 4YF
071 403 0888
This is a self-help group for the families of alcoholics. There are many local groups.

Alateen
61 Great Dover Street, London SE1 4YF
071 403 0888
A sub-group of Al-Anon: a support group for teenagers who are affected by *someone's else's* drinking.

Alcoholics Anonymous
PO Box 1, Stonebow House, Stonebow, York YO1 2NJ
0904 644026
This well-known organisation is for those who have problems with alcohol. There are many local groups.

ALLERGIES

AAA (Action Against Allergy)
Greyhound House, 23/24 George Street, Richmond, Surrey TW9 1JY
081-948 5771
National charity which provides information on allergies and allergy-related illnesses. It has a list of doctors who specialise in different types of allergy. Publishes *Allergy Newsletter*.

BACK AND NECK INJURIES

The Arthritis and Rheumatism Council for Research
Copeman House, St Mary's Court, St Mary's Gate Chesterfield, Derbyshire S41 7TD
A research charity whose aims include better understanding of these diseases. There are many local groups. They publish *Arthritis Research Today*.

The Association for Spina Bifida and Hydrocephalus
42 Park Road, Peterborough, Cambs PE1 2UQ
0733 555988
This offers practical support and assistance for sufferers and their families. There are a number of local groups and they publish a bulletin and magazine.

National Back Pain Association
31-33 Park Road, Teddington, Middx TW11 OAB
081 977 5474

This medical charity aims to educate people to use their bodies more appropriately in order to avoid back pain; there are a number of local groups. They publish *Talkback* quarterly.

National Association for the Relief of Paget's Disease
Teaching Unit 4, Withington Hospital, Nell Lane Manchester M20 8LR
061 445 8111 ext, 3781
To assist the relief of sufferers.

RSI Association
Christ Church, Redford Way, Uxbridge, Middx UB8 152
0895 38663
This association provides advice and information for sufferers about Repetitive Strain Injury.

Spinal Injuries Association
76 St James's Lane, London N10 3DF
081 444 2121
A self-help group run by those who have themselves had spinal injuries, it provides an information and welfare service.

COMPLEMENTARY MEDICINE

Academy of Systematic Kinesiology
39 Browns Road, Surbiton, Surrey KT5 8ST
081 399 2215
This association organises kinesiology 'workshops' and publishes a textbook on the subject.

British Acupuncture Association
34 Alderney Street, London SW14 4EM
071 834 1012/3350
This association publishes a register of members who have qualified in acupuncture skills. The register is a national standard, though its members are not necessarily medically qualified as well.

British Chiropractic Association
5 First Avenue, Chelmsford, Essex CM1 1RX
0245 353078/358487
This association will supply a list of local chiropractors and also produces leaflets.

British Herbal Medicine Association
Field House, Lye Hole Lane, Redhill, Avon RS18 7TB
0934 862994
This association for those who are involved with herbal medicine.

British Holistic Medical Association
179 Gloucester Place, London NW1
071 262 5299
This professional association publishes
information about complementary medicine.

British Homoeopathic Association
27A Devonshire Street, London W1N 1RJ
071 935 2163
The association has a reference library, provides
an information service, and a list of homeopathic
practitioners and pharmacists.

British Society of Medical and Dental Hypnosis
42 Links Road, Ashtead, Surrey KT21 2HJ
03722 73522
This professional group also publishes a list of
local practitioners.

Council for Acupuncture
10 Belgrave Square, London SW1X 8PH
There are three main acupuncture organisations
and the Council for Acupuncture publishes a
combined list of all British acupuncturists
registered with them.

Dietary Therapy Society
33 Priory Gardens, London N6 5QU
081 341 7260
Will supply a list of trained registered clinical
nutritionalists.

The General Council and Register of Osteopaths
1-4 Suffolk Street, London SW1Y 4HG
071 839 2060
The council publishes a register of qualified
osteopaths and will supply the names of local
registered osteopaths. MROs have had a long
period of traiing in osteopathy at the end of
which they have passed an examination.

Institute for Complementary Medicine
21 Portland Place, London W1N 3AS
071 636 9543
The institute publishes information about
complementary medicine.

**National Register of Hypnotherapists and
Psychotherapists**
*National College of Hypnotherapists and Psycho-
therapists, 25 Market Square, Nelson, Lancs*
0282 699378
This group will supply a list of qualified
practitioners.

The Register of Qualified Aromatherapists
54A Gloucester Avenue, London NW1 8JD
071 272 7403
A register of professional aromatherapists trained
to specific, high standards.

The Royal London Homoeopathic Hospital
Great Ormond Street, London WC1
071 837 3091
This is an NHS hospital; they will provide a list
of NHS and private homoeopathic doctors on
receipt of an sae. They also provide information
about homoeopathy in general.

The Society of Orthopaedic Medicine
19 Jesmond Road, Hove BN3 5LN
0273 410826
This is a professional association which can
provide lists of local physiotherapists, etc.

Society of Teachers of the Alexander Technique
*10 London House, 266 Fulham Road,
London SW10 9EL*
071 351 0828
This society will provide information and a list of
teachers in your locality – but you must send a
stamped addressed envelope.

EPILEPSY

British Epilepsy Associaiton
40 Hanover Square, Leeds, West Yorks LS3 1NE
0532 439393
This provides advice to people with epilepsy,
and their families. There are some local groups.
They publish *Epilepsy Today*.

National Society for Epilepsy
*Chalfont Centre for Epilepsy, Chalfont St Peter,
Gerrards Cross, Buckinghamshire SL9 ORJ*
02407 3991
This society consists of a number of community
network groups who offer support and
information, as well as sponsoring research.

EQUIPMENT

Equipment for the Disabled
*Mary Marlborough Lodge, Nuffield Orthopaedic
Centre, Headington, Oxford*
0865 750103
Publishes information on aids which can help
those who are disabled.

EYES

International Glaucoma Association
*c/o Kings College Hospital, Denmark Hill,
London SE5 9RS*
071 274 6222 ext. 2934/ 071 737 3265
This association mainly sends out information
booklets, as well as organising meetings and
distributing a newsletter.

Optical Information Council
57A Old Woking Road, West Byfleet, Surrey KT14 6LF
0923 53283
A voluntary body dedicated to promoting good
eye care. It sends out free information leaflets on
request.

Partially Sighted Society
Dean Clerk House, Southernhay East, Exeter EX1 1PE
0392 210656
This is an advice group to help and support those with poor eyesight; they have a number of self-help groups and can give advice about low-vision aids; they also have a mail-order service.

GENERAL HEALTH

Health Education Council
78 New Oxford Street, London WC1A 1AH
071 637 1881
Gives a general information service and publishes leaflets on aspects of health.

Intractable Pain Society of Great Britain and Ireland
Basingstoke District Hospital, Aldermaston Road, Basingstoke, Hants RG24 9NA
0256 473202
They hold a register of all pain clinics through the United Kingdom.

Royal Association for Disability and Rehabilitation
25 Mortimer Street, London W1N 8AB
071 637 5400
They publish information and offer advice, including legal advice.

HEAD INJURIES

The Amnesia Association (AMNASS)
St Charles Hospital, Exmoor Street, London W10 6D7
081 969 0796
A charity to help people who have memory problems as a result of brain damage. It provides information and advice, and publishes a newsletter called *Recall.*

Headway
National Head Injury Association Ltd, 200 Mansfield Road, Nottingham NG1 3HX
0602 622382
This organisation provides advice and counselling, together with local volunteer groups to help people with head injuries and their families. They publish *Headway News* quarterly.

ME (MYALGIC ENCEPHALOMYELITIS)

Myalgic Encephalomyelitis Association
PO Box 8, Stanford-le-Hope, Essex SS17 8EX
0375 642466
A network of self-help groups who aim to support sufferers and educate the general public about ME.

MENINGITIS

National Meningitis Trust
Fern House, Bath Road, Stroud, Gloucestershire GL5 3TJ
0453 751738

This group provides help and support for meningitis victims and aims to raise public awareness of the problem.

MIGRAINE

British Migraine Association
178A High Road, Byfleet, West Byfleet, Surrey KT14 7ED
09323 54268
This charity is run by migraine sufferers in order to provide a network of support, information, and advice for migraine sufferers. They publish a newsletter.

The City of London Migraine Clinic
22 Charterhouse Square, London EC1M 6DX
This is a medical charity linked to St Bartholomew's Hospital. You will need to be referred by your doctor.

The Princess Margaret Migraine Clinic
Department of Neurology, Charing Cross Hospital, Fulham Palace Road, London W6 8RF
You will need to be referred by your doctor to this clinic.

The Migraine Trust
45 Great Ormond Street, London WC1N 3HZ
071 278 2676

PSYCHIATRY

Anorexia and Bulimia Nervosa Association
Women's Health Centre, Tottenham Town Hall, Approach Road, London N15 4RB
081 885 3936
This group runs a helpline for those who are affected by anorexia and bulimia.

Depressives Associated
PO Box 5, Castletown, Portland, Dorset DT5 1BQ
This group aims to help depressed people and their families by putting them in touch with one another and setting up small self-help groups. They have a quarterly publication, *A Single Step.*

Manic Depression Fellowship Limited
13 Rosslyn Road, Twickenham, Middx TW1 2AR
081 892 2811
This is a network of self-help groups. It also aims to educate the general public about manic depression and support research into it.

Phobic Action
Greater London House, 547-551 High Road, Leytonstone, London E11 4PR
081 558 6012
A number of local groups which aim to overcome problems of anxiety and phobias through self-help.

SAD Association (SADA)
51 Bracewell Road, London W1D 6AF
081 962 7028 (answerphone)
A registered charity which gives publicity and advice about seasonal affective disorder. It has a quarterly publication.

The Samaritans
17 Uxbridge Road, Slough, Berks SL1 1SN
0753 32713
Look in your phone book for your local Samaritans branch. This well-known organisation offers support to thoise who are in difficulty, or feeling suicidal.

Tranx (UK) Ltd
25A Masons Avenue, Wealdstone, Harrow HA3 5AH
This self-help organisation is run by those who have previously experienced problems with the use of tranquillisers. They offer individual advice.

SLEEP

BM Cry-sis Support Group
London WC1N 3XX
071 404 5011
This self-help support group is run by those who have had personal experience of coping with crying and non-sleeping babies. They aim to give practical and emotional network support to parents in similar situations. There is a national network of volunteers.

TUMOURS

Cancer Aftercare and Rehabilitation Society
21 Zetland Road, Redland, Bristol BS6 7AH
0272 427419/232302
This society provides emotional support for cancer sufferers and their families. Telephone counselling is available.

CancerLink
17 Britannia Street, London WC1X 9JN
071 833 2451
This is a resource centre to a large number of self-help groups spread throughout the United Kingdom, and aims to provide emotional support and information. Telephone enquiries are welcome.

Cancer Relief Macmillan Fund
Anchor House, 15-19 Britten Street, London SW3 3TZ
071 351 7811
This is a charity concerned with providing staff to help those suffering from cancer.

GYNAECOLOGICAL PROBLEMS

Association for Post-natal Illness
7 Cowan Avenue, Fulham, London SW6 6RN
071 731 4867
This is a network of volunteers who have personal experience of post-natal illness and the intention is to support those who are depressed following childbirth by establishing a one-to-one relationship with them.

National Association for Pre-menstrual Syndrome
PO Box 72, Sevenoaks, Kent TN13 1XQ
This group aims to help those suffering from PMS. The aim is to help sufferers through personal advice and support.

Pre-Eclampsia Society
Eaton Lodge, 8 Southend Road, Hockley, Essex
0702 205088
This is a self-help group.

Pre-Menstrual Society (Premsoc)
PO Box 102, London SE1 7ES
Provides support and education for sufferers of PMS and has a number of local groups.

SAFETY AND QUALIFICATIONS OF COMPLEMENTARY PRACTITIONERS

Just because a practitioner is a member of a particular association does not guarantee that he or she knows anything about orthodox medicine, or that he or she knows anything about other therapies outside his/her discipline. Many complementary therapies do not have an adequate system of vetting to ensure that a particular standard is met. Indeed, in some areas you do not have to be a member of any professional body, nor even have had any training before setting up as a practitioner of some therapies.

Therefore if you're intending to consult a complementary medical practitioner *please* do your very best to find out about him or her beforehand. It's best to go by recommendation, if possible. Ask your doctor, who is likely to know whether the practitioners in your area get good results; write to the various associations asking for a list of their registered and recommended members. Ask around. See whether the practitioner has a good or a bad reputation. Remember, one in six conventional doctors also practice at least one complementary therapy and may well have close links with other practitioners.

INDEX

A

abcess, dental 111, 174, 175
ACE-inhibitors 147
acupressure:
arthritis 71, 81; depression 193;
drug withdrawal 232; high blood
pressure 149; infections 106;
migraine 26, 51-2; neck problems
66, 86; sex-related headaches
209; sinusitis 116; strokes 123;
sub-arachnoid haemorrhage 131;
temporal arteritis 163; tension
headache 60; toothache 175;
toxaemia 201
acupuncture:
arthritis 71, 81; caffeine-related
headaches 237; childhood
diseases 105; dental problems
175, 177; depression 193; drug
withdrawal 232; glaucoma 168;
head injury 140; high blood
pressure 149; immune system
160; infections 106; menopause
204; migraine 51-2; neck
problems 66, 75, 86, 91; post-
menstrual syndrome 196; shingles
108; sinusitis 116; strokes 123;
sub-arachnoid haemorrhage 131;
sub-dural haemorrhage 137;
temporal arteritis 163; tension
headache 60; toxaemia 200;
tumours 160
acyclovir 99
adenosine 108
adrenal glands 82
AIDS 65, 107
air-conditioning 115, 224-5, 239
alcohol 233-5; addiction 186, 233,
234, 235
Alexander technique 53, 66, 71, 81,
91, 143, 193, 245
allergies 221-2, 234;
desensitization 225, 230; tobacco
smoke 111, 113, 115, 236; see also
food allergies and under
chemicals; dust-mite; pollen
Amish people 186
anaemia 44
aneurysms, berry 127, 206
angina 231
angiogram 129-30
angiotensin 147
antibiotics 100, 101, 102, 103, 111,
117, 219;
viral infections immune 95, 96
anti-depressants 48, 113, 186, 187-
8, 196
antihistamines 33, 59, 112, 224, 225
anti-inflammatories 79, 80, 84, 86,
87, 90, 139;
herbal 116-17, 140; see also
NSAIDs
antrum 109, 113
anxiety 159, 184-93;
cause of headache 43, 59, 62,
183; after illness 122, 129, 130,

131; treatment 189
aromatherapy:
alcohol-related headaches 235;
arthritis 71, 82; bite abnormalities
177; blood pressure, high 149;
body clock problems 216;
depression 192-3; drug
withdrawal 232; epilepsy 182; eye
problems 168, 170; head injury
140; infections 105-6; meningitis
98; menopause 204; migraine 26,
52-3; neck problems 66, 91; post-
traumatic headache 143;
premenstrual syndrome 196-7;
respiratory failure 220; sex,
headache during 209; shingles
108; sinusitis 116; stroke 123;
temporal arteritis 163-4; tension
headache 61; tobacco-related
headaches 236; toxaemia 201;
tumours 160
art therapy 60, 98, 123, 187, 192,
232
arteriosclerosis 119, 123, 236
arthritis:
and atmosphere 239; of neck 12,
14, 15, 56, 68; rheumatoid 68, 77-
82; tempero-mandibular 176; see
also osteo-arthritis
aspirin:
contraindications 49, 103;
exertion headache 217; herbal
sources 116, 125-6; infections
101, 104; migraine 25, 26, 35, 49;
paracetamol alternation 103, 105;
stomach damage 234, 235; sun-
related headaches 242; TIA prevention 124, 125; tumour pain 159
assertiveness training 59, 61, 191
asthma 81, 103
atmosphere 238-42
atropine 168
auriculotherapy 60

B

Bach flower remedies:
alcohol-related headaches 235;
bite abnormalities 177; blood
pressure, high 149; childhood
diseases 105; depression 193;
drug withdrawal 232; epilepsy
182; fear 177; glaucoma 168; head
injury 140; infections 106;
meningitis 98; migraine 26; post-
traumatic headache 143; stopping
smoking 236; sub-arachnoid
haemorrhage 131; sub-dural
haemorrhage 137; temporal
arteritis 163; tension headache 60;
wry neck 66
back see neck; spine
bacteria see infections
beds 59, 89, 115
bending down 18; 43
beta-blockers 26, 48, 143, 147,
207,217
biofeedback:

blood pressure, high 148; dental
problems 177; depression 193;
drug withdrawal 232; head injury
140; migraine 52; pre-menstrual
syndrome 197; sub-dural
haemorrhage 137; tension
headache 60
biological agents 115, 224-5
biopsy 158, 162
bite 17, 19, 20, 21, 44, 77, 176-7
blindness 17, 31, 173
blood:
circulatory problems 49; structure
38, 49, 124; sugar 39, 40; tests 20-
1, 78, 152; see also blood pressure
blood pressure,high 9, 144-9;
contraceptive pill and 144;
hormone problems 149;
phaeochromocytoma 21;
pregnancy 144, 199, 200;
psychologically caused
headaches 193; stress and 19,
149; and stroke 126, 148, 149;
sub-arachnoid haemorrhage 129,
149, 210; symptoms 15, 16, 17,
19, 58, 111, 144-5, 157, 173;
tension headaches 62, 149;
treatment 122, 123, 145-9, 230-1;
uraemia 218, 219
body clock 19, 44, 215-16
boxing 133, 139
brain:
fag 42; see also head injury;
stroke; tumours
bromocriptine 196
bronchitis 219-20

C

C-Reactive Protein 78
caffeine:
alcohol-related headache 235;
cause of headache 41, 58, 236-7;
ergotamine combination 49; and
migraine 25, 41, 50; withdrawal
19, 237
calcitonin 218
calcium channel blockers 48, 54,
147
cancer:
HRT and 203, 204; of sinuses 111;
smoking and 236; see also
tumours
carbon monoxide 227, 228-9
cars:
comfort 82, 89, 223-4; fumes 228-
9; migraine trigger 43, 46; safety
restraints 79-80, 83, 85
cartilage 68, 70
CAT scans 21, 99, 152, 180
catarrh 116-17
cerebro-spinal fluid see CSF
cervical spondylosis 52, 69, 72-7,
126;
symptoms 16, 21, 72-3, 74, 75, 76-
7, 84, 88, 111, 173
chemicals 18, 224, 225, 226;
allergy 112, 186, 224, 226, 229-30;

and migraine 33, 45, 224
chemotherapy 158-9, 160
chest infections 101, 104, 219-20
chickenpox 106
children **211-14**;
 car restraints 85; complementary
 treatments 52, 53, 105; danger
 from drugs 65, 103; immune
 system 212; stomach aches 101,
 211; temperature 101, 103, 212;
 *see also under individual
 complaints*
chiropractic 52, 66, 81, 91, 123, 131,
 204, 209
cholesterol 123, 149
clonidine 26, 48, 203
cluster headache **53-4**;
 symptoms 15, 16, 17, 19, 53-4,
 167, 173, (migraine compared)
 18, 26, 46, 54
coital headache 18, 19, 47, 128,
 206, 208, 217
collars, cervical 77, 79-80, 85
colour therapy 60, 140
complementary medicine 11; *see
 also individual types*
Computerised Axial Tomography
 see CAT
computers: printer noise 223;
 VDUs 43, 172, 181-2, 222;
 working position 18, 56, 59, 83
concussion 16, 19, **132-3**, 137
connective tissue disorders 161
contraceptive pill 18, 144, 195, **198-
 9**;
 and migraine 31, 32-3, 43, 121,
 198-9, 231
contrast radiography 22-3
convulsions, febrile 96, 103-4, 105,
 180
copper 71, 80, 81
coproxamol 35, 49
cortisone 82
counselling 60, 186, 189-90, 191,
 193, 204, 232
cranio-sacral therapy 61
cribriform plate 93
CSF 22, 23, 92, 95, 130

D
dance therapy:
 depression 187, 192; drug
 withdrawal 232; epilepsy 182;
 neck problems 91; post-traumatic
 headache 143; strokes 123; sub-
 arachnoid haemorrhage 131;
 tension headache 60
decongestants 111, 112, 113, 117
dehydration 241-2
dental problems 14, 15, 44, 101,
 174-7;
 see also abcess; bite; toothache
depression **184-93:**
 causes 185-7; 5-HT reduction 50;
 after illness 98, 122, 126, 129, 130,
 131, 142, 143; and migraine 43;
 symptoms 16, 19; and tension
 headache 58, 59, 62; treatment
 98, 187-93; *see also* anti-
 depressants; SAD
desensitization 225, 230
dexamethasone 155, 159

diabetes 41, 103, 104, 145
diagnosis **9-10, 12-23**
diazepam 48, 59, 65
diet:
 arthritis 71. 80-1, 82; depression
 192; drug withdrawal 232; eating
 disorders 189; epilepsy 182; high
 blood pressure 149; menopause
 203, 204; migraine 25, 26, 39-42,
 53; pre-menstrual syndrome 196,
 197; shingles 108; temporal
 arteritis 164; tension headache 61;
 toothache 175; toxaemia of
 pregnancy 200; tumours 160; *see
 also* food; food allergies
dipyridamole 125
disc trouble *see* cervical
 spondylosis
disease-altering drugs 79
disorientation 16
diuretics 146, 149
DLPA 53
domperidone 48
drowsiness 137, 138
drugs:
 addiction 186, 189, 193, 226, 231-
 2; cause of headache 58;
 compounds, and overdose 50;
 side-effects 148, 168, 230-1;
 withdrawal 231-2
 duration of headache 19
dust-mite allergy 111, 112, 113-14,
 114-15

E
eclampsia 15, 17, 18, 19, 173, 199
ECT 189
EEG *see* electro-encephalogram
elderly:
 ECT 189; infections 104, 105;
 lighting for 171; migraines 28;
 osteo-arthritis 78; sub-dural
 haemorrhage 135; temperature
 101; temporal arteritis 161;
 tumours 160
electro-encephalogram 23, 47, 99,
 152, 180, 181
electro-convulsive therapy 189
embolus 119
emergencies:
 convulsion 96, 104; *see also*
 encephalitis; glaucoma (acute);
 meningitis; sub-arachnoid
 haemorrhage; temporal arteritis
emphysema 219, 220
encephalitis 16, 19, *98-9*, 181
endorphins 51, 53, 191, 204
epilepsy **178-82**;
 aura 179, 181; causes 180, 181;
 children 153, 180, 214; and
 migraine 45, 179, 181; prevention
 181-2; symptoms 15, 16, 23, 47,
 179; temporal lobe 47, 179, 181,
 196; treatment 180, 181-2; triggers
 181-2; and tumours 153, 156, 180
ergonomics *see* working practices
ergotamine 25, 49, 54
Erythrocyte Sedimentation Rate
 (ESR) 20, 58, 152, 162
examination, medical **19-23**
exercise:
 arthritis 81; depression 191; high

blood pressure 146, 148, 149;
 menopause 203, 204; migraine
 43; neck problems 63, 66, 67, 69;
 pre-menstrual syndrome 196;
 sub-arachnoid haemorrhage 127,
 131; tension headaches 19, 57,
 58, 62; toxaemia of pregnancy
 200
exercise *or* exertion headache 18,
 19, **216-17**
eye problems **165-73**;
 astigmatism 169, 170, 214;
 children 171, 211, 214; eye strain
 19, 55, 56, 169-73; focusing 169-
 70, 214; migraines 17, 30-1, 32,
 173; squint 170-1, 214; symptoms
 15, 16-17, 19, 20, 138; and tension
 headache 55, 56, 171; treatment
 170; *see also* blindness;
 glaucoma; light; spectacles;
 treatment

F
face, pain in 14, 15, 17
fasting, religious 41
fear:
 of dental treatment 175, 177; and
 depression 186-7; of serious
 illness 42, 129, 130, 131, 160, 163
Feldenkrais method 86, 123, 137
feverfew 26, 51, 52, 81, 209
5-HT 38, 185, 186, 189;
 agonists 25, 50; blockers 48, 50,
 189
flotation therapy 61, 140
flushes, hot 18
follicle-stimulating hormone *see*
 FSH
food **232-3**;
 addiction 39-40, 233; additives 53,
 186, 232-3; missed, and migraine
 25, 39, 40, 41, 42, 51, 233; *see also*
 diet; food allergies
food allergies 226, 232;
 and addiction 39-40, 233; to
 additives 186; arthritis 80;
 children 166; migraine 25, 33,
 39-42, 45, 51, 53, 213; sinusitis
 112, 116
forehead, pain in 14, 15, 17
FSH 194, 201, 202
fungi, air-borne 115, 224-5

G
gas, domestic 226-8
genetics *see* heredity
German measles 105
glare 173, 239-40, 242
glaucoma **165-9**;
 acute 47, 54, 166, 168, 173;
 chronic 166; symptoms 15, 16, 17,
 19, 47, 111, 167
gliomas 156
glyceryl trinitrate 231
gums 164, 175

H
Habnemann, Samuel 106
haemophilus influenzae 93, 97
haemorrhages *see* sub-arachnoid;
 sub-dural
hangovers 233, 234, 235

hayfever 111, 112, 113-14, 117
head injury **132-43**;
  aftermath 140-3; benign intra-
  cranial hypertension 217;
  bleeding, internal 133, 134-5, 137-
  8; children 134, 139; and epilepsy
  180, 181; and neck injury 139,
  141, 142, 143; prevention 138-9;
  sub-dural haemorrhage 135-7;
  symptoms 16, 19, 128-9, 142;
  treatment 137-40; see also
  concussion; skull
head restraints in car 79-80, 83, 85
headgear 83, 138
heart trouble 49, 104, 203, 220, 236
heat:
  migraine trigger 43, 44, 51;
  treatment with 59, 60, 65
herbalism:
  alcohol-related headaches 235;
  anti-inflammatories 140; arthritis
  71, 81-2; aspirin, natural 116, 125-
  6; blood pressure, high 123, 149;
  caffeine-related headaches 237;
  childhood diseases 105; dental
  problems 175, 177; depression
  192; drug withdrawal 232;
  epilepsy 182; eye problems 168,
  170; head injury 140; infections
  105, 106; meningitis 97-8;
  migraine 26, 51, 52; neck
  problems 66, 75-6, 86, 91; post-
  traumatic headache 143; pre-
  menstrual syndrome 197;
  respiratory failure 220; shingles
  108; sinusitis 116-17; strokes 123;
  sub-dural haemorrhage 137;
  tension headache 60-1; tobacco-
  related headaches 236; toxaemia
  of pregnancy 200; tumours 160
heredity:
  depression 185-6; glaucoma 165,
  167; high blood pressure 145;
  hydrocephalus 217; migraine 30,
  44-5; neck problems 64; osteo-
  arthritis 70
herpes zoster **106-8**, 173
holistic approach 243-6
home surroundings 115, 226-8, 229;
  see also beds; seating
homoeopathy:
  alcohol-related headaches 235;
  arthritis 81; blood pressure, high
  149; cervical spondylosis 75;
  children 53, 105; dental problems
  175, 177; desensitization 225, 230;
  drug withdrawal 232; epilepsy
  182; eye problems 168, 170; head
  injury 140; infections 105, 106,
  219; meningitis 98; menopause
  204; migraine 53; post-traumatic
  headache 143; pre-menstrual
  syndrome 197; respiratory failure
  220; shingles 108; sinusitis 117;
  sub-dural haemorrhage 137;
  tension headache 61; tobacco-
  related headaches 236; toxaemia
  of pregnancy 200; tumours 160;
  viruses 105
hormones:
  angiotensin 147; blood pressure,
  high 149; calcitonin 218; growth

20; melatonin 215, 216; and
migraine 25, 38, 43, 48, 53;
replacement 30, 32, 195-6, 201,
202, 203, 204; tumours and 20,
151, 159;see also FSH; oestrogen;
progesterone
HRT 30, 32, 195-6, 201, 202, 203,
204
humidity 239, 241
hydrocephalus 16, 19, 217;
  children 156, 212-13
hydrotherapy 79
hypertension:
  intra-cranial 16, **217-18**;
  malignant 147; see also blood
  pressure
hysterectomy 18, 34, 202-3

I

ibuprofen 25, 84, 139, 143, 213
immune system 93, 100, 107, 117,
160, 212
immunisation 97, 100
indomethacin 216-17
infections **100-8**;
  bacterial 16, 100, 101, 102, 103,
  104; brain 217; children 65, 101,
  104, 105, 211, 212, 219; neck 65;
  spirochaetes 100-1; treatment
  102-6; see also urinary tract; viral
  infections
influenza 9, 98, 103, 104-5
inhalations 116, 220
injections; auto-injector 50
ions 115, 225, 238-9

J

jaw see bite; tempero-mandibular
jet lag 19, 44, 215, 216

K

kidneys:
  disease 16, 17, 18, 102, 186, 218;
  and hypertension 145, 149
kinesiology 60, 137, 140, 193, 232

L

L-Tyrosine 61
lifting 43, 75, 89, 91
ligaments 83
light 18, 239-41;
  fluorescent 222, 225; glare 173,
  239-40, 242; and meningitis 167;
  and migraine 18, 25, 36, 43, 46,
  167; at work 171, 222, 225
liniments 85
liver 186, 234-5
lumbar puncture 23, 95, 99, **218**
lymph nodes 65
lymphatic glands 101

M

magnesium 38, 71
Magnetic Resonance Imaging see
  MRI
malaria 16, 101, 102, 106
MAOIs 113
massage 59, 78, 81, 193, 209
measles 98, 105
mefenamic acid 196
melatonin 215, 216
Menière's disease 45, 53

meninges 92, 156
meningism 16, 96
meningitis 9, **92-8**;
  bacterial 92, 93, 95-6, 97; children
  94, 97, 102, 104, 180, 212, 213;
  and epilepsy 181; first febrile
  convulsion to be treated as 104;
  headaches after 98; and
  hydrocephalus 213, 217;
  immunisation 97; localised
  concentrations 94, 97; rarity 93,
  94; symptoms 15, 16, 19, 23, 47,
  94, 95, 96, 102, 128, 157, (light
  sensitivity) 18, 167, (stiff neck) 16,
  94, 96, 97, 102, 212; treatment 94,
  95-7; viral 92-3, 96, 97
menopause 18, 20, 185, 194, **201-4**;
  migraine 28, 32, 43, 48, 201
menstruation 194-8;
  headaches 18, 20, 61, 197;
  migraine 8-9, 30, 32, 33-4, 48,
  197-8, 201; see also premenstrual
  syndrome
methotrexate 79
metoclopramide 48
migraine 8, 9, **24-54**;
  abdominal 25, 29-30, 32, 52, 53,
  211; alcohol and 234; aura 24, 27,
  29, 31, 35, 36, 38, 181; basilar 30,
  32; caffeine and 41, 50; causes 37-
  9; children 25, 28, 32, 42, 43,
  (abdominal pains) 30, 211, 213-
  14, (treatment) 49, 52, 53;
  classical 24, 29; and cluster
  headache 18, 26, 46, 54; and
  coital headache 206, 208;
  common 24, 28-9; complications
  31; contraceptive pill and 32-3,
  48, 198-9, 231, (danger of stroke)
  31, 121, 198, 231; dental
  problems 44, 176, 177; duration
  of headache 19; and epilepsy 179,
  181; exercise 43; and exertion
  headache 216, 217; eye
  symptoms 30-1, 167, 173; 5-HT
  and 50, 189; hemiplegic 30, 44-5,
  120-1; and hormones 25, 38, 43,
  48, 53; and neck 12, 26, 44, 52;
  ophthalmoplegic 30-1, 32; phases
  24, 34-7, 38; pregnancy 32;
  prevention 25-6, 35, 42, 47-8, 50,
  53; retinal 17, 31; site of headache
  15, 17, 18, 46; status migrainosus
  31; with stroke 31; symptoms 16,
  17, 18, 19, 26-7, **34-7**, 46, 96, 111,
  200, (see also under eyes; light);
  and tension headache 31, 46, 62;
  treatment 25, 26, 38, 47-53; trigger
  factors 25, 33, 39-44, 50-1, 53, (see
  also under chemicals; food; food
  allergies; oestrogen; sleep;
  stress); and tumours 153;
  weekend 41, 42, 44; at work 18,
  45-6; see also under menopause;
  menstruation; women
migraine equivalent 30
Migraleve 33, 48
minerals 106, 164, 182, 220, 235,
  236
monoamineoxidas inhibitors 113
monosodium glutamate 233
morphine 25, 48, 49

motion sickness 32, 37
moxibustion 81
MRI 22, 76, 152, 180
mumps 98, 105
muscle relaxants 59, 65, 69, 70, 87, 189
muscle spasm, neck 11; and coital headache 206; after head injury 139, 141; manipulation 126; and migraine 44; pain/spasm vicious circle 11, 90-1; physiotherapy 126; and stroke 121-2, 126; symptoms 10, 16, 17, 173; tension headaches 55-6, 56-7, 58-9; in viral infection 101; with other neck problems 63, 70, 78, 84
music therapy 61, 98, 123, 131, 143, 187, 192, 232

N
naturopathy 61, 232
neck problems **63-91**; chiropractic 66; and coital headache 18, 206, 210; congenital 64; diagnosis 14, 15, 17, 20, 21, 88; duration of headache 19; exercises 63, 66, 69; eye symptoms 167, 173; infection 65; injuries 17, 38, 47, 58, **82-7**, (and coital headache) 18, 206, (with head injury) 139, 141, 1452, 143, (psychologically-caused headaches) 183, 193, (and spine) 64, 73; manipulation 26, 44, 66, 69; and migraine 12, 26, 38, 44, 52; muscle spasm *see separate entry*; nerve entrapment 73-4; posture 56, 75, 82, 83, 88, 89-90, 91; and spine 64, 71, 73, 89; stiffness, (and meningitis) 94, 96, 97, 102, 212, (and sub-arachnoid haemorrhage) 128; and tension headache 55, 57, 59, 61; treatment 66, 75, 83, 86, 88-9, 90, 91; vibration 224; viral infections 65-8; wry 65-7; *see also* arthritis; cervical spondylosis
nerve impulse blockers 147
nerves, trapped 73-4, 78, 88
neuralgia 26, 178, 179; trigeminal 17, 18, 19
night shift 19, 44, 216
noise 18, 25, 36, 37, 43, 46, 223
NSAIDs (non-steroidal anti-inflammatories) 25, 78-9, 143, 213, 216-17
Nuclear Magnetic Resonance 22
numbness 17, 29, 36, 84
Nurofen 84, 139

O
obesity 61, 70-1, 144-5, 148, 217
odontoid peg 77-8, 79
oedema 149, 199, 201
oestrogen 159, 194, 195; and menopause 201, 202, 203, 204; and migraine 25, 30, 32, 34, 43, 198, 201
orgasmic cephalegia *see* coital headache
osmotherapy 193
osteo-arthritis 52, 68, **70-1**; with neck problems 84, 245; with

stroke 122, 126; symptoms 16, 17, 21, 73, 78, 84, 88, 173
osteopathy: arthritis 81; dental problems 177; head injury 140; menopause 204; migraine 52; neck problems 66, 75, 86, 91; sex, headache during 209; strokes 123; sub-arachnoid haemorrhage 131; sub-dural haemorrhage 137; and tension headache 60
osteopathy, cranial: children 52; dental problems 177; epilepsy 182; head injury 140; migraine 52; neck problems 66; post-traumatic headache 143; and strokes 123; sub-arachnoid haemorrhage 131; sub-dural haemorrhage 137
osteophytes 73
osteoporosis 201, 203

P
P, substance 81-2
Paget's disease 21, **218**
painkillers 10, 90-1, 159; herbal 53; *see also individual drugs*
pantothenic acid 71
paracetamol 25, 49, 101, 104, 242; /aspirin alternating 103, 105; dangers 103, 234-5
paralysis 29, 143
parasites 101
perfume allergy 230
periodic syndrome 32
pethidine 25, 49
phaeochromocytoma 21, 145
pharmacological effect 224, 226, 232
phenobarbitone 103, 181
phenylalanine 53, 160
physiotherapy:
neck problems 59, 75, 86, 126; respiratory failure 220; rheumatoid arthritis 78, 79, 81; stroke 121, 122, 123
pineal gland 215
pituitary gland:
hormones 20, 194, 201, 202, 204; tumours 17, 20, 21, 145, 151-2, 158, 173
pizotifen 26, 32, 48, 50
pollen allergy 111, 112, 113-14, 117
post-traumatic headache 19, **142-3**
posture 18;
arthritis 70, 79; neck problems 56, 75, 82, 83, 88, 91; tension headache 55, 59; *see also* lifting; working practices
pre-eclampsia 173, 199
pregnancy:
contraindicated treatments 21, 49, 59, 65, 71, 81, 103, 107, 117; benign intra-cranial hypertension 217; blood pressure 144, 149, 199, 200; migraine 32, 43; toxaemia **199-201**;*see also* eclampsia
pre-menstrual syndrome 18, 185, 186, 187, 194, **195-7**
progesterone 194, 195, 202
propranolol 26, 48, 54, 143, 207, 217
psychological causes 19, 183-93

psychotherapy 123, 137, 140, 186, 189-90, 209-10

R
radiotherapy 158-9, 159-60
referred pain 174, 175
reflexes 20, 74
reflexology:
children 53; depression 193; drug withdrawal 232; epilepsy 182; head injury 140; high blood pressure 149; migraine 53; neck problems 66, 75, 86, 91; post-traumatic headache 143; pre-menstrual syndrome 197; sex, headache during 209; shingles 108; stopping smoking 236; stroke 122, 123; sub-arachnoid haemorrhage 131; temporal arteritis 163; tension headache 61; toothache 175; tumours 160
relaxation therapy:
dental problems 177; depression 193; drug withdrawal 232; head injury 140; high blood pressure 148; migraine 52; neck problems 75; post-traumatic headache 143; pre-menstrual syndrome 196; rheumatoid arthritis 82; strokes 123; sub-arachnoid haemorrhage 131; temporal arteritis 163; tension headache 58, 59, 61
respiratory failure **219-20**
Reye's syndrome 103
rigors 102
Roosevelt, Franklin D. 147
routine 19, 44, 215-16
rubefacient creams 85
rubella 105

S
salt 148, 149, 196, 241, 242
sclerotomy 167
Seasonal Affective Disorder 186, 240-1
seating 59, 89
selenium 123, 160
serotonin 50
sex, headaches during 18, **205-10**; exertion headache 216; sub-arachnoid haemorrhage 127, 128, 205, 206; *see also* coital headache
shiatsu 168, 170, 177, 209
shingles **106-8**, 173
sick building syndrome **225**
sinuses, cancer of 111
sinusitis **109-17**;
and migraine 53; symptoms 14, 15, 17, 18, 19-20, 58, 110-11, 164, 167; treatment 111-17
site of headache **14-15**, **17-18**
skull, fractures of 133-5, 138, 140
sleep 16, 193;
blood pressure, high 144-5; clenching jaws during 44, 176; depression 184, 188, 189; menopause 204; migraine 19, 41, 42-3, 51, 145; tension headache 57, 61, 145
smells 25, 45, 230
smoking 25, 44, 113, 219, 220, **263**; passive 111, 113, 115, 225

sodium nitrite 233
spectacles 82, 170, 171, 170; sunglasses 240, 242
speech problems 29, 36, 119-20, 121
spine **63-91**; cancer 151; contrast radiography 23; injuries 18, 38, 82, 89, 193, 206, 207; neck problems affect 64, 71
spirochaetes 100-1
sponging, tepid 103, 105
sports injuries 82
squint 170-1, 214
status migrainosus 31
stellate ganglion 38
steroids 112, 159, 162, 163, 164, 220
stomach: aspirin 234, 235; children's pains 101, 211; *see also* migraine (abdominal)
straining 17, 43, 57, 127
stress 183, 193;
   and bite 177; and blood pressure 146, 149; children 214; heredity and 45; management 59, 123; and migraine 18, 19, 41, 42-3, 44, 45, 50; noise and 223; and stroke 123; and tension headache 55, 59; and toxaemia 200; work-related 59, **221, 225**, (withdrawal) 19, 21, 41, 42, 44, 144-5, 221
stroke 9, **118-26**;
   blood pressure 148, 149; and epilepsy 180, 181; and migraine 31, 120-1; prevention 122, 123; risk factors 31, 121, 198, 231, 236; symptoms 16, 17, 18, 19, 20, 47, 119-20, 128, 157; treatment 121-3; and tumours 153, 155, 157
sub-arachnoid haemorrhage 9, **127-31**; and blood pressure 129, 149, 210; migraines not connected 33, 34; during sex 18, 128, 205, 206; symptoms 14, 15, 16, 17, 18, 19, 47, 96, 127-30; treatment 129-31
sub-dural haemorrhage 19, 135-7
Sumatriptan 25, 50, 54
swimmimg 56, 59, 66, 116, 117, 216, 245
Syndol 59, 65, 90
synovium 68, 71, 78

T
TA *see* transactional analysis
T'ai Chi 66, 71, 76, 123, 131, 149, 193, 232
teeth *see* dental problems
television flicker 181
temperature, body 16, 20, 101, 102, 103, 212
tempero-mandibular joint 17, 19, 21, 77, 176-7
temples 14, 15, 17, 20, 133, 161
temporal arteritis **161-4**; symptoms 10, 12, 14, 15, 16-17, 19, 47, 58, 162, 171; treatment 162, 163-4
tension headaches 8, 9, **55-62**;
   associated conditions 61-2; blood pressure 149; causes 55-7; children 214; diagnoses, other possibile 10, 12, 46, 57-8, 88, 96,
111, 128, 157, 162, 164-5, 200; exacerbating factors 18, 19, 145, 206, 208, 209; eye sympto ms 56, 167, 171, 173, 239; and migraine 31, 46, 62; neck muscle spasm 55, 56-7, 58-9; symptoms 12, 14, 15, 16, 17, 18, 19, 57; treatment 58-61; working conditions and 18, 56
tests, diagnostic 20-3
thyroid malfunction 186, 187
TIAs 17, 119, 120,**124-6**, 153, 157
tobacco *see* smoking
tomograms 21
toothache 17, 18, 19, 21, 111, 164-5, 174-5
toxaemia of pregnancy **199-201**
tranquillisers 48-9, 189, 193
transactional analysis 190, 193
Transient Ischaemic Attacks *see* TIAs
travel 32, 37, 97, 101, 223-4, 228-9; *see also* cars
tryptophan 216
tuberculosis 65
tumours **150-60**: benign 150, 153, 156, 158; bone 159, 218; brain 21, 152, 173; children 153-4, 156, 212, 213; in elderly 153, 154-6; and epilepsy 153; 156, 180, 181; and exertion headache 216; headaches not early symptom 19, 150, 154, 155-6; hormone therapy 159; hormone-producing 145, 151; and hydrocephalus 213, 217; malignant 150-2, 153-6, 158-9; and migraine 153; *phaeochromocytoma* 21, 145; secondary 151, 156, 158, 159; and stroke 153, 155, 157; symptoms 14, 15, 16, 17-18, 19, 22, 47, 152-3, 155, 156-7, 173; temporal lobe 156; treatment 153-6, 158-60; *see also under* pituitary gland
tyramine 39, 40, 232

U
uraemia 16, 17, 18, 173, **218-19**
urinary tract infection 101, 102, 106, 211, 219

V
Valium (diazepam) 48, 59, 65
Vanillymandelic Acid 21
VDUs *see under* computers
ventricles 22
vibration 223-4
viral infections 8, **100-8**; brain 180; children 65, 101, 105, 211, 212; immunisation 97, 100; and neck problems 65-8; symptoms 16, 17, 19, 57-8, 61, 101; treatment 95, 96, 99, 101, 102-3, 104, 105, 106, 107; *see also individual infections*
vision disorders 16-17, 29, 36, 37-8
vitamins: and alcohol 235; arthritis 71, 80; depression 192; epilepsy 182; infections 105, 106; high blood pressure 149; and menopause 203, 204; for migraine 53; Paget's disease 218; pre-
menstrual syndrome 195, 196, 197; respiratory failure 220; shingles 108; sinusitis 117; stroke 123; temporal arteritis 164; tension headache 61; tobacco-related headaches 236; toothache 175; and tumours 160
vomiting; prevention 25, 48, 49

W
weakness, muscular 29, 30, 74, 75, 76
weather 43-4, 58, 114, 238-42
weekends 19, 41, 42, 44, 144-5, 221
whiplash injury 16, 52, 56, 79-80, **83-7**, 143
whooping cough 105
Wilson, Dr Edward Adrian 43
women **194-204**; migraine 25, 28, 32-4, 38, 43, 48; *see also* menopause; menstruation; pregnancy
work-related headaches 19, 45-6, 56, **221-5**
working conditions: air quality 115, 224-5, 238-9, 241-2; and epilepsy 181-2; head protection 138-9; lighting 171, 222, 225; shift working 19, 44, 216; sick building syndrome **225**; *see also* chemicals; computers; stress
working practices 18, 221, 225; arthritis 70, 79; neck problems 56, 59, 60, 73, 82, 88, 91, 89-90

X
X-rays 21, 72-3, 75, 110, 137, 152; contrast radiography 22-3; tomograms 21

Y
yoga 66, 71, 76, 123, 131